Handbook of
Fluid, Electrolyte, and
Acid-Base Imbalances

Second Edition

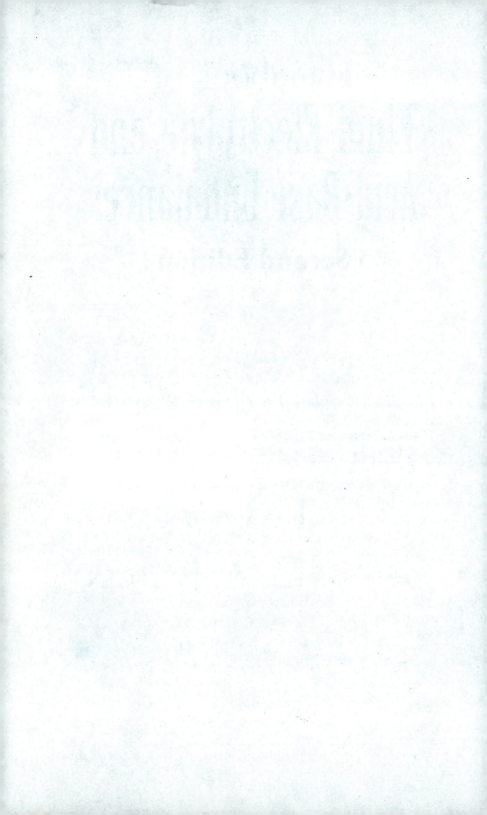

Handbook of
Fluid, Electrolyte, and Acid-Base Imbalances

Second Edition

Joyce LeFever Kee, RN, MS
Associate Professor Emerita
College of Health and Nursing Sciences
University of Delaware
Newark, Delaware

Betty J. Paulanka, RN, EdD
Dean and Professor
College of Health and Nursing Sciences
University of Delaware
Newark, Delaware

Larry D. Purnell, PhD, RN, FAAN
Professor of Nursing
College of Health and Nursing Sciences
University of Delaware
Newark, Delaware

THOMSON
™
DELMAR LEARNING

Australia   Canada   Mexico   Singapore   Spain   United   Kingdom   United States

THOMSON

DELMAR LEARNING

Handbook of Fluid, Electrolyte, and Acid-Base Imbalances
Second Edition
Joyce LeFever Kee, Betty J. Paulanka, Larry D. Purnell

Vice President, Health Care Business Unit:
William Brottmiller

Editorial Director:
Cathy L. Esperti

Acquisitions Editor:
Matthew Filimonov

Developmental Editor:
Patricia A. Gaworecki

Editorial Assistant:
Patricia Osborn

Marketing Director:
Jennifer McAvey

Marketing Coordinator:
Kip Summerlin

Art and Design Coordinator:
Jay Purcell

Project Editors:
Bryan Viggiani
Natalie Wager

Production Coordinator:
Kenneth McGrath

Kee, Joyce LeFever.
  Handbook of fluid, electrolyte, and acid-based imbalances/Joyce LeFever Kee, Betty J. Paulanka, Larry D. Purnell.–2nd ed.
    p.; cm.
  Includes bibliographical references and index.
  ISBN 1-4018-1033-0
  1. Body fluid disorders–Handbooks, manuals, etc. 2. Acid-base imbalances–Handbooks, manuals, etc. 3. Water-electrolyte imbalances–Handbooks, manuals, etc. I. Paulanka, Betty J. II. Purnell, Larry D. III. Kee, Joyce LeFever. Fluids and electrolytes with clinical applications. IV. Title.
  [DNLM: 1. Water-Electrolyte Imbalances–Handbooks. 2. Acid-Base Imbalance–Handbooks. 3. Body Fluids–Handbooks. WD 200.1 K26h 2004]
  RC630.H36 2004
  616.3'992–dc22   2003062678

Dedication

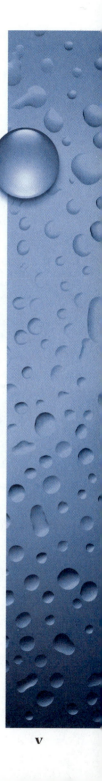

To
Joyce Kee for her consistent
support to faculty development in
the Department of Nursing in the
College of Health and Nursing Sciences
at the University of Delaware.

Contents

Preface

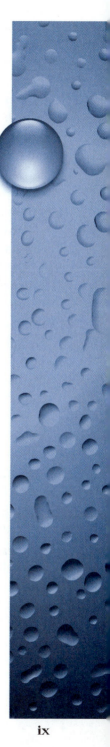

The *Handbook of Fluid, Electrolyte, and Acid-Base Imbalances,* Second Edition is developed from a parent text, *Fluids and Electrolytes with Clinical Applications: A Programmed Approach,* 7E by Joyce LeFever Kee, Betty J. Paulanka, and Larry D. Purnell. It is designed to be used in the clinical setting, both in conjunction with the parent text and as a stand-alone product. With a clear comprehensive approach, this quick reference pocket guide of basic principles of fluid, electrolyte, and acid-base balances, imbalances, and related disorders is a must-have for all who work in the field! The convenient handbook size enables readers to keep it handy for quick access to over 200 diagrams and tables containing valuable information. A developmental approach is used to provide examples across the life span that illustrate common health problems associated with imbalances. Three additional chapters have been added to address the fluid and electrolyte needs of clients suffering from serious burns, increased intracranial pressure, and cancer disorders. Nursing assessments, nursing diagnoses, interventions, and rationales are in a tabular format for quick retrieval and ease of comprehension. All the important information readers need is right at their fingertips!

ORGANIZATION

Handbook of Fluid, Electrolyte, and Acid-Base Imbalances comprises 22 chapters organized into five units:

Unit I lays the foundation for influence of fluids on the body. It covers fluid imbalances related to extracellular fluid volume deficit, excess, and fluid shift, and intracellular fluid volume excess.

Unit II builds upon this material and discusses six electrolyte imbalances—potassium, sodium, chloride, calcium, magnesium, and phosphorus.

Unit III provides a quick guide to determine the types of acid-base imbalances.

Unit IV covers intravenous therapy. The chapters on intravenous fluid therapy and total parenteral nutrition (TPN) include: calculation, monitoring IV fluids, and complications that may occur. With this strong foundation, the learner can then move on to the more complex issues found in the next unit.

Unit V focuses on Clinical Situations and outlines the causes of fluid, electrolyte, and acid-base imbalances in a brief reference style format. Chapters related to acute disorders (trauma and shock), burns and burn shock, gastrointestinal surgical interventions, increased intracranial pressure, and chronic diseases such as heart failure, diabetic ketoacidosis, and chronic obstructive pulmonary disease are included. Also addressed are the fluid problems of infants and children, and older adults.

Appendix contains three appendices. These act as invaluable reference tools for the user. Included are shock, clinical pathways for HF, and children with fluid and electrolyte imbalances; common laboratory tests and values for adults and children; foods rich in potassium, sodium, calcium, magnesium, chloride, and phosphorus; and so much more.

● SYMBOLS

Throughout the handbook the following symbols are used: ↑ (increased), ↓ (decreased), > (greater than), < (less than). A dagger (†) in tables indicates the most common signs and symptoms.

The content in this book is geared for nurses (students, licensed practitioners), laboratory personnel, technicians, and all health care professionals wanting to learn more about fluid, electrolyte, and acid-base imbalances that influence the health status of their clients.

Joyce L. Kee, RN, MS, Professor Emerita
Betty J. Paulanka, RN, EdD, Dean and Professor
Larry D. Purnell, RN, PhD, Professor of Nursing

Acknowledgments

We wish to extend our deepest appreciation to Department of Nursing faculty: Ingrid Aboff, Linda Bucher, Sheila Cushing, Judy Herrman, Lisa Plowfield, Carlee Polek, Kathy Schell, Gail Wade, Julie Waterhouse, Erlinda Wheeler, and a University of Delaware graduate, Linda Laskowski-Jones of Christiana Care Health Systems for their contributions and assistance; to St. Francis Hospital, Wilmington, Delaware, for the use of their Clinical Pathway for Clients with Heart Failure, and to Christiana Care, Visiting Nurse Association, Wilmington, Delaware, for the use of their Clinical Pathway for the Newborn with Hyperbilirubinemia.

We especially wish to thank Don Passidomo, head librarian at the V.A. Medical Center, Wilmington, Delaware, for his valuable assistance and service and for the literature search on fluids and electrolytes.

We also offer our thanks to our editors Matthew Filimonov and Patricia Gaworecki at Delmar Learning for their helpful suggestions and assistance.

Joyce LeFever Kee, RN, MS
Betty J. Paulanka, RN, EdD
Larry D. Purnell, RN, PhD, FAAN

Contributors and Consultants

Ingrid Aboff, RN, MA
Instructor—Department of Nursing
College of Health and Nursing Sciences
University of Delaware
Newark, Delaware

Linda Bucher, RN, DNSc
Associate Professor—Department of Nursing
College of Health and Nursing Sciences
University of Delaware
Newark, Delaware

Sheila Cushing, RN, MS
Assistant Professor, Department of Nursing
College of Health and Nursing Sciences
University of Delaware
Newark, Delaware 19716

Judith Herrman, RN, MS
Instructor, Department of Nursing
College of Health and Nursing
University of Delaware
Newark, Delaware 19716

Lisa Ann Plowfield RN, PhD
Associate Professor and
Chairperson, Dept of Nursing
College of Health and Nursing Sciences
University of Delaware
Newark, DE 19716

Carolee Polek RN, PhD
Assistant Professor Department of Nursing
College of Health and Nursing

Linda Laskowski-Jones, RN, MS, CS, CCRN
Trauma Clinical Specialist
Trauma Service
Christiana Care Health Systems
Wilmington, Delaware

Kathleen Schell, RN, DNSc
Assistant Professor, Department of Nursing
College of Health and Nursing Sciences
University of Delaware
Newark, Delaware

Gail H. Wade, RN, MS
Associate Professor, Department of Nursing
College of Health and Nursing Sciences
University of Delaware
Newark, Delaware

Julie Waterhouse, RN, PhD
Associate Professor—Department of Nursing
College of Health and Nursing Sciences
University of Delaware
Newark, Delaware

Erlinda Wheeler, RN, PhD
Assistant Professor—Department of Nursing
College of Health and Nursing Sciences
University of Delaware
Newark, Delaware

Reviewers

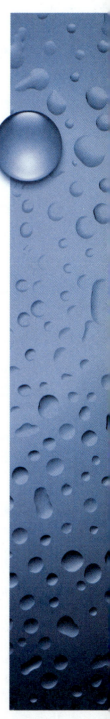

Sharon Abbatte, RN, MSN
Professor of Nursing
Middle Tennessee State University
Murfreesboro, Tennessee

Sandra Cawley Baird, EdD, RN, CNS
Director, Professor
School of Nursing
University of Northern Colorado

Mary Kathleen Doyle, RN, BSN, MS
Clinical Instructor of Nursing
Maria College of Nursing
Albany, New York

Carol Della Ratta, RN, MS, CCRN
Clinical Assistant Professor
State University of New York at Stony Brook

FLUIDS AND THEIR INFLUENCE ON THE BODY

INTRODUCTION

The human body is a complex machine that contains hundreds of bones and the most sophisticated inter-action of systems of any structure on earth. Yet, the substance that is basic to the very existence of the body is the simplest substance known, WATER. In fact, it makes up almost two-thirds of an adult's body weight.

Body water represents about 60% of the total body weight in the average adult, 45–55% of an older adult, 70–80% of a newborn infant, and 97% of the early human embryo. Figure U1-1 demonstrates the percentage of body water concentration across the life span. Many persons think the extra water in infants acts as a protective mechanism. Since infants have larger body surface in relation to their weight, extra water acts as a cushion against injury. Body fat is essentially free of water. An obese person has less body water than a thin person. The leaner the indi-vidual, the greater the proportion of water in total body weight.

BODY COMPARTMENTS

Body water is distributed among three body com-partments: intracellular (within the cells), intravas-cular (within the blood vessels), and interstitial (within the tissue spaces). Because fluids in the blood vessels and tissue spaces are outside the cells, they are referred to as extracellular fluid. Table U1-1 gives the proportion of intracellular and extracellu-lar fluid in the body.

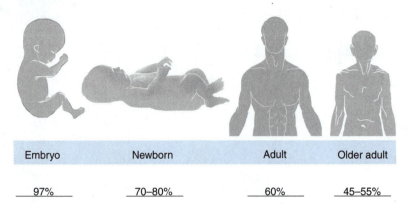

Embryo	Newborn	Adult	Older adult
97%	70–80%	60%	45–55%

FIGURE U1-1   Percentages of body fluid per body weight.

Table U1-1 Percentage of Body Fluids in Body Fluid Compartments		
Intracellular fluid (ICF) compartment $(\frac{2}{3})$		40%
Extracellular fluid (ECF) compartment $(\frac{1}{3})$		20%
Interstitial fluid	15%	
Intravascular fluid	5%	
	Total	60%

FUNCTIONS OF BODY WATER

Without water, the body is unable to maintain life. Five functions of water that the body needs to maintain a healthy state are stated in Table U1-2.

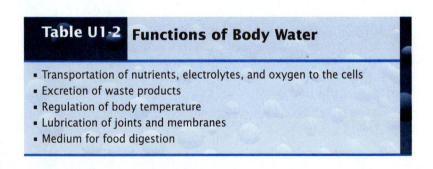

Table U1-2 Functions of Body Water
▪ Transportation of nutrients, electrolytes, and oxygen to the cells
▪ Excretion of waste products
▪ Regulation of body temperature
▪ Lubrication of joints and membranes
▪ Medium for food digestion

Table U1-3	Daily Body Fluid Intake and Losses		
Fluid Intake		**Fluid Losses**	
Liquid	1000–1200 mL	Urine	1000–1400 mL
Food	800–1000 mL	Feces	100 mL
Oxidation	200–300 mL	Lungs	400–500 mL
		Skin	300–500 mL
Total	2000–2500 mL		1800–2500 mL

When body water is insufficient and the kidneys are functioning normally, urine volume diminishes and the individual becomes thirsty. Therefore, the person drinks more water to correct the fluid deficit. When there is an excessive amount of water intake, the urine output increases proportionately.

Sources of fluid intake include liquids, foods, and products of the oxidation of food process. The average intake and output of fluid per day is 1800–2500 mL. Body fluids are lost daily through the urine, feces, lungs, and skin. Body water loss through the skin, which is not measurable, is called *insensible perspiration.* Appropriately 300–500 mL of fluid is lost daily through processes such as sweat gland activity. Table U1-3 lists the daily fluid intake and losses. Definitions related to fluid functions and movement are presented in the accompanying box.

Definitions Related to Fluid Function and Movement

Membrane. A layer of tissue covering a surface or organ or separating spaces.

Permeability. The capability of a substance, molecule, or ion to diffuse through a membrane.

Semipermeable membrane. An artificial membrane such as a cellophane membrane.

Selectively permeable membrane. Permeability of the human membranes.

Solvent. A liquid with a substance in solution.

Solute. A substance dissolved in a solution.

Osmosis. The passage of a solvent through a membrane from a solution of lesser solute concentration to one of greater solute concentration.

Note: Osmosis may be expressed in terms of water concentration instead of solute concentration. Water molecules pass from an area of higher water concentration (fewer solutes) to an area of lower water concentration (more solutes).

Diffusion. The movement of molecules such as gas from an area of higher concentration to an area of lesser concentration. Large molecules move less rapidly than small molecules.

Osmol. A unit of osmotic pressure. The osmotic effects are expressed in terms of osmolality. A **milliosmol (mOsm)** is 1/1000th of an osmol and determines the osmotic activity.

Osmolality. Osmotic pull exerted by all particles per unit of water, expressed as osmols or milliosmols per kilogram of water concentrate and body fluids.

Osmolarity. Osmotic pull exerted by all particles per unit of solution, expressed as osmols or milliosmols per liter of solution.

Ion. A particle carrying a positive or negative charge.

Plasma. Blood minus the blood cells (composed mainly of water).

Serum. Plasma minus fibrogen (obtained after coagulation of blood).

Tonicity. The effect of fluid on cellular volume concentration of IV solution.

● FLUID PRESSURES (STARLING'S LAW)

Extracellular fluid (ECF) shifts between the intravascular space (blood vessels) and the interstitial space (tissues) to maintain a fluid balance within the ECF compartment. There are four measurable pressures that determine the flow of fluid between the intravascular and interstitial spaces. These are the colloid osmotic (oncotic) pressures and the hydrostatic pressures that occur in both the vessels and the tissue spaces. The colloid osmotic pressure and the hydrostatic pressure of the blood and tissues influence the movement of fluid through the capillary membrane. Fluid exchange occurs only across the walls of capillaries and not across the walls of arterioles or venules. Therefore, fluid moves into the interstitial space at the arteriolar end of the capillary and out of the interstitial space into the capillary at the venular end of the capillary.

Fluid flows only when there is a difference in pressure at the two ends of the system. The difference in pressure be-

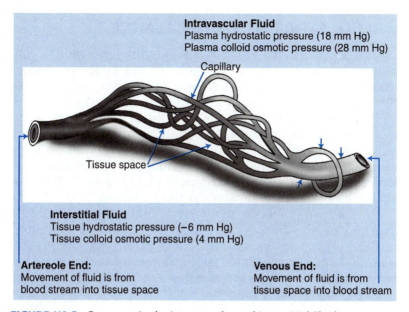

Intravascular Fluid
Plasma hydrostatic pressure (18 mm Hg)
Plasma colloid osmotic pressure (28 mm Hg)

Capillary

Tissue space

Interstitial Fluid
Tissue hydrostatic pressure (−6 mm Hg)
Tissue colloid osmotic pressure (4 mm Hg)

Artereole End:
Movement of fluid is from
blood stream into tissue space

Venous End:
Movement of fluid is from
tissue space into blood stream

FIGURE U1-2 Pressures in the Intravascular and Interstitial Fluid.

tween two points is known as the pressure gradient. If the pressure at one end is 32 mm Hg and at the other end is 26 mm Hg, the pressure gradient is 6 mm Hg. The plasma in the capillaries has hydrostatic pressure and colloid osmotic pressure. The tissue fluids have hydrostatic pressure and colloid osmotic pressure. The difference in pressure between the plasma colloid osmotic pressure and the tissue colloid osmotic pressure is known as the colloid osmotic pressure gradient; likewise, the difference in pressure between the plasma hydrostatic pressure and the tissue hydrostatic pressure is known as the hydrostatic pressure gradient. Figure U1-2 describes the fluid flow based upon the pressures in the intravascular and interstitial spaces.

Because the plasma hydrostatic pressure (18 mm Hg) in the arteriolar end of the capillary is higher than the tissue hydrostatic pressure (−6 mm Hg) in the tissue spaces, fluid moves out of the capillary and into the tissue spaces. The plasma colloid osmotic pressure (28 mm Hg) in the venular end of the capillary is higher than the tissue colloid osmotic pressure (4 mm Hg) in the tissue spaces, causing fluids to move from the tissue spaces into the capillary. Without the colloid osmotic forces, fluid is lost from circulation and remains in the tissues, causing swelling or edema.

REGULATORS OF FLUID BALANCE

Thirst, electrolytes, protein and albumin, hormones, enzymes, lymphatics, skin, and kidneys are major regulators that maintain body fluid balance. Thirst alerts the person that there is a fluid loss; thus, thirst stimulates the person to increase his or her oral intake. The thirst mechanism in the medulla may not respond effectively to a fluid deficit in the older adult or the very young child; therefore, these groups of individuals are prone to lose fluid and become easily dehydrated. Table U1-4 lists the various regulators of fluid balance. The body compensates for fluid changes.

If a person is febrile or there is an increase in humidity, diaphoresis may occur. This causes a fluid loss. The amount of fluid loss from the skin in this situation may be greater than 500 mL for the day. Deep and rapid breathing or hyperventilation can also increase fluid loss through the lungs in an amount greater than 500 mL.

OSMOLALITY

Osmolality (serum) is determined by the number of dissolved particles, mainly sodium, urea, and glucose, per kilogram of water. Sodium is the largest contributor of particles to osmolality. The normal serum osmolality range is 280–295 mOsm/kg (milliosmols per kilogram); serum osmolality values in this range are considered iso-osmolar since the serum concentration is similar to plasma. If the serum osmolality is less than (<) 280 mOsm/kg, the serum concentration of fluid is hypo-osmolar, and if the serum osmolality is greater than (>) 295 mOsm/kg, the serum concentration is hyperosmolar. The serum osmolality is "roughly" estimated by doubling the serum sodium level. For example, if the serum sodium is 142 mEq/L, the serum osmolality is 284 mOsm/kg. Doubling the serum sodium level provides a "rough estimate" of the serum osmolality. Another formula that is more accurate in determining the serum osmolality is displayed in the accompanying box. If the client's serum sodium is 140 mEq/L, blood urea nitrogen (BUN) is 12 mg/dL, and serum glucose is 99 mg/dL, the serum osmolality for this client is 289.5 mOsm/kg; the serum concentration is iso-osmolar or iso-osmolality.

Table U1-4 Regulators of Fluid Balance

Regulators	Actions
Thirst	An indicator of fluid need.
Electrolytes and Nonelectrolytes	
Sodium	Sodium promotes water retention. With a water deficit, less sodium is excreted via kidneys; thus, more water is retained.
Protein, albumin	Protein and albumin promote body fluid retention. These nondiffusible substances increase the colloid osmotic (oncotic) pressure in favor of fluid retention.
Hormones and Enzymes	
Antidiuretic hormone (ADH)	ADH is produced by the hypothalamus and stored in the posterior pituitary gland (neurohypophysis). ADH is secreted when there is an ECF volume deficit or an increased osmolality (increased solutes). ADH promotes water reabsorption from the distal tubules of the kidneys.
Aldosterone	Aldosterone is secreted from the adrenal cortex. It promotes sodium, chloride, and water reabsorption from the renal tubules.
Renin	Decreased renal blood flow increases the release of renin, an enzyme, from the juxtaglomerular cells of the kidneys. Renin promotes peripheral vasoconstriction and the release of aldosterone (sodium and water retention).

(continues)

Table U1-4	Regulators of Fluid Balance—*continued*
Regulators	**Actions**
Body Tissues and Organs	
Lymphatics	Plasma protein that shifts to the tissue spaces cannot be reabsorbed into the blood vessels. Thus, the lymphatic system promotes the return of water and protein from the interstitial spaces to the vascular spaces.
Skin	Skin excretes approximately 300–500 mL of water daily through normal perspiration.
Lungs	Lungs excrete approximately 400–500 mL of water daily through normal breathing.
Kidneys	The kidneys excrete 1000–1500 mL of body water daily. The amount of water excretion may vary according to the balance between fluid intake and fluid loss.

Formula for Calculating Serum Osmolality

$$2 \times \text{serum sodium} + \frac{\text{BUN}}{3} + \frac{\text{glucose}}{18} = \text{serum osmolality}$$

Rough Estimation of Serum Osmolality

$$2 \times \text{serum sodium} = \text{serum osmolality}$$

Use the formula in the accompanying box for clients A and B. Client A: The serum sodium is 145 mEq/L, BUN is 27 mg/dL, and the serum glucose is 120 mg/dL. Client A's serum osmolality is 305.7 or 306 mOsm/kg, which shows hyperosmolality. Client B: The serum sodium is 133 mEq/L, BUN is 9 mg/dL, and the serum glucose is 90 mg/dL. Client B's serum osmolality is 274 mOsm/kg, which shows hypo-osmolality.

The terms osmolality and tonicity have been used interchangeably; though similar, they are different. **Osmolality** is the concentration of body fluids and **tonicity** is the concentration of IV solutions. Increased osmolality (hyperosmolality) can result from impermeant solutes such as sodium and permeant solutes such as urea (blood urea nitrogen). Hypertonicity results from an increase of impermeant solutes such as sodium, but *not* of permeant solutes such as urea (BUN). Hyperosmolality of body fluid occurs with an increased serum sodium and BUN levels; however, it may also cause isotonicity since the BUN does not affect tonicity. Serum osmolality is a better indicator of the concentration of solutes in body fluids than tonicity measures. Tonicity is primarily used for the concentration of intavenous solutions.

● TONICITY OF INTRAVENOUS (IV) SOLUTION

The tonicity of an IV solution can be hypo-osmolar or hypotonic, iso-osmolar or isotonic, hyperosmolar or hypertonic. The tonicity of an IV solution is determined by the serum osmolality average, which is 290 mOsm/kg (280–295 mOsm/kg). The normal range for the tonicity of a solution is +50 mOsm or −50 mOsm of 290 mOsm, or 240–340 mOsm. Tonicity may be used to describe the concentration of IV solution because of the effect of impermeant solutes like sodium and chloride in the solution on the cellular volume. Since the solute concentration is determined by the number of osmols or milliosmols in solution, hypo-osmolar, iso-osmolar, and hyperosmolar are the suggested terms.

A liter of 5% dextrose in water (D_5W) is 250 mOsm, and a liter of 0.9% sodium chloride or normal saline is 310 mOsm; both solutions have somewhat the same tonicity as plasma. These solutions are iso-osmolar. However, in D_5W, the dextrose is metabolized quickly, causing the solution to become hypo-osmolar. The tonicity of a liter of 5% dextrose in water with 0.9% sodium chloride is 560 mOsm. This solution is hyperosmolar or hypertonic.

Many disease entities have some degree of fluid imbalance such as fluid loss, fluid excess, and/or fluid volume shift. The four major fluid imbalances: extracellular fluid volume deficit (ECFVD), extracellular fluid volume excess (ECFVE), extracellular fluid volume shift (ECFVS), and intracellular fluid volume excess (ICFVE) are discussed in Chapters 1, 2, 3, and 4.

CLINICAL PROBLEMS ASSOCIATED WITH FLUID IMBALANCES

Table U1-5 illustrates the most common clinical problems associated with fluid imbalances.

Table U1-5

Clinical Problems	ECFVD	ECFVE	ECFV Shift	ICFVE
Gastrointestinal				
Vomiting and diarrhea	+			
GI fistula	+			
GI suctioning	+			
Increased salt intake	+			
Intestinal obstruction	+		+	
Perforated ulcer	+		+	
Excessive hypotonic fluids, oral and intravenous				+
Renal				
Renal failure		+		
Renal disease		+		
Cardiac				
Heart failure		+		
Miscellaneous				
Brain tumor/injury				+
Fever	+			
Profused diaphoresis	+			
SIADH (syndrome of inappropriate antidiuretic hormone)		Initially +		+
Burns	+	+	+	
Diabetic ketoacidosis	+			
Ascites (cirrhosis)		+	+	
Venous obstruction		+		
Sprain			+	
Massive trauma	+		+	
Drugs				
Cortisone group of drugs		+		

Extracellular Fluid Volume Deficit (ECFVD)

Carolee Polek, RN, PhD

INTRODUCTION

Extracellular fluid volume deficit (ECFVD) indicates a loss of body fluid from the interstitial (tissue) and/or intravascular (vascular–blood vessel) spaces. When there is a *severe* extracellular fluid loss and the serum osmolality is increased (more solutes than water), the fluid in the intracellular (cells) is greatly decreased. Hyperosmolality pulls water out of the cells to maintain homeostasis (equilibrium) of the body fluid and cellular dehydration results. If serum osmolality remains normal (loss of water and the loss of solutes is equal), intracellular fluid loss is unlikely to occur.

Dehydration means lack of water. Dehydration may occur due to extracellular fluid loss or a decreased fluid intake. An elevated serum osmolality occurs frequently with dehydration. The serum osmolality can be closely estimated using the serum sodium, BUN, and glucose values presented in Unit I.

PATHOPHYSIOLOGY

A loss of the electrolyte sodium is usually accompanied by a loss of extracellular fluid. The extracellular fluid is usually decreased or moves from the ECF to the ICF (intracellular fluid) compartment. When fluid and sodium are lost in equal amounts, the type of fluid deficit that usually occurs is **iso-osmolar** (iso-osmolar fluid volume deficit). The serum osmolality remains in normal range between 280 and 295 mOsm/kg, as shown in the accompanying box. If the amount of water loss is in excess of the amount of sodium loss, the serum sodium level is increased. This type of fluid deficit is called a **hyperosmolar** fluid volume deficit. With the retention of sodium or loss of water, serum osmolality increases (>295 mOsm/kg). Hyperosmolar extracellular fluid causes intracellular dehydration because the increase in serum osmolality causes water to be drawn from the cells. With an iso-osmolar fluid volume loss, the loss of water and solute is equal. An iso-osmolar fluid volume loss is not classified as dehydration, although dehydration can occur with this type of fluid loss. Table 1-1 differentiates between iso-osmolar fluid volume deficit and hyperosmolar fluid volume deficit.

Normal serum osmolality: 280–295 mOsm/kg	
Hypo-osmolality:	<280 mOsm/kg
Iso-osmolality:	280–295 mOsm/kg
Hyperosmolality:	>295 mOsm/kg

Compensatory mechanisms such as increased heart rate and blood pressure attempt to maintain the fluid volume necessary for vital organs to receive adequate perfusion. When more than one-third of the body fluid is lost, vascular collapse occurs and shock results.

Table 1-1 Differentiation between Iso-osmolar and Hyperosmolar Fluid Volume Deficit

Situation	Iso-osmolar Fluid Volume Deficit	Hyperosmolar Fluid Volume Deficit
There is a proportional loss of both body fluids and solutes	X	
The loss of body fluid is greater than the loss of solutes		X
A serum osmolality of 282 mOsm/kg occurs with ECFVD	X	
A serum osmolality of 320 mOsm/kg occurs with ECFVD		X

● ETIOLOGY

The causes of hyperosmolar and iso-osmolar fluid volume deficits differ. Vomiting and diarrhea may cause both types of fluid volume deficits; however, in most cases, the severity of vomiting and diarrhea indicates which type of ECFVD occurs. Table 1-2 discusses the types, causes, and rationale for ECFVDs. Table 1-3 summarizes the pathophysiology and etiology related to extracellular fluid volume deficit.

Table 1-2 **Causes of Extracellular Fluid Volume Deficits**	
Types and Causes	**Rationale**
Hyperosmolar Fluid Volume Deficit	
Inadequate fluid intake	A decrease in water intake results in an increase in the numbers of solutes in body fluid. The body fluid becomes hyperosmolar.
Increased solute intake (salt, sugar, protein)	An increase in solute intake increases the solute concentration in body fluid; the body fluids can become hyperosmolar with a normal or decreased fluid intake.
Severe vomiting and diarrhea	Cause a loss of body water greater than the loss of solutes such as electrolytes, resulting in hyperosmolar body fluid.
Diabetes ketoacidosis	An increase in glucose and ketone bodies can result in body fluids becoming more hyperosmolar, thus causing diuresis. The resulting fluid loss is greater than the solute loss (sugar and ketones).
Sweating	Water loss is usually greater than sodium loss.
Iso-osmolar Fluid Volume Deficit	
Vomiting and diarrhea	Usually result in fluid losses that are in proportion to electrolyte (sodium, potassium, chloride, bicarbonate) losses.
Gastrointestinal (GI) fistula or draining abscess and GI suctioning	The GI tract is rich in electrolytes. With a loss of GI secretions, fluid and electrolytes are lost in somewhat equal proportions.

(continues)

Table 1-2 Causes of Extracellular Fluid Volume Deficits—*continued*	
Types and Causes	**Rationale**
Iso-osmolar Fluid Volume Deficit	
Fever, environmental temperature, and profuse diaphoresis	Result in fluid and sodium losses via the skin. With profuse sweating, the sodium is usually lost in proportions equal to water losses. Depending upon the severity of the sweating and fever, symptoms of mild, moderate, or marked fluid loss may be observed.
Hemorrhage	Excess blood loss is fluid and solute loss from the vascular fluid. If hemorrhage occurs rapidly, fluid shifts to compensate for blood losses can be inadequate.
Burns	Burns cause body fluid with solutes to shift from the vascular fluid to the burned site and surrounding interstitial space (tissues). This may result in inadequate circulating fluid volume.
Ascites	Fluid and solutes (protein, electrolytes, etc.) shift to the peritoneal space, causing ascites (third-space fluid). A decrease in circulating fluid volume may result.
Intestinal obstruction	Fluid accumulates at the intestinal obstruction site (third-space fluid), thus decreasing the vascular fluid volume.

● CLINICAL MANIFESTATIONS

The clinical manifestations (signs and symptoms) of ECFVDs are listed in Table 1-4. The table describes the degrees of ECF loss, percentage of body weight loss, symptoms, and body water deficit by liter for a man weighing 150 pounds.

Thirst is a symptom that occurs with mild, marked, and severe fluid loss. Lack of water intake is the main contributing cause of mild dehydration. In the elderly, the thirst mechanism in the medulla does not alert the older person that there is a water deficit. Common symptoms of marked ECF loss include decreased skin turgor, dry mucous mem-

Table 1-3	Summary of Pathophysiology and Etiology Related to Extracellular Fluid Volume Deficit (ECFVD)
Pathophysiology	**Etiology**
↓ ECF + ↓ Na = *Iso-osmolar FVD*	*Iso-osmolar FVD*
Proportional equal loss of fluid and sodium	Vomiting and diarrhea
	Fever, profuse diaphoresis
	GI losses (suctioning, fistula, draining abscess)
↓ ECF + ↑ Na = *Hyperosmolar FVD*	Excess blood loss
Fluid loss is greater than sodium loss	Burns
	Ascites
	Intestinal obstruction
Compensatory Mechanisms to ECFVD	*Hyperosmolar FVD*
↑ Blood Pressure	Vomiting and diarrhea (SEVERE)
↑ Pulse	Inadequate fluid intake
	↑ Solute intake (sodium, sugar, protein)
	Diabetic ketoacidosis
One-third of ECFV loss = vascular collapse	

branes, increased pulse rate, weight loss, and decreased urine output. With marked and severe body fluid loss, the hematocrit, hemoglobin, and blood urea nitrogen (BUN) are generally increased.

During early dehydration, the serum osmolality may not show signs of significant change. As dehydration continues, fluid is lost in greater quantities from the extracellular space than from the intracellular space. This results in an ECF deficit. When dehydration is severe, the serum osmolality increases, causing water to leave the cells. This results in cellular dehydration. A severe ECF deficit can lead to an ICF deficit.

The health professional can make a quick assessment of dehydration caused by hypovolemia by checking the peripheral veins in the hand. First hold the hand above the heart level for a short time and then lower the hand below the heart level. With a normal blood volume and circulating blood flow, the peripheral veins in the hand held below the heart level should be engorged within 5–10 seconds. If the peripheral

Table 1-4 Degrees of Dehydration

Degrees of Dehydration	Percentage of Body Weight Loss (%)	Symptoms	Body Water Deficit by Liter
Mild dehydration	2	1. Thirst	1–2
Marked dehydration	5	1. Marked thirst	3–5
		2. Dry mucous membranes	
		3. Dryness and wrinkling of skin—poor skin turgor	
		4. Hand veins: slow filling with hand lowered	
		5. Temperature—low-grade elevation, e.g., 99°F (37.2°C)	
		6. Tachycardia (pulse greater than 100) as blood volume drops	
		7. Respiration >28	
		8. Systolic BP 10–15 mm Hg ↓ in standing position	
		9. Urine volume <25 mL/h	
		10. Specific gravity >1.030	
		11. Body weight loss	
		12. Hct ↑, Hgb ↑, BUN ↑	
		13. Acid-base equilibrium toward greater acidity	
Severe dehydration	8	1. Same symptoms as marked dehydration, plus:	5–10
		2. Flushed skin	
		3. Systolic BP <60 mm Hg	
		4. Behavioral changes, e.g., restlessness, irritability, disorientation, and delirium	
Fatal dehydration	22–30 total body water loss can prove fatal	1. Anuria	
		2. Coma leading to death	

Abbreviations: BP, blood pressure; Hg, mercury; Hct, hematocrit; Hgb, hemoglobin; BUN, blood urea nitrogen

veins do not engorge in 10 seconds, this may be indicative of dehydration or low blood volume. Body weight is another important tool for assessing fluid imbalance. Two and two-tenths (2.2) pounds of body weight loss or gain is equivalent to 1 liter of water loss or gain. Of course, in order to make an accurate assessment, the health professional needs to know the baseline body weight prior to the fluid loss.

● CLINICAL MANAGEMENT

In replacing body water loss, the total fluid deficit is estimated according to the percentage of body weight lost. The health care provider computes the fluid replacement for his or her client. To determine the total fluid loss, multiply the percentage of body weight loss by kilograms of body weight. If the client's weight loss is 10 pounds and his original weight was 154 pounds or 70 kg, the client has a 6% body weight loss, which totals 4.2 liters of total fluid loss. Table 1-5 gives a formula for estimating total fluid loss.

Table 1-5 **Estimation of Total Fluid Loss**

Formula:
a. Pounds to kilograms:
    Previous weight in pounds ÷ 2.2 = kg   (2.2 pounds = 1 kilogram)
b. Percent of body weight lost:
    Weight loss ÷ Previous weight   (subtract present weight from previous weight to obtain weight loss)

c. Total fluid deficit/loss:
    Percentage of body weight loss × Kilograms of body weight = *Total fluid loss*

Example:
The client's weight loss is 10 pounds and his original weight was 154 pounds. What is the client's total body fluid loss? How many liters (milliliters) are needed to replace the client's fluid loss? Use the formula for determining body fluid loss.
a. 154 lb ÷ 2.2 = 70 kg
b. 10 lb of weight loss ÷ 154 lb = 0.06 or 6% body weight loss
c. 0.06 × 70 kg = 4.2 liters (4200 mL) of total fluid loss

One-third of the body water deficit is from ECF (extracellular fluid) and two-thirds of the body water deficit is from ICF (intracellular fluid). The daily fluid loss that needs replacement is 2.5 liters or 2500 mL. During the first day the patient should receive:

$\frac{1}{3} \times 4.2$ L = 1.4 L or 1400 mL (ECF replacement)

$\frac{2}{3} \times 4.2$ L = 2.8 L or 2800 mL (ICF replacement)

2.5 L or 2500 mL to replace the current day's losses

Note: The amount for fluid replacement can vary according to the client's physical health and age. Clients with heart failure cannot receive huge fluid replacements.

Table 1-6 lists suggested solution and potassium replacement for an ECF deficit. The amount of fluid replacement might change according to the client's health status. According to Table 1-6, as potassium enters the cells, fluid flows into the cells with the potassium replacement. Cellular fluid increases and the cells become hydrated. When potassium is being administered intravenously, the client's urinary output must be closely monitored. The urine output should be at least 250 mL per 8 hours; since 80–90% of potassium is excreted by the kidneys, poor urine output results in a potassium excess.

The health care provider must also consider the electrolyte balance with different types of fluid replacement. If

Table 1-6	Suggested Solution Replacement for ECF Deficit

1. Lactated Ringer's, 1500 mL, to replace ECF losses (varies according to the serum potassium and calcium levels).
2. Normal saline solution (0.9% NaCl solution), 500 mL.
3. Five percent dextrose in water (D_5W), 4700 mL, to replace the water deficit and increase urine output.
4. Potassium chloride, 40–80 mEq, may be divided into 3 liters to replace potassium loss. The serum potassium level must be closely monitored.
5. Bicarbonate as needed if an acidotic state exists.

dextrose in water is administered without any other electrolyte content such as sodium, the dextrose is metabolized quickly, leaving only water and a resulting hypo-osmolar or hypotonic condition. An electrolyte solution such as lactated Ringer's and/or saline solution (0.9% or 0.45%) should be included as part of the replacement formula.

CLINICAL CONSIDERATIONS: ECFVD

1. Thirst is an early symptom of ECFVD or dehydration. Encourage fluid intake.

2. The serum osmolality is one method to detect dehydration. A serum osmolality of >300 mOsm/kg indicates dehydration.

3. Decreased skin turgor, dry mucous membranes, an increased pulse rate, and a systolic blood pressure (while standing) <10–15 mm Hg of the regular blood pressure are some signs and symptoms of dehydration.

4. Urine output less than 25 mL/h or 600 mL/day should be reported. A decrease in urine output can indicate insufficient fluid intake, hypovolemia, or renal dysfunction.

5. A quick assessment of hypovolemia or dehydration can be accomplished by checking the peripheral veins in the hand. First hold the hand above the heart level for 10 seconds and then lower the hand below the heart level. The peripheral veins in the hand below the heart level become engorged within 5–10 seconds with a normal blood volume. If the peripheral veins are not engorged, hypovolemia or dehydration is present.

6. Lactated Ringer's and 5% dextrose in $\frac{1}{3}$ or $\frac{1}{2}$ normal saline are solutions that are helpful for treating ECFVD.

CLIENT MANAGEMENT

Assessment

● Obtain a client history identifying factors that may cause a fluid volume deficit (ECFVD).

- Assess for signs and symptoms associated with body fluid loss or dehydration. These may include poor skin turgor, dry mucous membranes, slow filling of hand veins, a decrease in urine output, and tachycardia.
- Check vital signs. Heart compensates for fluid loss by increasing the heart rate. Check blood pressure while the client is sitting and again if the client is able to stand without difficulty (a fall of 10–15 mm Hg in systolic pressure can indicate marked ECFVD). A narrow pulse pressure of less than 20 mm Hg can indicate severe hypovolemia.
- Check the urine output for volume and concentration. A decrease in urine output may be due to a lack of fluid intake or excess body fluid loss.
- Assess weight gain/loss to assist in accurate fluid replacement.
- Check laboratory results of BUN and hematocrit. Elevated levels might indicate fluid loss.

Nursing Diagnoses

- *Deficient Fluid Volume,* related to inadequate fluid intake, vomiting, diarrhea, hemorrhage, or third-space fluid loss (burns or ascites)
- *Risk for Impaired Skin Integrity,* related to a fluid deficit in body tissues
- *Ineffective Tissue Perfusion, renal,* related to decreased renal blood flow and poor urine output secondary to ECFVD, or hypovolemia

Interventions

- Monitor vital signs at least every 4 hours. Check the blood pressure in lying, sitting, and standing positions.
- Routinely check body weight. *Remember:* 2.2 pounds equals 1 kilogram, which is equivalent to 1 liter (1000 mL) of fluid loss.
- Monitor skin turgor, mucous membranes, lips, and tongue for dryness or improvement.

- Promote adequate fluid replacements, oral and intravenous.
- Monitor urine output. Report if urine output is below 250 mL per 8 hours.
- Provide oral hygiene several times a day.
- Monitor laboratory results such as elevated BUN and hematocrit.
- Provide comfort.
- Listen to client's concerns. Answer questions or refer the questions to appropriate health professionals.

Evaluation/Outcome

- Evaluate that the cause of extracellular fluid volume deficit (ECFVD) has been controlled or eliminated.
- Remain free of signs and symptoms of dehydration; skin turgor improved, moist mucous membranes, vital signs within normal range, and body weight increased.
- Evaluate the effects of clinical management for ECFVD; fluid deficit is lessened.
- Urine output is within normal range: 600–1400 mL/24 hours.
- Evaluate the laboratory test results; serum osmolality and electrolytes are within normal range.

CHAPTER 2

Extracellular Fluid Volume Excess (ECFVE)

Carolee Polek, RN, PhD

INTRODUCTION

Extracellular fluid volume excess (ECFVE) is increased fluid in either the interstitial (tissues) and/or intravascular (vascular or vessel) spaces. Usually it relates to the excess fluid in tissues of the extremities (peripheral edema) or lung tissues (pulmonary edema). Terms for ECFVE are hypervolemia, overhydration, and edema. Hypervolemia and overhydration contribute to fluid excess in tissue spaces. Fluid overload is another term for overhydration and hypervolemia.

Usually edema is the abnormal retention of fluid in the interstitial spaces in the ECF compartment, but it can occur in serous cavities such as the peritoneal cavity. In edema, sodium retention is the frequent cause of the increased extracellular fluid volume. Figure 2-1 demonstrates the changes in body fluid compartments as edema occurs.

PATHOPHYSIOLOGY

When sodium and water are retained in the same proportion, the fluid volume excess is referred to as **iso-osmolar** fluid volume excess. Usually the serum sodium level is within the normal range. If only free water is retained, the fluid volume excess is referred to as **hypo-osmolar** fluid volume excess. The serum sodium level is decreased. When there is fluid volume excess, the fluid pressure is greater than the oncotic pressure; therefore, more fluid is pushed into the tissue

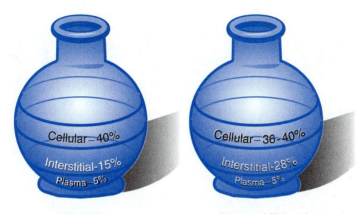

Cellular—40%
Interstitial-15%
Plasma—5%

Cellular—36–40%
Interstitial-28%
Plasma—5%

Normal
Fluid percent of Body Weight

Abnormal (Edema)
Fluid percent of Body Weight

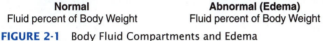

FIGURE 2-1 Body Fluid Compartments and Edema

spaces. Table 2-1 differentiates between iso-osmolar and hypo-osmolar fluid volume excess.

If the kidneys cannot excrete the excess intravascular fluid, fluid is frequently pushed into the tissue spaces and into the lung tissue spaces. Peripheral and/or pulmonary edema results. Fluid overload in the periphery will settle in the most dependent region: for example, feet and ankles when standing and sacrum when lying supine. When excess fluid crosses the alveolar-capillary membrane of the lungs, pulmonary edema results.

● ETIOLOGY

Edema is commonly associated with excess extracellular body fluid or excess fluid. Physiologic factors leading to edema may be caused by various clinical conditions, such as heart failure (HF), renal failure, cirrhosis of the liver, steroid excess, and allergic reaction. Table 2-2 lists the physiologic factors for edema, the rationale, and the clinical conditions associated with each physiologic factor.

Table 2-1	Differentiation Between Iso-osmolar and Hypo-osmolar Fluid Volume Excess	
Situation	**Iso-osmolar Fluid Volume Excess**	**Hypo-osmolar Fluid Volume Excess**
There is a proportional gain of both body fluids and solutes (sodium)	X	
The gain of body fluid is greater than the gain of sodium		X
A serum osmolality of 284 mOsm/kg occurs with ECFVE	X	
A serum osmolality of 273 mOsm/kg occurs with ECFVE		X

Table 2-2	Physiologic Factors Leading to Edema	
Physiologic Factors	**Rationale**	**Clinical Conditions**
Plasma hydrostatic pressure in the capillaries	↑ Increased Blood dammed in the venous system can cause "back" pressure in capillaries, thus raising capillary pressure. Increased capillary pressure will force more fluid into tissue areas, thus producing edema.	1. Heart failure with increased venous pressure. 2. Kidney failure resulting in sodium and water retention. 3. Venous obstruction leading to varicose veins. 4. Pressure on veins because of swelling, constricting bandages, casts, tumor, pregnancy. *(continues)*

Table 2-2	**Physiologic Factors Leading to Edema—*continued***

Physiologic Factors	Rationale	Clinical Conditions
Plasma colloid osmotic pressure	↓ Decreased plasma colloid osmotic pressure results from diminished plasma protein concentration. Decreased protein content may cause water to flow from plasma into tissue spaces, thus causing edema.	1. Malnutrition due to lack of protein in diet. 2. Chronic diarrhea resulting in loss of protein. 3. Burns leading to loss of fluid containing protein through denuded skin. 4. Kidney disease, particularly nephrosis. 5. Cirrhosis of liver resulting in decreased production of plasma protein. 6. Loss of plasma proteins through urine.
Capillary permeability	↑ Increased permeability of capillary membrane will allow plasma proteins to leak out of capillaries into interstitial space more rapidly than lymphatics can return them to circulation. Increased capillary permeability is predisposing factor to edema.	1. Bacterial inflammation causes increased porosity. 2. Allergic reactions. 3. Burns causing damage to capillaries. 4. Acute kidney disease, e.g., nephritis.

(continues)

Table 2-2	Physiologic Factors Leading to Edema—*continued*	
Physiologic Factors	**Rationale**	**Clinical Conditions**
Sodium retention	↑ Increased Kidneys regulate level of sodium ions in extracellular fluid. Kidney function will depend on adequate blood flow. Inadequate blood flow, presence of excess aldosterone or glucocorticosteroids, and diseased kidneys are predisposing factors to edema since they cause sodium, chloride, and retention.	1. Heart failure causing inadequate circulation of blood. 2. Renal failure—inadequate circulation of blood through kidneys. 3. Increased production of adrenal cortical hormones—aldosterone, cortisone, and hydrocortisone—will cause retention of sodium. 4. Cirrhosis of liver. Diseased liver cannot destroy excess production of aldosterone. 5. Trauma resulting from fractures, burns, and surgery.
Lymphatic drainage	↓ Decreased Blockage of lymphatics will prevent return of proteins to circulation. Obstructed lymph flow is said to be high in protein content. With inadequate return of proteins to circulation, plasma colloid osmotic pressure will be decreased, thus causing edema.	1. Lymphatic obstruction, e.g., cancer of lymphatic system. 2. Surgical removal of lymph nodes. 3. Elephantiasis, which is parasitic invasion of lymph channels, resulting in fibrous tissue growing in nodes, obstructing lymph flow. 4. Obesity because of inadequate supporting structures for lymphatics in lower extremities. Muscles are considered the supporting structures.

As blood is "backed up" in the venous system, capillary pressure is increased, forcing more fluid into the tissue spaces. A decrease in plasma/serum protein results in a decrease in plasma colloid osmotic (oncotic) pressure. This causes water to move from the vessels into the tissue spaces. An increase in the capillary membrane permeability permits plasma proteins to escape from the capillaries; thus, more water moves into the interstitial spaces. The kidneys regulate the gain/loss of sodium, chloride, and water via the renin-angiotensin-aldosterone system. With inadequate blood flow to the kidney or renal dysfunction or the presence of excess aldosterone, sodium retention occurs. Sodium retention results in water retention.

Clients with limited cardiac or renal reserve frequently develop pulmonary edema. When the heart is not able to function adequately and the kidneys cannot excrete a sufficient amount of urine, the fluid backs up into the pulmonary circulatory system; fluid moves from the vessels into the lung tissues. Administering an excessive amount of intravenous fluids to a person in pulmonary edema will further worsen the edema in the lungs. Intravenous infusions should be restricted in clients with pulmonary edema.

CLINICAL MANIFESTATIONS

There are numerous clinical manifestations (signs and symptoms) of ECFVE that relate to pulmonary edema and peripheral edema. When the fluid volume excess (hypervolemia or overhydration) causes a backup of fluid that seeps into the lung tissue, pulmonary edema results. An early symptom of pulmonary edema is a constant, irritating, nonproductive cough. Table 2-3 lists the clinical signs and symptoms of ECFVE related to pulmonary and peripheral edema. Laboratory test results influenced by ECFVE are included. The rationale for each sign or symptom is given.

Table 2-3	Clinical Manifestations of ECFVE—Hypervolemia, Overhydration, Edema

Signs and Symptoms	Rationale
Pulmonary Edema	
Constant, irritating, nonproductive cough	An irritating cough is frequently the first clinical symptom of hypervolemia. It is caused by fluid "backed up" into the lungs (fluid is in the alveoli).
Dyspnea (difficulty in breathing)	Breathing is labored and difficult due to fluid congestion in lungs.
Neck vein engorgement	Jugular vein remains engorged when the patient is in semi-Fowler's or sitting position.
Sublingual vein engorgement	Engorged veins under the tongue may indicate hypervolemia.
Hand vein engorgement	Peripheral veins in the hand remain engorged with hand elevated above heart level for 10 seconds.
Moist crackles in lung	Lungs are congested with fluid. Moist crackles in lung can be heard with the stethoscope.
Bounding pulse	A full, bounding pulse may be present with hypervolemia. The pulse rate may increase.
Cyanosis	Can be a late symptom of pulmonary edema as a result of impaired gas exchange caused by fluid in the alveolar space.
Peripheral Edema	
Pitting edema in extremities	Peripheral edema present in the morning may result from inadequate heart, liver, or kidney function. A positive test of pitting edema is a finger indentation on the edematous area.
Tight, smooth, shiny skin over edematous area	Excess fluid in the peripheral tissues may cause the skin to be tight, smooth, and shiny.
Pallor, cool skin at edematous area	Excess fluid causes a decrease in circulation. The skin becomes pale, shiny, and cool.
Puffy eyelids (periorbital edema)	Swollen eyelids occur with generalized edema.
Weight gain	A gain of 2.2 pounds is equivalent to a gain of 1 liter of body water.

(continues)

Table 2-3	Clinical Manifestations of ECFVE— Hypervolemia, Overhydration, Edema—*continued*
Signs and Symptoms	**Rationale**
Laboratory Tests Decreased serum osmolality	Excess fluid dilutes solute concentration; thus, serum osmolality is below 280 mOsm/kg.
Decreased serum protein and albumin, BUN, Hgb, Hct	Serum protein, albumin, BUN, and Hgb and Hct levels can be decreased due to excess fluid volume (hemodilution).
Increased CVP (central venous pressure)	An increase in CVP measurement of more than 12–15 cm H_2O is indicative of hypervolemia, evidenced as an increase in the fluid pressure.

A quick assessment for hypervolemia, or overhydration, can be done by checking the peripheral veins in the hand. Instruct the client to hold a hand above the heart level. If the peripheral veins of the hand remain engorged after 10 seconds, this can be an indication of hypervolemia. When the jugular vein remains engorged after a person is in semi-Fowler's position, the cause is most likely hypervolemia. Lungs should be checked for the presence of moist crackles. Cyanosis is a late symptom of pulmonary edema.

Gravity has an effect on the distribution of fluid in the edematous person. In a lying position, there is more equal distribution of edema, whereas in an upright position the edema is more prevalent in the lower extremities. This is called *dependent edema.* Dependent edema should not be present after the client has been in a prone or supine position for the night. If edema is present in the morning, it is most likely due to cardiac, renal, or liver disease and can be called *nondependent edema.* Edema that does not respond to diuretics is called *refractory edema.*

● CLINICAL MANAGEMENT

Normally, water alone does not cause or increase edema. Salt and water intake increases fluid retention and can cause edema. The three D's—diuretics, digoxin, and diet

Table 2-4	Basic Management for ECFVE or Edema
Correction Measures	**Rationale**
Diuretics: thiazides, high ceiling (loop)	Potassium-wasting diuretics are potent and promote the loss of sodium, water, and unfortunately, potassium. Diuretics cause a decrease in fluid volume excess via kidneys.
Digoxin	This cardiac glycoside causes the heart to beat more forcefully; thus, it improves heart function and circulation. Increased circulation promotes water loss through the kidneys.
Diet	A diet low in sodium decreases sodium and water retention.
Increased protein intake for a malnourished person	Protein increases the oncotic pressure in the vessels, thus pulling water out of the tissues.

(low sodium)—are frequently prescribed for the clinical management of clients with ECFVE and with heart failure (HF). Table 2-4 presents the basic management with rationale for correcting edema.

● CLINICAL CONSIDERATIONS: ECFVE

1. ECFVE, overhydration or hypervolemia, usually relates to excess fluid in tissues of the extremities (peripheral edema) or lungs (pulmonary edema).
2. Body water retention (edema) usually results from sodium retention. If only free water is retained, the excess is referred to as hypo-osmolar (hypotonic) fluid volume excess.
3. A constant, irritating, nonproductive cough is frequently the first clinical symptom of hypervolemia. It is caused by excess fluid "backed up" into the lungs.
4. For quick assessment of ECFVE, check for hand vein engorgement. If the peripheral veins in the hand remain

engorged when the hand is elevated above the heart level for 10 seconds, ECFVE or hypervolemia is present.

5. Moist crackles in the lung usually indicate that the lungs are congested with fluid.

6. Peripheral edema present in the morning may result from inadequate heart, liver, or kidney function. Peripheral edema in the evening may be due to fluid stasis— dependent edema. Peripheral edema should be assessed in the morning before the client gets out of bed.

7. A weight gain of 2.2 pounds is equivalent to the retention of 1 liter of body water.

8. Excess fluid dilutes solute concentration in the vascular space. A serum osmolality of <280 mOsm/kg indicates an ECFVE.

● CLIENT MANAGEMENT

Assessment

● Obtain a client history to identify typical health problems that may contribute to the development of ECFVE, such as heart failure (HF), kidney or liver disease, infection, and malnutrition.

● Obtain a dietary history that emphasizes sodium, protein, and water intake.

● Assess vital signs and urinary output. Report a bounding pulse.

● Check client's weight. Present weight is a baseline for comparison with daily weight.

● Assess for signs and symptoms of hypervolemia: constant, irritating, nonproductive cough, dyspnea, neck and hand vein engorgement, chest crackles.

● Check laboratory test results; a decreased hematocrit and hemoglobin level that had previously been normal may indicate ECFVE. Serum sodium levels may or may not be elevated because of hemodilution.

● Assess urine output; decreased urinary output may be a sign of body fluid retention and/or renal dysfunction.

● Auscultate the lungs for diminished breath sound and crackles, which could be due to pulmonary edema.

- Assess extremities for peripheral edema. Assessment for pitting edema in the lower extremities should be performed in the morning before the client arises.
- Make a quick assessment for hypervolemia by checking the peripheral veins in the hand, first lowering the hand and then raising the hand above the heart level.

Nursing Diagnoses

- *Excess Fluid Volume, Edema*, related to body fluid overload secondary to heart, renal, or liver dysfunction
- *Ineffective Breathing Pattern*, related to increased capillary permeability causing fluid overload in the lung tissue (pulmonary edema)
- *Ineffective Tissue Perfusion: Decreased*, related to hypervolemia as manifested by peripheral edema

Interventions

- Monitor vital signs with particular attention to respiratory status. Report abnormal findings, i.e., crackles, diminished breath sound.
- Monitor weight daily before breakfast. A weight gain of 2.2 pounds (1 kg) is equivalent to 1 liter of water. Usually edema does not occur unless there are 2 or more liters of excess body fluids.
- Monitor diet. Instruct the client to avoid excess use of salt on foods. Sodium retains water.
- Observe for the presence or decline of edema on a daily basis. Check for pitting edema in the morning.
- Check laboratory test results that are pertinent to electrolyte status and fluid balance.
- Monitor urine output. Urine output should be at least 250 mL per 8 hours.
- Administer diuretics as ordered. Assess fluid and electrolyte balance.
- Listen to client's concerns. Answer questions or refer questions to appropriate health professionals.

Evaluation/Outcome

● Evaluate that the cause of extracellular fluid volume excess (ECFVE) has been controlled or eliminated.

● Remain free of signs and symptoms of overhydration/hypervolemia; dyspnea, neck vein engorgement, moist crackles in the lung, and peripheral edema are absent.

● Evaluate the effects of clinical management for ECFVE; pulmonary edema and/or peripheral edema are absent or decreased because of clinical management.

● Urine output is increased to baseline measurement; vital signs are within normal range.

● Maintain a patent airway and the breath sounds are improved.

● Determine that the serum electrolytes are within normal range.

CHAPTER 3

Extracellular Fluid Volume Shift (ECFVS)

Carolee Polek, RN, PhD

INTRODUCTION

In the extracellular fluid compartment, ECF is constantly shifting between the intravascular and interstitial spaces for the purpose of maintaining fluid balance. When fluid volume with electrolytes and protein shifts from the intravascular to the interstitial spaces and remains there, this fluid is referred to as **third-space fluid.** This fluid is nonfunctional and is considered to be physiologically useless. Later, third-space fluid shifts back from the interstitial space to the intravascular space.

PATHOPHYSIOLOGY

Refer to the Pathophysiology section in Chapters 1 (ECFVD) and 2 (ECFVE).

ETIOLOGY

Clinical causes of ECFV shift can be as simple as a blister or sprain or as serious as massive injuries, burns, ascites, abdominal surgery, a perforated peptic ulcer, intestinal obstruction, or severe infections. Burns, massive injuries, and abdominal surgery are the most common causes of third-space fluid.

Fluid shift occurs in two phases. The first phase is when fluid shifts from the intravascular to the interstitial (vessel/plasma to tissue) space. For example, with burns, fluid loss occurs at the burned area and surrounding tissues. Fluid from the vascular space "pours" into the burned site and remains there for 3–5 days. When massive amounts of fluid shift to the tissues and remain there, fluid in the vascular space decreases and hypovolemia occurs. In the second phase of fluid shift, fluid then shifts from the injured tissue space back to the vascular space (vessels); hypervolemia may result.

●CLINICAL MANIFESTATIONS

In a fluid shift due to tissue injury, it takes approximately 24–48 hours for the fluid to leave the blood vessels and accumulate in the injured tissue spaces. Edema may or may not be visible. When fluid (massive amounts) shifts out of the vessels, changes in vital signs occur that are similar to symptoms of shock. Vital sign measures are similar to those of a fluid volume deficit (marked dehydration). These measures include increased pulse rate, increased respiration, and decreased systolic blood pressure (depending on the severity of fluid loss to the injured site). Other shock-like symptoms include cold extremities, pallor, confusion, and disorientation. In severe cases the hemoglobin and hematocrit can be increased.

After 3–5 days following severe tissue injury, fluid shifts from the injured site to the vascular space or blood vessels. If the kidneys cannot excrete the excess fluid from the vascular space, ECFVE or hypervolemia results. Symptoms related to intravascular overload include constant, irritating, nonproductive cough, dyspnea, moist chest crackles, full bounding pulse, and hand and neck vein engorgement. Table 3-1 lists the two phases of fluid shifts, signs and symptoms, and fluid correction ratio.

● CLINICAL MANAGEMENT

An assessment must be completed in order to determine the cause of the third-space fluid. If the cause is due to a minor injury such as a sprain or blisters, the amount of fluid shift is usually minor. Ice packs applied periodically to the sprained area can decrease the amount of fluid shift during the first 24 hours. Fluid replacement is not necessary. However, when there is severe tissue destruction, the fluid shift may be so severe that hypovolemia results from the massive amount of fluid shifting from the vascular space into the injured tissue areas. During the first phase of fluid shift to the injured tissue site, intravenous (IV) infusion in the amount of two to three times the urine output may be necessary to maintain the circulating fluid volume. The ratio is three times the intake to one time the output.

During the second phase of fluid shift, less IV fluid is needed. This fluid reduction is because a large quantity of fluid shifts back into the vascular space, and too much IV fluid may cause a fluid overload. In the second phase of fluid shift with normal renal function, the urine output increases. Excreting excess fluid prevents fluid overload. The amount of IV fluid administered should decrease by a ratio of 1 : 3 (one time the intake to three times the urine output) (see Table 3-1).

Table 3-1	ECFV Shift: Signs, Symptoms, and Corrections	
Phase of Fluid Shift	**Signs and Symptoms**	**Fluid Correction Ratio**
Phase 1	Shock-like Symptoms— Severe ECFVD	IV Intake to Urine Output 3 : 1
	Pulse, respiration, BP	
	Cold, clammy skin, pallor, confusion, disorientation	Three times more IV intake to urine output
Phase 2	Overhydration-like Symptoms	IV Intake to Urine Output 1 : 3
	Constant, irritating, nonproductive cough, dyspnea, bounding pulse, vein engorgement, moist chest crackles	One to three ratio: IV intake to urine output

● CLIENT MANAGEMENT

Assessment

● For extracellular fluid volume shift, refer to Chapter 1 (ECFVD) and Chapter 2 (ECFVE).

Nursing Diagnoses

● For extracellular fluid volume shift, refer to Chapter 1 (ECFVD) and Chapter 2 (ECFVE).

Interventions

● For extracellular fluid volume shift, refer to Chapter 1 (ECFVD) and Chapter 2 (ECFVE).

Evaluation/Outcome

● For extracellular fluid volume shift, refer to Chapter 1 (ECFVD) and Chapter 2 (ECFVE).

CHAPTER 4

Intracellular Fluid Volume Excess (ICFVE)

Carolee Polek, RN, PhD

INTRODUCTION

Intracellular fluid volume excess (ICFVE), also referred to as water intoxication, results from an excess of water or a decrease in the solute concentration in the intravascular system. Fluid in the blood vessels is hypo-osmolar. As a result of this excess water, the serum osmolality is decreased.

Hypo-osmolar fluid (decreased solute concentration in the circulating vascular fluid) moves by the process of osmosis from areas of lesser concentration of solutes to areas of greater concentration of solutes. Since intracellular fluid (cells) is iso-osmolar, the hypo-osmolar fluid from the vascular space moves into the cells.

PATHOPHYSIOLOGY

In ICFVE, the cerebral cells are usually the first cells involved in the fluid shift from the vascular to the cellular space. As fluid shifts into the cells, the cells swell, causing cellular edema. An excess secretion of the antidiuretic hormone (ADH) causes water to be reabsorbed from the renal tubules. This results in an increase in diluted fluid volume (hypo-osmolar vascular fluid), which causes additional fluid to move from the vascular space into the cells, causing cerebral edema.

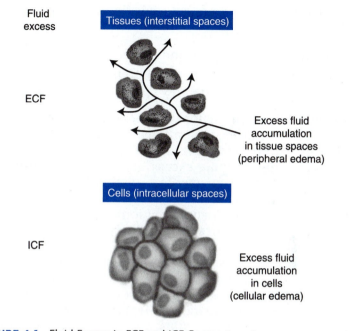

FIGURE 4-1 Fluid Excess in ECF and ICF Compartments

Edema may result from an excess of sodium, whereas water intoxication results from an excess of water. With edema there is excessive fluid in the extracellular fluid compartment, and with water intoxication (ICFVE) there is excess fluid in the intracellular fluid compartment. Edema is the accumulation of fluid in the interstitial spaces, and water intoxication is the excess of hypo-osmolar fluid in the vessels moving into the cells. Figure 4-1 shows the differences between the two fluid imbalances, ECFVE and ICFVE.

● ETIOLOGY

Intracellular fluid volume excess is not as common as ECFVD and ECFVE, but if untreated, it can cause serious health problems. Common causes of water intoxication are the intake of water-free solutes and the administration of hypo-osmolar intravenous fluids such as 0.45% sodium chloride (1/2 normal saline solution) and 5% dextrose in water (D_5W). Dextrose 5% in water is an iso-osmolar IV solution; however, the dextrose is metabolized quickly, leaving water or a hypo-osmolar solution.

There are four major conditions that may cause ICFVE:

1. Excessive nonsolute water intake
2. Solute deficit (electrolyte and protein)
3. Increased secretion of the antidiuretic hormone (ADH)
4. Kidney dysfunction (inability to excrete excess water)

Table 4-1 lists four major conditions and laboratory tests for ICFVE, their causes, and rationale.

It is difficult for a person to drink himself or herself into intracellular fluid volume excess or water intoxication unless the renal mechanisms for elimination fail or psychogenic polydipsia occurs. If excessive water has been given and the kidneys are not functioning properly, water retention and water intoxication are likely to occur.

The most common occurrence of ICFVE is seen in postoperative clients when oral and intravenous fluids have been forced without compensatory amounts of salt. In these situations, the amount of water taken in exceeds that which the kidneys excrete. A postoperative client receiving several liters of 5% dextrose in water, ice chips, and sips of water by mouth can develop water intoxication (ICFVE). The dextrose in D_5W is metabolized rapidly and the solution in the vascular space becomes hypo-osmolar. After major surgery, there is frequently an overproduction of the antidiuretic hormone (ADH), known as the syndrome of inappropriate ADH secretions (SIADH). This is partly due to tissue trauma, anesthesia, pain, and narcotics. Because of SIADH, water excretion decreases, causing the urine volume to drop and the vascular fluid volume to increase. The vascular fluid is mainly hypo-osmolar; this diluted vascular fluid moves to the cells that have a higher solute concentration, thus water intoxication results.

● CLINICAL MANIFESTATIONS

An early sign/symptom of ICFVE is headaches. As the hypo-osmolar body fluids continue to pass into cerebral cells, the swollen cerebral cells cause behavioral changes such as apprehension, irritability, confusion, and disorientation. The intracranial pressure is increased. With progressive intracellular fluid volume excess, the blood pressure increases, pulse rate decreases, and respirations increase. The clinical signs, symptoms, and rationale of ICFVE are explained in Table 4-2.

Table 4-1	Causes of Intracellular Fluid Volume Excess: Water Intoxication	
Conditions	**Causes**	**Rationale**
Excessive water intake	Excessive plain water intake	Water intake with few or no solutes dilutes the vascular fluid.
	Continuous use of IV hypo-osmolar solutions (0.45% saline, D_5W)	Overuse of hypo-osmolar solutions can cause hypo-osmolar vascular fluid. Dextrose is metabolized rapidly, leaving water.
	Psychogenic polydipsia	Compulsive drinking of plain water can result in water intoxication.
Solute deficit	Diet low in electrolytes and protein	Decrease in electrolytes and protein may cause hypo-osmolar vascular fluids.
	Irrigation of nasogastric tube with water (not saline)	GI tract is rich in electrolytes. Plain water can wash out the electrolytes.
	Plain water enema	Plain water can wash out the electrolytes.
Excess ADH secretion	Stress, surgery, drugs (narcotics, anesthesia), pain, and tumors (brain, lung)	Overproduction of ADH is known as secretion (syndrome) of inappropriate antidiuretic hormone (SIADH), which causes mass amounts of water reabsorption by the kidneys and results in hypo-osmolar fluids.
	Brain injury or tumor	Cerebral cell injury may increase ADH production, causing excessive water reabsorption.
Kidney dysfunction	Renal impairment	Kidney dysfunction can decrease water excretion.
Abnormal laboratory tests	Decreased serum sodium level and decreased serum osmolality	Because of hemodilution, the solutes in the vascular fluid are decreased in proportion to water.

Table 4-2	Clinical Signs and Symptoms of Intracellular Fluid Volume Excess—Water Intoxication	
Type of Symptoms	**Signs and Symptoms**	**Rationale**
Early	Headache Nausea and vomiting Excessive perspiration Acute weight gain	Cerebral cells absorb hypo-osmolar fluid more quickly than other cells.

Progressive
Central nervous system (CNS)
	Behavioral changes:
	  progressive
	  apprehension,
	  irritability,
	  disorientation,
	  confusion
	Drowsiness,
	  incoordination
	Blurred vision
	Elevated intracranial
	  pressure (ICP)
		Hypo-osmolar body fluids usually pass into cerebral cells first. Swollen cerebral cells can cause behavioral changes and elevate ICP.

Vital signs (VS)	Blood pressure ↑ Bradycardia (slow pulse rate) Respiration ↑	VS are the opposite of shock. VS are similar to those in increased ICP.
Later (CNS)	Neuroexcitability (muscle twitching) Projectile vomiting Papilledema Delirium Convulsions, then coma	Severe CNS changes occur when water intoxication is not corrected.
Skin	Warm, moist, and flushed	

● CLINICAL MANAGEMENT

The overall objectives for clinical management of ICFVE are to reduce excess water intake and to promote water excretion. In less severe cases, water restriction may be sufficient or an extracellular replacement solution such as lactated Ringer's or normal saline solution can increase the osmolal-

Table 4-3	Clinical Management for Clients Having ICFVE
Stage of ICFVE	**Corrective Measures**
Early stage	Restrict plain water intake and ice chips. Administer balanced electrolyte solution (BES) such as lactated Ringer's solution, normal saline solution, 5% dextrose in 0.45% normal saline solution. Avoid using only 5% dextrose in water.
Moderate stage without severe behavioral changes	Same as the early stage. Five percent dextrose in 0.9% NaCl may be needed.
Moderate to severe stage with behavioral changes and elevated intracranial pressure (ICP)	Restrict plain water intake and ice chips. Discontinue 5% dextrose in water for replacement therapy. Administer concentrated saline (3%) solution and monitor for fluid overload. Administer osmotic diuretic such as mannitol.

ity of the extracellular fluid. A concentrated saline solution (3%) may be given in severe cases of water intoxication in order to raise the extracellular electrolyte concentration in order to draw the water out of the intracellular space and increase urine output.

However, administration of additional salt to a person who already has too much water can expand the blood volume and the interstitial fluid resulting in edema. An osmotic diuretic induces diuresis and promotes the loss of retained fluid, especially from the cells. Table 4-3 lists the methods in promoting water excretion for correcting ICFVE.

● CLINICAL CONSIDERATIONS: ICFVE

1. ICFVE is also known as water intoxication—excess water in the cells. It usually results from an excess of hypoosmolar (hypotonic) vascular fluid. Water intoxication is not the same as edema. Edema usually results from sodium retention, whereas water intoxication results from excess water.

2. In ICFVE, cerebral cells are usually the first cells involved in the fluid shift from the vascular to the cellular (cell) space. Large amounts of fluid shifting into the cerebral cells can result in cerebral edema.

3. Continuous administration of intravenous solutions that are hypotonic or the continuous use of 5% dextrose in water can result in ICFVE. In the latter case, dextrose is metabolized rapidly in the body; thus water remains. At least 1 or 2 liters of the dextrose solution should contain a percentage of a saline solution or be administered in combination with solutes such as lactated Ringer's.

4. Headache, nausea, and vomiting are early signs and symptoms of ICFVE. As ICFVE progresses, behavioral changes such as irritability, disorientation, and confusion may occur. Drowsiness and blurred vision may result.

5. Changes in vital signs are similar to those of cerebral edema: increased blood pressure, decreased pulse rate, and increased respirations.

6. A concentrated saline solution (3% NaCl) can be administered for severe ICFVE. It is given if the serum sodium is less than 115 mEq/L. Also, it draws the water out of the swollen cells.

7. Water restriction is suggested for mild ICFVE.

● CLIENT MANAGEMENT

Assessment

● Obtain a history to identify the possible cause(s) of ICFVE such as continuous use of D_5W without solutes (saline), excessive intake of oral fluid without solutes, or major surgical procedure that might cause SIADH.

● Assess vital signs (VS) by obtaining a baseline of VS that can be compared with past and future VS. Note the VS typical for cerebral edema, i.e., increased blood pressure, decreased pulse rate, and increased respirations.

● Assess for behavioral changes, such as apprehension, irritability, confusion, and/or disorientation. Headache is an early symptom of ICFVE.

● Assess for weight changes. With ICFVE, there is usually an acute weight gain; however, with peripheral edema, the weight gain occurs more slowly.

Nursing Diagnoses

● *Excess Fluid Volume, Water Intoxication,* related to excessive ingestion and infusion of hypo-osmolar fluids and solutions, and major surgical procedure causing SIADH

● *Risk for Injury,* related to confusion from cerebral edema secondary to ICFVE

Interventions

● Monitor fluid replacement. Report if the client is receiving ONLY 5% dextrose in water continuously without any solutes such as sodium chloride.

● Offer fluids that contain solutes to the postoperative client. Giving only plain water and ice chips increases the hypo-osmolar state.

● Monitor urine output. This is especially important postoperatively.

● Monitor vital signs and observe for behavioral changes.

● Protect the client from injury during periods of confusion and disorientation.

● Listen to client's and family's concerns. Refer unknown answers to appropriate health professionals.

Evaluation/Outcome

● Evaluate that the cause of intracellular fluid volume excess (ICFVE) has been corrected or controlled.

● Remain free of signs and symptoms of ICFVE or water intoxication; vital signs return to normal ranges, headaches have been lessened or absent.

● Evaluate the effects of clinical management of ICFVE; hypotonic/hypo-osmolar solutions discontinued, solutes offered with fluids.

● Responds clearly without confusion.

ELECTROLYTES AND THEIR INFLUENCE ON THE BODY

INTRODUCTION

Chemical compounds develop a tiny electrical charge when dissolved in water. The compounds break into separate particles known as ions; this process is referred to as ionization, and the compounds are known as electrolytes. Some electrolytes develop a positive charge (cations) when placed in water; others develop a negative charge (anions).

In this unit, six electrolytes [potassium, sodium, chloride, calcium, magnesium, and phosphorus (phosphate)] are discussed in relation to basic information associated with each electrolyte in terms of pathophysiology, etiology, clinical manifestations, and clinical management issues. Health assessment and intervention guidelines follow the presentation of each electrolyte.

ELECTROLYTES: CATION AND ANION

Electrolytes are compounds that when placed in solution, conduct an electric current and emit dissociated particles of electrolytes (ions) that carry either a positive charge (cation) or a negative charge (anion). Table U2-1 gives the principal cations and anions in human body fluids. Note the symbols for each electrolyte (e.g., K, Na) and their charge ($^+$ and $^-$).

The term *milliequivalents* is used to express the number of ionic charges of each electrolyte. Serum electrolyte values are expressed in milliequivalents and milligrams. The milliequivalents of electrolytes are the chemical activity of the ion rather than their weight. Table U2-2 gives the weights and equivalences of four cations and an anion. Note how the weights of the named ions differ but the equivalences remain the same according to their ionic charge.

Table U2-1 Cations and Anions

Cations		Anions	
Na^+	(Sodium)	Cl^-	(Chloride)
K^+	(Potassium)	HCO_3^-	(Bicarbonate)
Ca^{2+}	(Calcium)	HPO_4^{2-}	(Phosphate)
Mg^{2+}	(Magnesium)		

TABLE U2-1 Principle cations and anions in the Human Body

Table U2-2 Electrolyte Equivalents

Ion	Weight (mg)	Equivalence (mEq)
Na^+	23	1
K^+	39	1
Cl^-	35	1
Ca^{++}	40	2
Mg^{++}	24	2

TABLE U2-2 Weight and equivalence of the Four Cations and One Anion

The electrolyte composition of fluid differs within the two main classes of body fluid (intracellular, fluid and the extracellular fluid); refer to Unit I. Table U2-3 gives the ion concentrations of the intravascular fluid (referred to as plasma), interstitial fluid, and intracellular fluid. Note that sodium (Na) is more plentiful in the extracellular fluid (plasma and interstitial fluid) and potassium (K) is more plentiful in the intracellular fluid. Figure U2-1 shows the various cations and anions in extracellular and intracellular fluids.

Table U2-3	Electrolyte Composition of Body Fluid (mEq/L)		
	Extracellular		
Ions	**Intravascular or Plasma**	**Interstitial**	**Intracellular**
Na^+	142	145	10
K^+	5	4	141-150
Ca^{++}	5	3	2
Mg^{++}	2	1	27
Cl^-	104	116	1
HCO_3^-	27	30	10
HPO_4^{--}	2	2	100

TABLE U2-3 Electrolyte Concentrations in Body Fluids

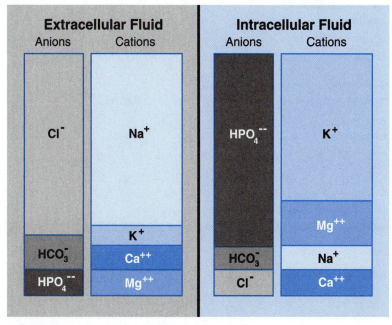

FIGURE U2-1 Anions and cations in body fluid.

CLINICAL PROBLEMS ASSOCIATED WITH ELECTROLYTE IMBALANCES

Table U2-4 illustrates the most common clinical problems associated with electrolyte imbalances.

Table U2-4	Unit II Clinical Problems Associated with Electrolyte Imbalances and Their Influence on the Body				
Clinical Problems	**Potassium**	**Sodium**	**Calcium**	**Magnesium**	**Phosphorus**
Gastrointestinal					
Vomiting and diarrhea	K↓	Na↓	Ca↓	Mg↓	P↓
Malnutrition	K↓	Na↓	Ca↓	Mg↓	P↓
Anorexia nervosa	K↓	Na↓	Ca↓	Mg↓	P↓
Intestinal fistula	K↓	Na↓		Mg↓	P↓
GI surgery	K↓	Na↓		Mg↓	P↓
Chronic alcoholism	K↓	Na↓	Ca↓	Mg↓	P↓
Lack of vitamin D			Ca↓		
Hyperphosphatemia			Ca↓		
Transfusion of citrated blood			Ca↓		
Cardiac					
Myocardial infarction	K↓	Na↓ Hypervolemia		Mg↓	
Heart failure (HF)	K↓/N	Na↑		Mg↓/N	
Endocrine					
Cushing's syndrome	K↓	Na↑		Mg↓	
Addison's disease	K↑	Na↓		Mg↓	
Diabetic ketoacidosis	K↑ Diuresis K↓	Na↑/↓	Ca↓ (ionized)	Mg↑ Diuresis Mg↓	P↓/N
Parathyroidism					
Hypo:			Ca↓		P↑
Hyper:			Ca↑		P↓
Renal					
Acute renal failure	Oliguria K↑ Diuresis K↓	Na↑		Mg↑	P↑
Chronic renal failure	K↑	Na↑	Ca↑/↓	Mg↑	P↑

(continues)

Table U2-4	**Unit II Clinical Problems Associated with Electrolyte Imbalances and Their Influence on the Body—*continued***				
Clinical Problems	**Potassium**	**Sodium**	**Calcium**	**Magnesium**	**Phosphorus**
Miscellaneous					
Cancer	K↓/↑	Na↓	Ca↑	Mg↓	P↓
Bone destruction			Ca↑		
Burns	K↓/↑	Na↓	Ca↓	Mg↓	P↓
Acute pancreatitis			Ca↓		
SIADH (syndrome of inappropriate antidiuretic hormone)		Na↓			
Metabolic acidosis	K↑		Ca↓		
Metabolic alkalosis	K↓				
Drugs					
Diuretics					
Potassium wasting	K↓	Na↓	Ca↑/↓	Mg↓	
Potassium sparing	K↑/N	Na↓		Mg↓	
ACE inhibitors	K↑	Na↓/N			

Potassium Imbalances

Joyce LeFever Kee, RN, MS

INTRODUCTION

Potassium (K), a cation, is the most abundant cation in the body cells. Ninety-seven percent of the body's potassium is found in the intracellular fluid (ICF) and 2–3% is found in the extracellular fluid (ECF), which comprises the intravascular (in vessels) and interstitial fluids (between tissues). Potassium is also plentiful in the gastrointestinal tract. The potassium level in the cells is approximately 150 mEq, and the potassium level in the ECF is 3.5–5.3 mEq. Because potassium levels cannot be measured within the cells, the potassium level is monitored by obtaining intravascular fluid or blood plasma specimens.

The normal plasma/serum potassium range is narrow; therefore, a serum potassium level outside the normal range may be life threatening. A serum potassium level less than 2.5 mEq/L or greater than 7.0 mEq/L can cause cardiac arrest. Thus, serum potassium values need to be closely monitored.

Basic information related to potassium balance is summarized in Table 5-1. Deviations from the normal result in a potassium imbalance.

PATHOPHYSIOLOGY

The assimilative processes involved in the formation of new tissue are referred to as **anabolism,** and the reactions concerned with tissue breakdown are referred to as **catabolism.**

Table 5-1	Basic Information Related to Potassium Balance
Categories	**Potassium Data**
Distribution	Ninety-seven percent of potassium is located within the cells (intracellular fluid). Two to 3% of potassium is located within the extracellular fluid. Potassium is most plentiful in the GI tract.
Functions	Potassium (1) promotes the transmission and conduction of nerve impulses and the contraction of skeletal, cardiac, and smooth muscles; (2) assists in the regulation of intracellular osmolality; (3) promotes enzyme action for cellular metabolism; and (4) assists in maintenance of acid-base balance. A potassium deficit is associated with alkalosis and a potassium excess is related to acidosis.
Normal serum value	3.5–5.3 mEq/L. A potassium deficit (hypokalemia) is less than 3.5 mEq/L and a potassium excess (hyperkalemia) is greater than 5.3 mEq/L.
Normal potassium excretion (urine)	Twenty to 120 mEq of potassium per day is excreted by the kidneys.
Food sources	Foods rich in potassium include vegetables, fruits, dry fruits, nuts, and meat. Foods rich in sodium promote a potassium loss.
Dietary requirements	Normal daily potassium intake is 40–60 mEq. Potassium is poorly stored in the body, so a daily potassium intake is essential.
Excretion	Eighty to 90% of the body's potassium is excreted through the kidneys. Ten to 20% is excreted in the feces.

When cellular activity is anabolic (building up), potassium enters the cells. When cellular activity is catabolic (breaking down), potassium leaves the cells. When tissues are destroyed as a result of trauma, starvation, or wasting diseases, large quantities of potassium leave the cells. If the kidneys are functioning, potassium is excreted and hypokalemia results. The pathophysiology related to potassium loss and retention is summarized in Table 5-2.

Table 5-2	Pathophysiology Related to Potassium Loss and Retention
Potassium Imbalance	**Pathophysiology**
Potassium loss	*Cellular Potassium Loss*
	Tissue injury: trauma, malnutrition
	Muscle contraction: continuous or strenuous exercise
	GI losses: vomiting, diarrhea
	Hormonal Influence
	Aldosterone promotes sodium retention and potassium excretion.
	Insulin promotes potassium leaving the ECF and moving into cells.
	Renal Potassium Loss
	Normal kidney function excretes excess potassium from the ECF.
Potassium retention	*Renal Dysfunction*
	Decreased renal function causes a buildup of potassium in the ECF, resulting in hyperkalemia.

During exercise, when muscles contract, the cells lose potassium and absorb a nearly equal quantity of sodium from the extracellular fluid. After exercise, when the muscles are recovering from fatigue, potassium reenters the cells and most of the sodium returns to the extracellular fluid. The cations potassium and sodium have an opposing effect on each other in the extracellular fluid. When one is retained, the other is excreted.

Hormonal influences affect serum potassium levels. Physiologic or psychologic stress causes a release of an excessive amount of potassium that is then lost through the kidneys. This potassium loss depletes the cells' supply. Stress also stimulates the adrenal gland to overproduce **aldosterone,** an adrenal cortical hormone. This hormone influences the kidneys to excrete potassium and to retain sodium, chloride, and water.

Insulin production or administration promotes glucose and potassium uptake by the cells and thus decreases the serum potassium level. Insulin administration may be used to temporarily correct a mild hyperkalemic state by forcing the potassium back into the cells. It is believed that glucagon increases the serum potassium level by releasing potassium from the liver and muscle cells.

When renal function is normal, the excess potassium is slowly excreted by the kidneys. However, if potassium intake is decreased without oral or intravenous supplements, potassium excretion by the kidneys can lead to potassium depletion or hypokalemia. If the kidneys are injured or diseased and the urine output is markedly decreased, potassium concentration increases in the extracellular fluid and hyperkalemia results.

ETIOLOGY

Daily potassium intake is necessary because potassium is poorly conserved within the body. Inadequate intake through a balanced diet may result in a potassium deficit. The elderly and the young tend to lose potassium faster than healthy adults; thus the potassium level must be monitored closely.

Causes of hypokalemia include dietary changes, gastrointestinal losses, renal losses, hormonal influence, and cellular damage. Summary data of these losses are presented in Table 5-3. Causes of hyperkalemia include excessive potassium intake, decreased renal function, altered cellular function, hormonal deficiency, and pseudohyperkalemia. Summary data are presented in Table 5-4.

CLINICAL MANIFESTATIONS

Clinical manifestations of hypokalemia and hyperkalemia can be determined by the serum potassium level, electrocardiography (ECG/EKG) tracings, and specific signs and symptoms related to gastrointestinal, cardiac, renal, and neurologic abnormalities. The serum potassium level and the ECG play a critical role in determining the severity of the potassium imbalance. Mild hypokalemia may go undetected until the serum potassium level is less than 3.2 mEq/L. Signs and symptoms of hyperkalemia may not be noted until the serum potassium level exceeds 5.6 mEq/L.

A potassium deficit slows muscular contraction; thus skeletal muscle contraction and GI smooth muscle activity are slowed. Hypokalemia decreases GI motility, which when severe may result in a paralytic ileus.

Table 5-3 — Causes of Hypokalemia (Serum Potassium Deficit)

Etiology	Rationale
Dietary Changes Malnutrition, starvation, alcoholism, unbalanced reducing diets, anorexia nervosa, crash diets	Potassium is poorly conserved in the body. For a potassium deficit to occur, a prolonged, inadequate potassium intake must occur.
Gastrointestinal Losses Vomiting, diarrhea, gastric/ intestinal suctioning, intestinal fistula, laxative abuse, bulimia, enemas	Potassium is plentiful in the GI tract. With the loss of GI secretions, large amounts of potassium ions are lost.
Renal Losses Diuretics, diuretic phase of acute renal failure, hemodialysis and peritoneal dialysis	The kidneys excrete 80–90% of the potassium lost. Diuretics are the major cause of hypokalemia, especially potassium-wasting diuretics [thiazides, loop (high-ceiling), osmotic].
Hormonal Influence Steroids, Cushing's syndrome, stress, excessive intake of licorice	Steroids, especially cortisone and aldosterone, promote potassium excretion and sodium retention. Stress increases the production of steroids in the body. In Cushing's syndrome, there is an excess production of adrenocortical hormones (cortisol and aldosterone). Licorice contains glyceric acid, which has an aldosterone-like effect.
Cellular Damage Trauma, tissue injury, surgery, burns	Cellular and tissue damage cause potassium to be released in the intravascular fluid. More potassium is needed to repair injured tissue.
Drugs Promoting Hypokalemia Epinephrine, decongestants, bronchodilators, and beta$_2$-adrenergic agonists	These drugs promote potassium excretion.
Redistribution of Potassium Insulin, alkalotic state	Insulin moves glucose and potassium into cells. Metabolic alkalosis promotes the movement of potassium into cells.

Table 5-4 Causes of Hyperkalemia (Serum Potassium Excess)

Etiology	Rationale
Excessive Potassium Intake	
Oral potassium supplements and salt substitutes	A potassium consumption rate greater than the potassium excretion rate increases the serum potassium level.
IV potassium infusions	Adequate urinary output must be determined when giving a potassium supplement.
Decreased Renal Function	
Acute renal failure	Because potassium is generally excreted in the urine, anuria and oliguria cause a potassium buildup in the plasma.
Chronic renal failure	
Drugs	
Potassium-sparing diuretics	Potassium-sparing diuretics can cause an aldosterone deficiency, promoting potassium retention.
ACE inhibitors, beta blockers	These drugs affect potassium balance.
Altered Cellular Function	
Severe traumatic injury	Cellular injury increases potassium loss due to cell breakdown. Potassium excretion may be greater than cellular K reabsorption. Potassium can accumulate in the plasma.
Metabolic acidosis	In acidosis, the hydrogen ion moves into the cells and potassium moves out of the cells, increasing the serum potassium level.
Blood for transfusion that is 1–3 weeks old	As stored blood for transfusion ages, hemolysis (breakdown of red blood cells) occurs; potassium from the cells is released into the ECF.
Hormonal Deficiency	
Addison's disease	Reduced secretion of the adrenocortical hormones causes a retention of potassium and a loss of sodium.
Pseudohyperkalemia	
Hemolysis	With hemolysis, ruptured red blood cells release potassium into the ECF.
Tourniquet application Phlebotomy, clenching of the fist	A tourniquet that has been applied too tightly or rapidly drawing blood with a small needle lumen (<21 gauge) can cause a falsely elevated potassium level in the blood specimen.

Mild to moderate hyperkalemia causes muscle irritability, while severe hyperkalemia causes muscle weakness. When a serum potassium level reaches 6.0 mEq/L, paresthesia (numbness, tingling) and an increased heart rate may be apparent. Table 5-5 lists specific signs and symptoms indicative of hypokalemia and hyperkalemia.

Potassium is abundant in cardiac muscle, and a deficit may result in cardiac dysrhythmias. Clients with cardiac ischemia, heart failure, and left ventricular hypertrophy who have a mild to moderate potassium loss are likely to develop cardiac dysrhythmias. Common ECG changes associated with hypokalemia include premature ventricular contractions (PVCs), a flat or inverted T wave, and a depressed ST segment. Figure 5-1 displays the ECG results related to hypokalemia, and Figure 5-2 includes the ECG changes resulting from hyperkalemia. A serum potassium level >6.0 mEq/L causes the my-

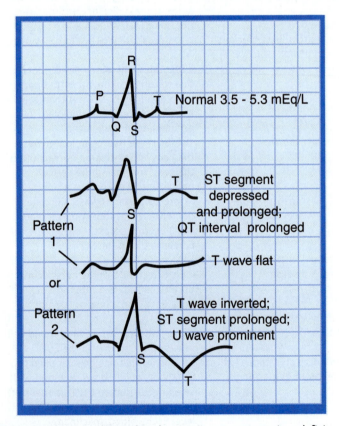

FIGURE 5-1 Electrocardiographic changes in serum potassium deficit.

Table 5-5	Clinical Manifestations of Potassium Imbalances	
Body Involvement	**Hypokalemia**	**Hyperkalemia**
Gastrointestinal Abnormalities	*Anorexia Nausea *Vomiting Diarrhea †Abdominal distention †Decreased peristalsis or silent ileus	*Nausea *Diarrhea †Abdominal cramps

Cardiac Abnormalities	†Dysrhythmias
	†Vertigo
	Cardiac arrest when severe
		Tachycardia, later
		  †bradycardia, and finally
		  cardiac arrest (severe)

ECG/EKG	†Flat or inverted T wave
	Depressed ST segment
		†Peaked, narrow T wave
		Shortened QT interval
		Prolonged PR interval
		  followed by
		  disappearance of P wave
		Prolonged QRS interval if
		  level continues to rise

Renal Abnormalities	Polyuria	†Oliguria or anuria
Neuromuscular Abnormalities	†Malaise Drowsiness †Muscular weakness Confusion Mental depression Diminished deep tendon reflexes Respiratory paralysis	Weakness, numbness, or tingling sensation Muscle cramps
Laboratory Values Serum potassium	<3.5 mEq/L	>5.3 mEq/L

†Most commonly seen symptoms of hypo-hyperkalemia
*Commonly seen symptoms of hypo-hyperkalemia

ocardium to become flaccid and dilate; an atrial or ventricular dysrhythmia is likely to occur. ECG changes usually do not occur until the serum potassium level approaches 7.0 mEq/L. ECG findings for hyperkalemia include narrow peaked T waves, a widened QRS complex, a depressed ST segment, and a widened P-R interval. These heart changes result in a decreased cardiac output.

● CLINICAL MANAGEMENT

Successful clinical management of a potassium imbalance requires immediate intervention if the potassium is less than 3.0 mEq/L or more than 5.8 mEq/L. Oral potassium replacement therapy is frequently ordered for a mild potassium deficit (3.3–3.4 mEq/L) or for preventive purposes. Potassium is irritating to the GI tract and should be ingested with at least 6–8 ounces of fluid. Intravenous (IV) potassium chloride (KCl) is suggested for a moderate to severe potassium deficit (<3.2 mEq/L). Intravenous KCl should NEVER be administered as a bolus or IV push. Cardiac arrest can result.

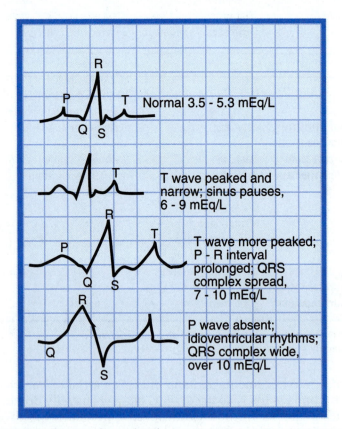

FIGURE 5-2 Electrocardiographic changes in serum potassium concentration.

Table 5-6	Oral Potassium Supplements
Preparation	**Drug**
Liquid	Potassium chloride 10% = 20 mEq/15 mL; 20% = 40 mEq/15 mL
	Kay Ciel (potassium chloride)
	Kaochlor 10% (potassium chloride)
	Kaon Cl 20 (potassium chloride)
	Potassium Triplex (potassium acetate, bicarbonate, citrate)
Tablet/capsule	Potassium chloride (enteric-coated tablet)
	Kaon—plain (potassium gluconate)
	Kaon Cl (potassium chloride)
	Slow K (potassium chloride—8 mEq)
	Kaochlor (potassium chloride)
	K-Lyte—plain (potassium bicarbonate-effervescent tablet)
	K-Lyte/Cl (potassium chloride)

Intravenous KCl must be well diluted in an IV solution. Table 5-6 lists selected potassium replacement drugs. Serum levels of magnesium, chloride, and protein should be checked when correcting hypokalemia. Low values of Mg, Cl, and protein can inhibit potassium utilization by the body.

Temporary interventions to correct hyperkalemia include the use of sodium bicarbonate and insulin and glucose infusion. These agents initially move potassium back into the cells; however, if the drugs are repeated for the purpose of decreasing the potassium level, they may not be effective. Calcium gluconate infusions may be prescribed to decrease the antagonistic effect of potassium excess on the myocardium when the cardiac disturbance is due to hyperkalemia.

With severe hyperkalemia (>6.8 mEq/L), polystyrene sulfonate (Kayexalate), a cation exchange resin, may be given orally or rectally. A potassium ion is exchanged for a sodium ion in the intestinal tract, and the potassium ion is excreted in the stool. Because Kayexalate is constipating, sorbitol may be given with Kayexalate to prevent constipation and induce diarrhea. A retention enema is the mode for administering rectal Kayexalate and sorbitol. Table 5-7 lists interventions to reduce potassium levels.

Table 5-7	Correction of Potassium Excess (Hyperkalemia)
Treatment Methods	**Rationale**
Potassium restriction	Restriction of potassium intake will slowly lower the serum level. For mild hyperkalemia (slightly elevated K levels), i.e., 5.4–5.6 mEq/L, potassium restriction is normally effective.
IV sodium bicarbonate ($NaHCO_3$)	By elevating the pH level, potassium moves back into the cells, thus lowering the serum level. This is a temporary treatment.
10% Calcium gluconate	Calcium decreases the irritability of the myocardium resulting from hyperkalemia. It is a temporary treatment and does not promote K loss. *Caution:* Administering calcium to a client on digitalis can cause digitalis toxicity.
Insulin and glucose (10–50%)	The combination of insulin and glucose moves potassium back into the cells. It is a temporary treatment, effective for approximately 6 hours, and is not always as effective when repeated.
Kayexalate (sodium polystyrene) and sorbitol 70%	Kayexalate is used as a cation exchange for severe hyperkalemia and can be administered orally or rectally. Approximate dosages are as follows: *Orally:* Kayexalate—10–20 g 3 to 4 times daily Sorbitol 70%—20 mL with each dose *Rectally:* Kayexalate—30–50 g Sorbitol 70%—50 mL; mix with 100–150 mL water (Retention enema—20–30 minutes)

Drugs and Their Effect on Potassium Balance

Potassium-wasting diuretics are a major cause of hypokalemia. Diuretics are divided into two categories: potassium-wasting and potassium-sparing drugs. Potassium-wasting diuretics ex-

Table 5-8	**Potassium-Wasting and Potassium-Sparing Diuretics**

Potassium-Wasting Diuretics	Potassium-Sparing Diuretics
Thiazides	Aldosterone antagonist
Chlorothiazide/Diuril	Spironolactone/Aldactone
Hydrochlorothiazide/HydroDIURIL	Triamterene/Dyrenium
Loop diuretics	Amiloride/Midamor
Furosemide/Lasix	
Ethacrynic acid/Edecrin	*Combination: K-Wasting and*
Carbonic anhydrase inhibitors	*K-Sparing Diuretics*
Acetazolamide/Diamox	Aldactazide
Osmotic diuretic	Spironazide
Mannitol	Dyazide
	Moduretic

crete potassium and other electrolytes such as sodium and chloride in the urine. Potassium-sparing diuretics retain potassium but excrete sodium and chloride in the urine. Table 5-8 lists the trade and generic names of potassium-wasting and potassium-sparing diuretics and a combination of potassium-wasting and potassium-sparing diuretics.

Laxatives, corticosteroids, antibiotics, and potassium-wasting diuretics are the major drug groups that can cause hypokalemia. The drug groups attributed to hyperkalemia include oral and intravenous potassium salts, central nervous system (CNS) agents, potassium-sparing diuretics, ACE inhibitors, and beta blockers. Table 5-9 lists the drugs that affect potassium balance.

● CLINICAL CONSIDERATIONS: POTASSIUM

1. Oral potassium should be taken with food and/or 8 ounces of fluid. Potassium is irritating to the gastric mucosa and can cause a gastric ulcer.
2. Mild hypokalemia, 3.4 mEq/L, can be avoided by eating foods rich in potassium, i.e., fresh fruits, dry fruits, fruit juices, vegetables, meats, nuts.
3. Intravenous potassium should be well diluted in IV solution. NEVER administer IV potassium as a bolus (IV push). It can cause cardiac arrest.

Table 5-9	Drugs Affecting Potassium Balance	
Potassium Imbalance	**Substances**	**Rationale**
Hypokalemia (serum potassium deficit)	Laxatives	Laxative abuse can cause potassium depletion.
	Enemas (hyperosmolar)	
	Corticosteroids	
	Cortisone	Ion exchange agent.
	Prednisone	Steroids promote potassium loss and sodium retention.
	Kayexalate	Exchange potassium ion for a sodium ion.
	Licorice	Licorice action is similar to aldosterone, promoting K loss and Na retention.
	Levodopa/L-dopa	Increases potassium loss via urine.
	Lithium	
	Antibiotic I	
	Amphotericin B	Toxic effect on renal tubules, thus decreasing potassium reabsorption.
	Polymyxin B	
	Tetracycline (outdated)	
	Gentamicin	
	Neomycin	
	Amikacin	
	Tobramycin	
	Cisplatin	
	Antibiotic II	
	Penicillin	Potassium excretion is enhanced by the presence of nonreabsorbable anions.
	Ampicillin	
	Carbenicillin	
	Ticarcillin	
	Nafcillin	
	Piperacillin	
	Azlocillin	
	Alpha-adrenergic blockers	These agents promote movement of potassium into cells, thus lowering the serum potassium level.
	Insulin and glucose	

(continues)

Table 5-9	Drugs Affecting Potassium Balance—*continued*	
Potassium Imbalance	**Substances**	**Rationale**

	Beta₂ agonists
	  Terbutaline
	  Albuterol
	Estrogen
		Beta₂ agonists promote potassium loss.

	Potassium-wasting diuretics	See Table 5–8

Hyperkalemia
(serum
potassium
excess)
	Potassium chloride
	  (oral or IV)
	Potassium salt
	  substitutes
	K penicillin
	KPO₄ enema
		Excess ingestion or infusion of these agents can cause a potassium excess.

	Angiotensin-converting
	  enzyme (ACE)
	  inhibitors
	  Captopril (Capoten)
	  Quinapril HCl (Accupril)
	  Ramipril (Altace)
	  and others
		Increase the state of hypoaldosteronism (decrease sodium and increase potassium) and impair renal potassium excretion.

	Angiotensin II receptor
	  antagonists
	  Losartan potassium
	  (Cozaar)
		Decrease adrenal synthesis of aldosterone; potassium is retained and sodium excreted.

	Beta-adrenergic
	  blockers
	  Propranolol (Inderal)
	  Nadolol (Corgard)
	  and others
		Decrease cellular uptake of potassium and decrease Na-K-ATPase function.

	Digoxin	Therapeutic dose is not affected; however, with overdose, potassium excess may occur.
	Heparin (>10,000 units/d)	Inhibits adrenal aldosterone production.

(continues)

Table 5-9	Drugs Affecting Potassium Balance—*continued*	
Potassium Imbalance	**Substances**	**Rationale**
	Low-molecular-weight heparin (LMWH)	Decreases potassium homeostasis; renal excretion of potassium is reduced.
	Immunosuppressive drugs Cyclosporine Tacrolimus Cyclophosphamide	Reduce potassium excretion by induction of hypoaldosteronism; loss of potassium from cells.
	Nonsteroidal anti-inflammatory drugs (NSAIDs) Ibuprofens and others Indomethacin	Impair potassium homeo. stasis and block cellular potassium uptake.
	Succinylcholine: intravenous	Allows for leakage of potassium out of cells.
	CNS agents Barbiturates Sedatives Narcotics Heroin Amphetamines	These CNS agents are usually characterized by muscle necrosis and cellular shift of potassium from cells to serum.
	Potassium-sparing diuretics	See Table 5–8.

4. The normal dose for IV potassium is 20–40 mEq in a liter of IV fluids to run for 8 hours.

5. Infiltration of IV potassium salt in solution causes sloughing of the subcutaneous tissues. IV potassium is irritating to blood vessels, and with prolonged use, phlebitis might occur.

6. Potassium should NOT be administered if the urine output is below 400 mL/day. Eighty to 90% of potassium is excreted in the urine.

7. Potassium deficit can enhance the action of digoxin; digitalis toxicity could result.

8. Potassium-wasting diuretics, i.e., thiazides [hydrochlorothiazide (hydrodIURIL)], and loop/high ceiling [furosemide (Lasix)] cause potassium loss via kidneys. Steroids promote potassium loss and sodium retention.

9. ACE inhibitors, beta blockers, NSAIDs, and potassium sparing diuretics increase the serum potassium level. The serum potassium levels should be monitored when taking these drug groups, especially in older adults and those with renal insufficiency.

10. Increasing the serum potassium level to >4.0 mEq/L can aid in lowering blood pressure and reduce the risk of stroke and cardiovascular diseases.

11. A high-sodium diet can cause an increase in urinary potassium loss.

12. Magnesium is a cofactor for potassium uptake. It is also impossible to correct a potassium deficit when there is a magnesium deficit. Both serum electrolytes need to be checked.

● CLIENT MANAGEMENT

Assessment

● Obtain a health history for clinical health problems that may cause hypokalemia or hyperkalemia.

● Assess for signs and symptoms of hypokalemia and hyperkalemia. Refer to Table 5–5.

● Check the serum potassium level that can be used as a baseline for comparison of future serum potassium levels. Recognize that a serum potassium value below 2.5 mEq/L may cause cardiac arrest.

● Check ECG strips for changes that denote hypokalemia or hyperkalemia.

● Assess vital signs and urine output. Report abnormal findings.

● Assess for signs and symptoms of digitalis toxicity, i.e., nausea, vomiting, anorexia, bradycardia, and dysrhythmias when a client is receiving a potassium-wasting diuretic and/or steroids with digoxin. Hypokalemia enhances the action of digoxin.

Nursing Diagnoses

● *Imbalanced Nutrition, less than body requirements,* related to insufficient intake of foods rich in potassium or potassium losses (gastric suctioning)

● *Risk for Injury, Vessels, Tissues, or Gastric Mucosa,* related to phlebitis from concentrated potassium solution, infiltration of potassium solution into subcutaneous tissues, or ingestion of concentrated oral potassium irritating and damaging to the gastric mucosa

● *Risk for Cardiac Output Decreased,* related to dysrhythmia secondary to hyperkalemia

● *Impaired Urinary Elimination,* related to renal dysfunction, cardiac insufficiency

Interventions

Hypokalemia

● Monitor vital signs and ECG findings.

● Monitor serum potassium values. Report serum potassium levels below 3.5 mEq/L.

● Dilute oral potassium supplements in at least 6–8 ounces of water or juice. Concentrated potassium is irritating to the gastric mucosa.

● Check infusion site for phlebitis or infiltration when KCl is administered intravenously. NEVER administer potassium intravenously as a bolus or IV push.

● Instruct clients to eat foods rich in potassium when hypokalemia is present or when the client is taking potassium-wasting diuretics and steroids. Examples of foods rich in potassium include fresh fruits, fruit juices, dry fruits, vegetables, meats, nuts, cocoa, and cola.

● Recognize other drugs and substances that decrease serum potassium levels, i.e., glucose, insulin, laxatives, licorice, lithium carbonate, salicylates, and tetracycline.

- Monitor serum magnesium, chloride, and protein when hypokalemia is present. Attempts to correct the potassium deficit may not be effective when hypomagnesemia, hypochloremia, and hypoproteinemia are present.

Hyperkalemia

- Monitor vital signs and ECG strips. Report abnormal results. Presence of peaked T wave, wide QRS complex, and prolonged P-R interval is indicative of hyperkalemia.
- Monitor serum potassium levels. Report values greater than 5.3 mEq/L.
- Monitor daily urine output. Report urine output that is less than 250 mL per 8 hours.
- Regulate IV flow rate with solution containing potassium so that no more than 10 mEq of KCl is administered per hour.
- Administer fresh blood (blood transfusion) to clients with hyperkalemia. When blood is 2–3 weeks old, the serum potassium of that blood can be very high and thus increase the risk of severe hyperkalemia.
- Monitor medical treatments for hyperkalemia. Know which corrective treatments are used for mild, moderate, and severe hyperkalemia.
- Recognize that ACE inhibitors, beta blockers, and potassium-sparing diuretics increase serum potassium levels and should be monitored in older adults and those with renal insufficiency.

Evaluation/Outcome

- Evaluate that the cause of potassium imbalance has been corrected.
- Evaluate the effect of the therapeutic regimen in correcting potassium imbalance; serum potassium levels within normal range.
- Remain free of signs and symptoms of hypokalemia or hyperkalemia; ECG, vital signs, and muscular tone are normal in pattern, range, and tone.

● Diet includes foods rich in potassium while the client is taking drugs that promote potassium loss.

● Urine output is adequate: >600 mL/day.

● Document compliance with the prescribed drug therapy and medical and dietary regimen.

Sodium and Chloride Imbalances

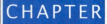

CHAPTER

6

Joyce LeFever Kee, RN, MS

INTRODUCTION

Sodium (Na) and chloride (Cl) are the principal cation and anion in the extracellular fluid (ECF). Sodium and chloride levels in the body are regulated by the kidneys and are influenced by the hormone aldosterone. Sodium is mainly responsible for water retention and the serum osmolality level. The chloride ion frequently appears in combination with the sodium ion.

The normal concentration of sodium in the extracellular fluid is 135–146 mEq/L. The normal serum chloride range is 95–108 mEq/L. A decreased serum sodium level is known as sodium deficit or **hyponatremia,** and an elevated serum sodium level is known as sodium excess or **hypernatremia.** A decreased serum chloride level is called a chloride deficit or **hypochloremia,** and an elevated serum chloride level is known as chloride excess or **hyperchloremia.** Table 6-1 includes the basic information related to sodium and chloride.

The two most important functions of sodium are water balance and neuromuscular activity. Table 6-2 explains the multiple functions of sodium, including the sodium pump action, which is also known as the sodium-potassium pump action. The functions of chloride are given in Table 6-3. The chloride ion is an important factor in acid-base balance and the acidity of gastric juice. Chloride, like sodium, changes the serum osmolality.

Table 6-1	Basic Information Related to Sodium and Chloride Balance
Categories	**Sodium and Chloride Data**
Distribution	Sodium concentration is in the extracellular fluid (ECF). Bones contain 800–1000 mEq of sodium, but only a portion of sodium is available for exchange in other parts of the body. Chloride concentration is greater in the ECF.
Functions	Sodium is important in neuromuscular activity and sodium-potassium pump action. Sodium and chloride are largely responsible for the osmolality of vascular fluids and in regulating acid-base balance. Chloride is partly responsible for the acidity in gastric juices.
Normal serum values	Sodium range is 135–146 mEq/L or 135–146 mmol/L; chloride range is 95–108 mEq/L or 95–108 mmol/L.
Normal urine value	Sodium: 40–220 mEq/L daily.
Dietary requirement	Sodium: 2–4 grams daily. Chloride: 3–9 grams daily.
Food sources	Sodium in high concentration: bacon, corned beef, ham, catsup, potato chips, pretzels with salt, pickles, olives, soda crackers, tomato juice, beef cube, dill, decaffeinated coffee. Chloride in high concentration: cheese, milk, crab, fish, dates.
Excretion	Sodium and chloride are primarily excreted via kidneys. Other avenues in excretion of Na and Cl are GI secretions and sweat.

● PATHOPHYSIOLOGY

Hyponatremia frequently occurs because of:

1. Sodium loss through the skin, GI tract, or kidneys
2. An increased amount of sodium shift into cells when there is a cellular potassium deficit
3. An excessive ADH release (SIADH) causing water retention and sodium dilution

Hypernatremia can occur because of:

1. Excess secretion of aldosterone or cortisol
2. Excess sodium intake

Table 6-2 Sodium and Its Functions

Body Involvement	Functions
Neuromuscular	Transmission and conduction of nerve impulses (sodium pump—see Cellular).
Body fluids	Largely responsible for the osmolality of vascular fluids. Doubling Na level gives the approximate serum osmolality. Regulation of body fluid (increased sodium levels cause water retention).
Cellular	Sodium pump action. Sodium shifts into cells as potassium shifts out of the cells, repeatedly, to maintain water balance and neuromuscular activity. When Na shifts into the cell, depolarization occurs (cell activity); and when Na shifts out of the cell, K shifts back into the cell, and repolarization occurs. Enzyme activity.
Acid-base levels	Assist with the regulation of acid-base balance. Sodium combines readily with chloride (Cl) or bicarbonate (HCO_3) to regulate the acid-base balance.

Table 6-3 Chloride and Its Functions

Body Involvement	Functions
Osmolality (tonicity) of ECF	Chloride, like sodium, changes the serum . osmolality. When serum osmolality is increased, > 295 mOsm/kg, there are more sodium and chloride ions in proportion to the water. A decreased serum osmolality, < 280 mOsm/kg, results in less sodium and chloride ions, and a lower serum osmolality.
Body water balance	When sodium is retained, chloride is frequently retained, causing an increase in water retention.
Acid-base balance	The kidneys excrete the anion chloride or bicarbonate, bicarbonate, and sodium reabsorbs either chloride or bicarbonate to maintain the acid-base balance.
Acidity of gastric juice	Chloride combines with the hydrogen ion in the stomach to form hydrochloric acid (HCl).

Table 6-4	Pathophysiology of Sodium and Chloride Imbalances
Sodium Imbalances	**Explanation**
Hyponatremia	
Central nervous system (CNS)	The CNS is most sensitive to a decrease in the sodium level. Excess water moves into the cerebral tissues, which can result in increased intracranial pressure.
Gastrointestinal tract	Loss of sodium and chloride from the GI tract can cause acid-base imbalances.
Kidneys	Renal dysfunction promotes sodium and water retention, resulting in a diluted sodium level.
Cellular activity	A sodium deficit decreases the sodium pump action; thus, there is a decrease in cellular activity.
Hypernatremia	
Overproduction of adrenal hormones	Excess secretions of aldosterone and cortisol promote an increase in the sodium level.
Cellular activity	A sodium excess increases the sodium pump action, which can increase cellular irritability. As the hypernatremic state intensifies, less sodium passes across the cell membrane; thus, less cellular activity occurs.

Table 6-4 describes the pathophysiology related to hyponatremia and hypernatremia.

● ETIOLOGY

The general causes of hyponatremia and hypochloremia are gastrointestinal losses, altered cellular function, renal losses, electrolyte-free fluids, and hormonal influences. Metabolic alkalosis can occur with hypochloremia. Table 6-5 lists the various causes and gives the rationale concerning sodium and chloride losses.

Table 6-5	Causes of Hyponatremia and Hypochloremia (Serum Sodium and Chloride Deficit)
Etiology	**Rationale**

Dietary Changes	
Low-sodium diet	A low-sodium intake over several months
Excessive plain water intake	can lead to hyponatremia. Drinking large quantities of plain water dilutes the ECF.
"Fad" diets/fasting	Administration of continuous IV D_5W
Anorexia nervosa	dilutes the ECF and can cause water
Prolonged use of IV D_5W	intoxication. Gastric juice is composed of the acid hydrogen chloride (HCl).
Gastrointestinal Losses	
Vomiting, diarrhea	Sodium and chloride are in high
GI suctioning	concentration in the gastric and intestinal
Tap-water enemas	mucosas. Sodium and chloride losses
GI surgery	occur with vomiting, diarrhea, GI
Bulimia	suctioning, and GI surgery.
Loss of potassium	Loss of potassium is accompanied by loss of chloride.
Renal Losses	
Salt-wasting kidney disease	In advanced renal disorders, the tubules do not respond to ADH; therefore, there is a
Diuretics	loss of sodium, chloride, and water. The extensive use of diuretics or excessively potent diuretics can decrease the serum sodium and chloride levels.
Hormonal Influences	
Antidiuretic hormone (ADH), syndrome of inappropriate ADH (SIADH)	ADH promotes water reabsorption from the distal renal tubules. Surgical pain, increased use of narcotics, and head trauma cause more water to be reabsorbed, thus diluting the ECF.
Decreased adrenocortical hormone: Addison's disease	Decreased adrenocortical hormone production related to decreased adrenal gland activity (Addison's disease) causes sodium loss and potassium retention.

(continues)

Table 6-5	Causes of Hyponatremia and Hypochloremia (Serum Sodium and Chloride Deficit)—*continued*
Etiology	**Rationale**
Altered Cellular Function	
Hypervolemic state: HF, cirrhosis	In hypervolemic states due to HF, cirrhosis, and nephrosis, the ECF is increased, thus diluting the serum sodium and chloride levels.
Burns	Great quantities of sodium and chloride are lost from burn wounds and from oozing burn surface areas.
Skin	Large amounts of sodium and chloride are lost from the skin due to increased environmental temperature, fever, and large skin wounds.
Acid-Base Imbalance	
Metabolic alkalosis	An increase in the concentration of bicarbonate ions is associated with a decrease in the concentration of chloride ions.

In hypernatremia and hyperchloremia, the general causes include dietary changes such as increased sodium intake with a decreased water intake, gastrointestinal disorders, decreased renal function, environmental changes, hormonal influence (excess adrenocortical hormone production), and altered cellular function. With hyperchloremia, metabolic acidosis can occur. Table 6-6 lists the causes and gives the rationale for sodium and chloride excesses.

A 24-hour urine sodium test is helpful in determining sodium retention or loss. The normal range for a 24-hour urine sodium is 40–220 mEq/L. If a client's 24-hour urine sodium is 32 mEq/L, the serum sodium level is 133 mEq/L, and the client has symptoms of heart failure, the likely cause is sodium retention.

When the client experiences severe vomiting without water replacement, the client is at risk for a sodium excess. Persistent vomiting and/or gastric suction can cause a loss of hydrogen and chloride ions; hypochloremic alkalosis can result.

Table 6-6	Causes of Hypernatremia and Hyperchloremia(Serum Sodium and Chloride Excess)
Etiology	**Rationale**
Dietary Changes Increased sodium intake Decreased water intake Administration of 3% saline solutions	Inadequate fluid intake and increased use of table salt, canned vegetables, and soups can increase the serum sodium and chloride levels. Administration of concentrated 3% saline solutions can cause hypernatremia and hyperchloremia.
GI Disorders Vomiting (severe) Diarrhea	With severe vomiting, water loss can be greater than sodium loss, causing a dangerously high serum sodium level. This is particularly true in babies who have diarrhea. Their loss of water can be greater than their loss of sodium.
Decreased renal function	Reduced glomerular filtration causes an excess of sodium in the body.
Environmental Changes Increased temperature and humidity Water loss	Increased environmental and body temperatures may cause profuse perspiration. Water loss can be greater than sodium and chloride losses.
Hormonal Influence Increased adrenocortical hormone production: oral or IV cortisone	Excess adrenocortical hormone can cause a sodium and chloride excess in the body whether it is due to cortisone ingestion or hyperfunction of the adrenal gland (Cushing's syndrome).
Altered Cellular Function HF, renal diseases	Usually with HF and renal disease, the body's sodium and chloride are greatly increased. If water retention is greatly enhanced, pseudohyponatremia may result.
Trauma: head injury	Chloride ions are frequently retained with the sodium.
Acid-base imbalance: metabolic acidosis	Increased chloride (Cl) ion concentration is associated with a decreased bicarbonate ion concentration.

Table 6-7	Fluid Volume Imbalances with Hypo-osmolar Hyponatremia
Fluid Volume Imbalances	**Associated Conditions**
Hypovolemic Hyponatremia	Diuretics, hypoaldosteronism, vomiting, diarrhea, gastric suction, burns, peritonitis
Euvolemic Hyponatremia	Syndrome of inappropriate ADH (SIADH), pain, postoperative state, cortisol deficiency, psychogenic polydipsia, decreased solute intake
Hypervolemic Hyponatremia	HF, cirrhosis of the liver, nephrotic syndrome, acute and chronic renal failure

The three types of hyponatremia are hypo-osmolar hyponatremia (most common), iso-osmolar hyponatremia, and hyperosmolar hyponatremia. The serum osmolality aids in identifying the type of hyponatremia. Refer to "osmolality" in Chapter 1.

The body fluid volume status with hyponatremia should also be considered in order to correct the underlying cause of hyponatremia. There are three types of body fluid volume imbalances associated with hyponatremia: hypovolemic (decrease volume), euvolemic (normal volume), and hypervolemic (increased volume). If the urine sodium spot testing is < 30 mEq/L, hypovolemic and hypervolemic hyponatremia are likely; however, if the urine sodium spot testing is > 30 mEq/L, euvolemic hyponatremia is likely.

Table 6-7 lists some of the causes of the three types of body fluid volume imbalances with hyponatremia.

⬤ CLINICAL MANIFESTATIONS

The severity of clinical manifestations of hypo-hypernatremia varies with the onset and extent of sodium deficit or excess. Mild hypernatremia is normally asymptomatic, and early non-specific symptoms such as nausea and vomiting may be overlooked. Table 6-8 gives the signs and symptoms associated with hypo-hypernatremia. Clinical manifestations of chloride

Table 6-8	Clinical Manifestations of Sodium Imbalances	
Body Involvement	**Hyponatremia**	**Hypernatremia**
Gastrointestinal Abnormalities	*Nausea, vomiting, diarrhea, abdominal cramps	*Nausea, vomiting, anorexia *Rough, dry tongue
Cardiac Abnormalities	Tachycardia, hypotension	*Tachycardia, possible hypertension
Central Nervous System (CNS)	*Headaches, apprehension, lethargy, confusion, depression, seizures	*Restlessness, agitation, stupor, elevated body temperature
Neuromuscular Abnormalities	*Muscular weakness	Muscular twitching, tremor, hyperreflexia
Integumentary Changes	Dry skin, pale, dry mucous membrane	*Flushed, dry skin, dry, sticky membrane
Laboratory Values		
Serum sodium	< 135 mEq/L	< 146 mEq/L
Urine sodium		< 40 mEq/L
Specific gravity	< 1.008	> 1.025
Serum osmolality	< 280 mOsm/kg	> 295 mOsm/kg

Note: *Most common clinical manifestations of hyponatremia and hypernatremia.

imbalances are given in Table 6-9. Hypochloremic symptoms are similar to metabolic alkalosis, and hyperchloremic symptoms are similar to metabolic acidosis.

● CLINICAL MANAGEMENT

The majority of Americans consume 3–5 grams of sodium per day; some consume 8–15 grams daily. The daily sodium requirements are 2–4 grams. A teaspoon of salt has 2.3 grams of sodium. When sodium intake increases, the water

Table 6-9	Clinical Manifestations of Chloride Imbalances	
Body Involvement	**Hypochloremia**	**Hyperchloremia**
Neuromuscular Abnormalities	Hyperexcitability of the nerves and muscles (tremors, twitching)	Weakness Lethargy Unconsciousness (later)
Respiratory Abnormalities	Slow and shallow breathing	Deep, rapid, vigorous breathing
Cardiac Abnormalities	↓ Blood pressure with severe Cl and ECF losses	
Laboratory Values Milliequivalent per liter	<95 mEq/L	>108 mEq/L

intake also tends to increase. As a result of the sodium and water increase, extracellular fluid is increased.

When the serum sodium level is < 130 mEq/L (hyponatremia), a saline solution to restore sodium balance is usually administered. The suggested sodium replacement includes:

Sodium Replacement According to the Serum Sodium Level
Serum sodium: < 130 mEq/L = normal saline solution (0.9% NaCl)
Serum sodium: < 115 mEq/L = 3% saline solution

When giving 3% saline solution, the client should be closely monitored for a fluid overload and pulmonary edema.

To correct hypernatremia, the cause should be known and corrected. If the client is consuming an excess amount of salt, then salt restriction should be enforced. If the cause of hypernatremia is heart failure (HF), medical treatment should be prescribed.

Drugs and Their Effect on Sodium Balance

The drug categories of certain antidepressant groups, certain anticancer drugs, oral antidiabetics, and certain CNS depressants (morphine, barbiturates) can cause hyponatremia. Corticosteroids, certain antibiotics, and ingestion and infusion of sodium are causes of hypernatremia. Table 6-10 lists the drugs that affect sodium balance.

Table 6-10	Drugs Affecting Sodium Balance	
Sodium Imbalance	**Drugs**	**Rationale**
Hyponatremia (serum sodium deficit)	Diuretics	Diuretics, either K- wasting or K- sparing, cause sodium excretion.
	Lithium	Lithium promotes urinary sodium loss.
	Antineoplastics/ Anticancer Vincristine Cyclophosphamide Cisplatin Antipsychotics Amitryptyline (Elavil) Thioridazine (Mellaril) Thiothixene (Navane) Tranylcypromine (Parnate) Antidiabetics Chlorpropamide (Diabenase) Tolbutamide (Orinase) CNS depressants Morphine Barbiturates Ibuprofens (Motrin) Nicotine Clonidine (Catapres)	Anticancer drugs, antipsychotics, and antidiabetics stimulate ADH release and cause hemodilution and decrease sodium level.

(continues)

Table 6-10	Drugs Affecting Sodium Balance—*continued*	
Sodium Imbalance	**Drugs**	**Rationale**

Hypernatremia (serum sodium excess)	Corticosteroids
	  Cortisone
	  Prednisone
		Steroids promote sodium retention and potassium excretion.

	Hypertonic saline
	  Sodium salicylate
	  Sodium phosphate
	  Sodium bicarbonate
	  Cough medicines
		Administration of sodium salts in excess.

	Antibiotics
	  Azlocillin Na
	  Penicillin Na
		Many of the antibiotics contain the sodium salt, which increases drug absorption.

	Mezlocillin Na Carbenicillin Ticarcillin disodium	Ion exchange.
	Cholestyramine Amphotericin B Demeclocycline Propoxyphene (Darvon)	These miscellaneous drugs promote urinary water loss without sodium.
	Lactulose	Water loss in excess of sodium via GI tract.

⬤ CLINICAL CONSIDERATIONS: SODIUM AND CHLORIDE

1. Serum osmolality of body fluids (ECF) can be estimated by *doubling the serum sodium level.* For a more accurate serum osmolality level, use the formula

$$2 \times \text{serum Na} + \frac{\text{BUN}}{3} + \frac{\text{glucose}}{18} = \text{serum osmolality (mOsm/kg)}$$

The normal serum osmolality range is 280–295 mOsm/kg.

2. Sodium causes water retention.

3. One teaspoon of salt is equivalent to 2.3 grams of sodium. Daily sodium requirement is 2–4 grams. Most Americans consume 3–5 grams of sodium per day, and some consume 8–15 grams daily.

4. Vomiting causes sodium and chloride losses, and diarrhea causes sodium, chloride, and bicarbonate losses.

5. A 3% saline solution should be given when there is a severe serum sodium deficit, e.g., < 115 mEq/L. When administering a 3% saline solution, check for signs and symptoms of pulmonary edema.

6. A serum potassium deficit cannot be fully corrected until the chloride deficit is corrected.

7. Sodium and potassium have opposite effects on cellular activity. The sodium pump effect causes sodium to shift into the cells, resulting in depolarization. When sodium shifts out of the cells, potassium shifts into cells and repolarization occurs. The sodium pump action is continuously repeated.

8. Continuous use of a saline solution causes a calcium loss.

9. Steroids promote sodium retention and, thus, water retention. Cough medicine, sulfonamides, and some antibiotics containing sodium can increase the serum sodium level.

10. If hypovolemic hyponatremia is present, normal saline solution is usually given. If hypervolemic hyponatremia occurs, salt and water restriction is ordered and loop diuretics may also be prescribed. If euvolemic hyponatremia occurs, water restriction is necessary.

11. Clients with heart failure (HF) or cirrhosis of the liver usually have hypervolemic hyponatremia.

● CLIENT MANAGEMENT

Assessment

● Obtain a history of high-risk factors for decreased and increased serum sodium and chloride levels. Examples of hyponatremia include GI losses, eating disorders such as anorexia nervosa and bulimia, continuous use of 5% dextrose in water, and potent diuretics. Examples of hypernatremia include increased salt intake, renal and cardiac diseases, and increased production of aldosterone.

● Assess for signs and symptoms of hyponatremia or hypernatremia.

● Obtain serum sodium and chloride levels that can be used as baseline values for future comparison.

● Check the serum osmolality level. A serum osmolality value of <280 mOsm/kg indicates hyponatremia and a serum osmolality of >295 mOsm/kg indicates hypernatremia.

Nursing Diagnoses

● *Impaired Electrolyte, Sodium,* related to vomiting, diarrhea, gastric suction, SIADH resulting from surgery, potent diuretics

● *Imbalanced Nutrition, more than body requirements,* related to excess intake of foods rich in sodium

● *Impaired Skin Integrity,* related to peripheral edema secondary to sodium and water excess

Interventions

Hyponatremia

● Monitor the serum sodium and chloride levels. Sodium replacement with chloride may be needed if the serum sodium deficit is due to GI losses. Hypervolemic conditions such as HF can indicate pseudohyponatremia.

● Keep an accurate intake and output record. Excess water intake can cause hyponatremia and hypochloremia related to hemodilution.

● Observe changes in vital signs, i.e., pulse rate. Shocklike symptoms can occur if hyponatremia is due to hypovolemia.

● Restrict water when hyponatremia is due to hypervolemia.

- Administer a 3% saline solution (for severe sodium deficit) cautiously. Check for signs of fluid overload and pulmonary edema.

Hypernatremia

- Instruct the client with hypernatremia to avoid foods rich in salt, i.e., canned foods, lunch meats, ham, pickles, and salted potato chips and pretzels.
- Monitor the serum sodium level. Check for chest crackles and for edema in the lower extremities.
- Identify drugs the client is taking that could have a sodium-retaining effect, such as cortisone preparations, cough medicines, and certain laxatives containing sodium.

Hypochloremia and Hyperchloremia

- Monitor arterial blood gases when an acid-base imbalance is suspected. With hypochloremia, metabolic alkalosis can result, and with hyperchloremia, metabolic acidosis can occur.

Evaluation/Outcome

- Evaluate that the cause of sodium and chloride imbalances has been corrected or controlled.
- Evaluate the effect of the therapeutic regimen on the correction of sodium and chloride imbalances; serum sodium and chloride levels should be periodically checked.
- Remain free of signs and symptoms of hyponatremia and hypernatremia.
- Check that fluid imbalances are not contributing to sodium and chloride imbalances; the client is not dehydrated or overhydrated.
- Determine that the urine output has been adequate, >600 ml/day.

Calcium Imbalances

Joyce LeFever Kee, RN, MS

INTRODUCTION

Calcium (Ca) is found in both the extracellular and intracellular fluids; however, it is somewhat more concentrated in the extracellular fluid. Approximately 55% of serum calcium is bound to protein and 45% is free ionized calcium. It is the free calcium that is physiologically active.

The serum calcium concentration range is 4.5–5.5 mEq/L, 9–11 mg/dl, or 2.23–2.57 mmol/L. A decrease in the serum calcium level is known as **hypocalcemia,** and an increase in serum calcium level is called **hypercalcemia.** Today's blood analyzers allow the ionized calcium (iCa) level to be measured. The normal serum ionized calcium range is 2.2–2.5 mEq/L, 4.25–5.25 mg/dl, or 1.15–1.30 mmol/L. Certain changes in the blood composition can either increase or decrease the serum iCa level. When an individual is acidotic, calcium is released from the serum protein and increases the serum iCa level. During alkalosis, calcium is bound to protein and there is less iCa.

Vitamin D is needed for calcium absorption from the gastrointestinal tract. The anion phosphorus (P) inhibits calcium absorption. Thus, the actions of these two ions on the body have an opposite physiologic effect. Both calcium and phosphorus are stored in the bones and excreted by the kidneys. Table 7-1 includes the basic information regarding calcium balance.

The parathyroid glands secrete the parathyroid hormone (PTH), which is responsible for the homeostatic regulation of the calcium ion in body fluids. The parathyroid glands are

Table 7-1	Basic Information Related to Calcium Balance
Categories	**Calcium Data**
Distribution	Ninety-nine percent of calcium is in teeth and bones; 1% is in the extracellular fluid (ECF) and intracellular fluid (ICF), with the greater concentration of the 1% in the ECF.
Functions	Includes neuromuscular activity, maintaining cardiac contraction and cellular permeability, promoting blood clotting and the formation of teeth and bone.
Normal serum values	Calcium (Ca): 4.5–5.5 mEq/L, 9–11 mg/dL Ionized calcium (iCa): 2.2–2.5 mEq/L, 4.25–5.25 mg/dl
Normal excretion (urine)	Two hundred milligrams per day.
Dietary requirement	Eight hundred milligrams daily.
Food sources	Milk, cheese, vegetables (baked beans, kale, greens, broccoli), meats, salmon.
Excretion	Urine: 200 mg/day; bile: 200 mg/day; others: pancreatic and intestinal (feces) secretions.

located on the posterior thyroid gland. When the serum calcium level is low, the parathyroid glands secrete more parathyroid hormone (PTH); PTH increases the calcium level by promoting calcium release from the bone as needed. Calcitonin from the thyroid gland increases calcium return to the bone, decreasing the serum calcium level. Figure 7-1 diagrams the sequence and actions of PTH and calcitonin from the parathyroid and thyroid glands on the bone.

Calcium is needed for neuromuscular activity, contraction of the myocardium, normal cellular permeability, coagulation of blood, and bone and teeth formation. Table 7-2 explains the functions of calcium.

● PATHOPHYSIOLOGY

A serum calcium level less than 4.5 mEq/L, or 9 mg/dl, is known as hypocalcemia and a serum calcium level greater than 5.5 mEq/L, or 11 mg/dl, is known as hypercalcemia.

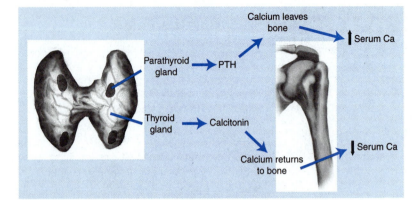

FIGURE 7-1 Functions of PTH and calcitonin.

Table 7-2	Calcium and Its Functions
Body Involvement	**Functions**
Neuromuscular	Normal nerve and muscle activity. Calcium causes transmission of nerve impulses and contraction of skeletal muscles.
Cardiac	Contraction of heart muscle (myocardium).
Cellular and Blood	Maintenance of normal cellular permeability. ↑ calcium decreases cellular permeability and ↓ calcium increases cellular permeability. Coagulation of blood. Calcium promotes blood clotting by converting prothrombin into thrombin.
Bones and Teeth	Formation of bone and teeth. Calcium and phosphorus make bones and teeth strong and durable.

Muscles (skeletal, smooth, and cardiac) and nerves (peripheral) are affected by hypocalcemia. Table 7-3 explains the pathophysiologic effects of calcium imbalances.

ETIOLOGY

The causes of hypocalcemia include dietary changes, renal dysfunction, hormonal and electrolyte influences, and multiple citrated blood transfusions. Table 7-4 lists these causes

Table 7-3	Pathophysiology of Calcium Imbalances
Calcium Imbalance	**Explanations**
Hypocalcemia	
Parathyroid hormone (PTH)	Decreased PTH level causes calcium release from bones to be inhibited.
Neuromuscular	Excitability of the skeletal, smooth, and cardiac muscles.
Bone	A prolonged serum calcium deficit leads to osteoporosis.
Clotting time	A marked serum calcium deficit impairs the clotting time and clot formation. A decrease in blood coagulation results in bleeding.
Electrolyte: magnesium	A severe magnesium deficit results in a calcium deficit. PTH secretions are decreased when there is a magnesium deficit; thus, the serum calcium level is decreased.
Hypercalcemia	
Gastrointestinal	Hypercalcemia decreases GI peristalsis and GI motility. An increased calcium level enhances hydrochloric acid, gastrin, and pancreatic enzyme release.
Cardiac	A calcium excess decreases cardiac activity. Dysrhythmias, heart block, and ECG/EKG changes can occur.
Altered cellular changes	Hypercalcemia decreases cellular permeability.
Bones	A calcium excess frequently results in calcium loss from the bones. An elevated serum calcium level usually results from bone loss because of malignancy or prolonged immobilization.

and the rationale. Lack of calcium intake, inadequate vitamin D, hypoalbuminemia, and a decreased parathyroid hormone (PTH) are some major causes of hypocalcemia.

The total serum calcium level may be low because of hypoalbuminemia, and the ionized calcium level could be within normal range. With a low albumin or protein level there is more free ionized calcium available. Hypomagnesemia

Table 7-4	Causes of Hypocalcemia (Serum Calcium Deficit)
Etiology	**Rationale**
Dietary Changes	
Lack of calcium intake, inadequate vitamin D, and/or lack of protein in diet	A calcium (Ca) deficit resulting from lack of Ca intake is rare. Vitamin D must be present for calcium absorption from GI tract. Inadequate protein intake inhibits the body's utilization of calcium.
Chronic diarrhea	Chronic diarrhea interferes with adequate calcium absorption.
Hypoalbuminemia (low albumin level)	The most common cause of low total serum calcium level.
Renal Dysfunction	
Renal failure	Renal failure causes phosphorus and calcium retention. Lack of PTH decreases renal calcium absorption.
Hormonal and Electrolyte Influence	
Decreased parathyroid hormone (PTH)	With hypoparathyroidism, there is less PTH secreted. PTH deficiency decreases renal production of calcitriol, which causes a decrease in calcium absorption from the intestines.
Increased serum phosphorus (phosphate)	
Increased serum magnesium	Secondary hypoparathyroidism may be caused by sepsis, burns, surgery, or pancreatitis.
Severe decreased magnesium	
Increased calcitonin	Overuse of phosphate laxatives can decrease calcium retention. Magnesium imbalances inhibit PTH secretion.
Calcium Binders or Chelators	
Citrated blood transfusions	Rapid administration of citrated blood binds with calcium, inhibiting ionized (free) Ca.
Alkalosis	Alkalosis increases calcium protein binding.
Increased serum albumin level	With an increase in serum albumin, more calcium is bound and less calcium is free and active.

inhibits PTH secretion, and normal saline solution (NSS, 0.9% NaCl) promotes renal calcium excretion.

Calcitriol has a synergistic effect with PTH on bone absorption and it increases calcium absorption from the intestines. With calcitriol deficiency, there would be less calcium absorption. The causes of hypercalcemia include dietary changes, renal impairment, cellular destruction, and hormonal and drug influence. Hypercalcemia occurs in 10–20% of clients with malignancies. Hyperparathyroidism is a cause of hypercalcemia in 80–90% of ambulatory clients. It increases the production of PTH, which promotes the release of calcium from the bone. Table 7-5 lists these causes and the rationale. The thiazide diuretics promote calcium retention; however, the loop diuretics cause calcium loss.

Table 7-5	Causes of Hypercalcemia (Serum Calcium Excess)
Etiology	**Rationale**
Dietary Changes: Increased Calcium Salts (supplements)	Excessive use of calcium supplements, calcium salts, and antacids can increase the serum calcium level.
Renal Impairment, Diuretics: Thiazides	Kidney dysfunction and use of thiazide diuretics decrease the excretion of calcium.
Cellular Destruction Bone Immobility Malignancies	A malignant bone tumor, a fracture, and/or a prolonged immobilization can cause loss of calcium from the bone. Some malignancies cause an ectopic PTH production. Increased immobility promotes calcium loss from the bone.
Hormonal and Drug Influence Increased PTH	Hyperparathyroidism increases the production of PTH, and increased PTH then promotes the release of calcium from the bone.
Decreased serum phosphorus	A decreased phosphorus level can increase the serum calcium level to the extent that the kidneys are unable to excrete excess calcium.
Steroid therapy	Steroids such as cortisone mobilize calcium absorption from the bone.
Thiazide diuretics	Thiazides increase the action of PTH on kidneys, promoting calcium reabsorption.

● CLINICAL MANIFESTATIONS

Signs of hypocalcemia and hypercalcemia are ECG/EKG changes, the serum calcium level, and the serum ionized calcium level. A commonly seen clinical manifestation of hypocalcemia is tetany. Positive Chvostek's and Trousseau's signs indicate hypocalcemia. Figure 7-2 describes the technique for checking Chvostek's and Trousseau's signs. Table 7-6 lists the clinical manifestations for hypocalcemia and hypercalcemia.

Figure 7-3 displays two ECG strips that reflect the ECG/EKG changes resulting from either hypocalcemia or hypercalcemia.

● CLINICAL MANAGEMENT

Clinical management of hypocalcemia consists of oral supplements and intravenous calcium diluted in 5% dextrose in water (D_5W). Calcium should NOT be diluted in a normal saline solution (0.9% NaCl) because the sodium encourages calcium loss. Table 7-7 lists the oral and intravenous

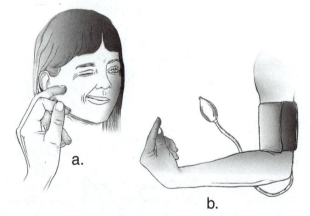

FIGURE 7-2 Testing for Chvostek's and Trousseau's Signs (a) Chvostek's sign: The face is tapped over the facial nerve (2 cm anterior to the earlobe). A positive test results when the facial muscle twitches. (b) Trousseau's sign: Inflate a blood pressure cuff (20–30 mm Hg) on the upper arm to constrict circulation. A positive Trousseau's is evidenced as the occurrence of a carpopedal spasm of the finger and hands within 1–5 minutes.

Table 7-6	Clinical Manifestations of Calcium Imbalances	
Body Involvement	**Hypocalcemia**	**Hypercalcemia**
CNS and Muscular Abnormalities	Anxiety, irritability Tetany 　Twitching around 　　mouth 　Tingling and numbness 　　of fingers 　Carpopedal spasm 　Spasmodic contractions 　Laryngeal spasm 　Convulsions 　Abdominal cramps 　Muscle cramps	Depression/apathy Muscles are flabby
Chvostek's Sign	Positive	
Trousseau's Sign	Positive	
Cardiac Abnormalities	Weak cardiac contractions	Signs of heart block Cardiac arrest in systole
ECG/EKG	Lengthened ST segment Prolonged QT interval	Decreased or diminished ST segment Shortened QT interval
Blood Abnormalities	Blood does not clot normally, reduction of prothrombin.	
Skeletal Abnormalities	Fractures occur if deficit persists.	Pathologic fractures Deep pain over bony areas Thinning of bones apparent
Renal Abnormalities		Flank pain Calcium stones formed in the kidney
Laboratory Values Serum Ca Ionized serum Ca Serum Ca Ionized serum Ca	<4.5 mEq/L <2.2 mEq/L <9.0 mg/dl <4.25 mg/dl	>5.5 mEq/L >2.5 mEq/L >11.0 mg/dl >5.25 mg/dl

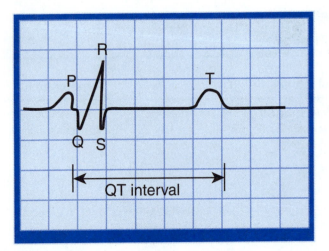

FIGURE 7-3A   Lengthened ST segment.
Prolonged QT interval.

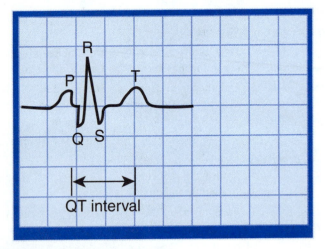

FIGURE 7-3B   Decreased ST segment.
Shortened QT interval.

preparations of calcium salts and their dosages and drug form. Calcium carbonate can cause GI upset because it produces carbon dioxide. For better calcium absorption, calcium supplements should contain vitamin D and oral calcium should be taken 30 minutes before meals.

Table 7-8 gives guidelines for the suggested clinical management for hypocalcemia.

Table 7-7	Calcium Preparations	
Calcium Name	**Drug Form**	**Drug Dose**
Orals		
Calcium carbonate	650–1500-mg tablets	400 mg/g*
Calcium citrate	950-mg tablet	211 mg/g*
Calcium lactate	325–650-mg tablets	130 mg/g*
Calcium gluconate	500–1000-mg tablets	90 mg/g*
Intravenous		
Calcium chloride	10 ml size	272 mg/g*; 13.5 mEq
Calcium gluceptate	5 ml size	90 mg/g*; 4.5 mEq
Calcium gluconate	10 ml size	90 mg/g*; 4.5 mEq

*Elemental calcium is 1 gram (1g).

Table 7-8	Suggested Clinical Management for Hypocalcemia
Calcium Deficit	**Suggested Clinical Management**
Mild	Oral calcium salts with vitamin D, take twice a day. 10% IV calcium gluconate (10 ml) in D_5W solution. Administer slowly, 1–3 ml/min.
Moderate	10% IV calcium gluconate (10–20 ml) in D_5W solution. Administer slowly, 1–3 ml/min.
Severe	10% IV calcium gluconate (100 ml) in 1 liter of D_5W. Administer over 4 hours.

To treat hypercalcemia, expanding the fluid volume is important to increase renal calcium excretion. The use of normal saline solution (NSS) to increase volume expansion decreases calcium reabsorption in the renal proximal tubules. Sodium in NSS promotes calcium loss. Also a loop diuretic such as furosemide (Lasix) is prescribed to prevent fluid overload. Table 7-9 lists suggested treatments for correcting mild to moderate and severe hypercalcemia. The goal for managing hypercalcemia is to correct the underlying cause of the serum calcium excess.

Table 7-9	Suggested Treatments for Correcting Hypercalcemia
Mild to Moderate Hypercalcemia (11–14 mg/dL)	**Severe Hypercalcemia (>14 mg/dL)**
Normal saline solution (NSS, 0.9% NaCl)	Normal saline solution (NSS, 0.9% NaCl)
Loop diuretics, e.g., furosemide (Lasix)	Loop diuretics, e.g., furosemide (Lasix)
	Calcitonin, 4 units/kg, SC
	Others:
	Corticosteroids
	Antitumor antibiotics, e.g., plicamycin (Mithracin, Mithramycin)

Malignancies are a common cause of hypercalcemia. A metastatic bone lesion can destroy the bone, which releases calcium into the circulation, thus elevating the serum calcium level. Some cancers promote the secretion of the parathyroid hormone (PTH) and may be referred to as tumor-secreting (ectopic) PTH production. The most common types of cancer that cause hypercalcemia are lung, breast, ovary, prostate, leukemia, and gastrointestinal cancers. The antitumor antibiotic plicamycin (Mithramycin) inhibits the action of PTH on osteoclasts in the bone and decreases the serum calcium level.

Drugs and Their Effect on Calcium Balance

Phosphate preparations, corticosteroids, loop diuretics, aspirin, anticonvulsants, magnesium sulfate, and Mithramycin are some of the groups of drugs that can lower the serum calcium level. Excess calcium salt ingestion and infusion and thiazide and chlorthalidone diuretics can increase the serum calcium level. Table 7-10 lists the drugs that affect calcium balance.

Table 7-10 Drugs Affecting Calcium Balance

Calcium Imbalance	Drugs	Rationale
Hypocalcemia (serum calcium deficit)	Magnesium sulfate Propylthiouracil/Propacil Colchicine Plicamycin/Mithracin Neomycin Excessive sodium citrate	These agents inhibit parathyroid hormone/PTH secretion and decrease the serum calcium level.

	Acetazolamide
	Aspirin
	Anticonvulsants
	Glutethimide/Doriden
	Estrogens
	Aminoglycosides
	  Gentamicin
	  Amikacin
	  Tobramycin
		These agents can alter the vitamin D metabolism that is needed for calcium absorption.

	Phosphate preparations:
	Oral, enema, and
	  intravenous
	    Sodium phosphate
	    Potassium phosphate
		Phosphates can increase the serum phosphorus level and decrease the serum calcium level.

	Corticosteroids
	  Cortisone
	  Prednisone
		Steroids decrease calcium mobilization and inhibit the absorption of calcium.

	Loop diuretics Furosemide/Lasix	Loop diuretics reduce calcium absorption from the renal tubules.
Hypercalcemia (serum calcium excess)	Calcium salts Vitamin D	Excess ingestion of calcium and vitamin D and infusion of calcium can increase the serum Ca level.
	IV lipids	Lipids can increase the calcium level.

	Kayexalate, androgens
	Diuretics
	  Thiazides
	  Chlorthalidone/
	    Hygroton
		These agents can induce hypercalcemia.

● CLINICAL CONSIDERATIONS: CALCIUM

1. Administer an oral calcium supplement containing vitamin D. Vitamin D is necessary for intestinal absorption of calcium.
2. Oral calcium supplements with vitamin D should be given 30 minutes before meals to improve GI absorption.
3. Intravenous calcium salts should be diluted in 5% dextrose in water (D_5W). Do NOT dilute calcium salts in a saline solution; sodium promotes calcium loss.
4. The suggested IV flow rate for a calcium solution is 1–3 ml/min (average: 2 ml/min).
5. Infiltration of calcium solution, especially calcium chloride, can cause sloughing of the subcutaneous tissues.
6. An elevated serum calcium level can enhance the action of digoxin, causing digitalis toxicity.
7. Diuretics such as furosemide (Lasix) can decrease the serum calcium level, and thiazide diuretics tend to increase the serum calcium levels. Steroids decrease serum calcium levels.

● CLIENT MANAGEMENT

Assessment

● Obtain a health history to identify potential causes of hypocalcemia or hypercalcemia; see Tables 7-4 and 7-5.
● Assess for signs and symptoms of hypocalcemia or hypercalcemia. Tetany symptoms (twitching around mouth, carpopedal spasms, laryngospasms) occur with a severe calcium deficit.
● Obtain a serum calcium level that can be used as a baseline for comparison of future serum calcium levels. A serum calcium level <4.5 mEq/L or <9 mg/dl or iCa<2.2 mEq/L indicates hypocalcemia. A serum calcium level >5.5 mEq/L or >11 mg/dl or iCa >2.5 mEq/L indicates hypercalcemia.
● Check ECG/EKG strips for changes that are indicative of a calcium imbalance.

● Determine the acid-base status when hypocalcemia is present. In an acidotic state, calcium is ionized and can be utilized by the body even though there is a calcium deficit.

● Assess for positive Trousseau's or Chvostek's signs when hypocalcemia is suspected.

● Identify drugs that the client is taking that contribute to a calcium imbalance.

Nursing Diagnoses

● *Imbalanced Nutrition, less than body requirements,* related to insufficient calcium intake, poor calcium absorption due to insufficient vitamin D and protein intake, or drugs (antacids, cortisone preparations) that interfere with calcium ionization

● *Risk for Injury, bleeding,* related to the interference with blood coagulation secondary to calcium loss

● *Risk for Injury,* related to pathologic fractures due to bone destruction from bone cancer, prolonged immobilization, and hypercalcemia

● *Impaired Urinary Elimination,* related to causes of hypercalcemia

Interventions

Hypocalcemia

● Monitor serum calcium levels, vital signs, and ECG strips for changes.

● Monitor intravenous solutions that contain calcium; infiltration can cause sloughing of the subcutaneous tissues.

● Administer oral calcium supplements at least 30 minutes prior to a meal to enhance intestinal absorption.

● Regulate IV 10% calcium gluconate or chloride in a liter of 5% dextrose in water to run 1–3 ml/min. Do not administer calcium salts in an IV normal saline solution. Sodium encourages calcium loss.

- Teach clients to eat foods rich in calcium, vitamin D, and protein, especially the older adult. Tell the client that protein is needed to aid in calcium absorption.

- Explain to persons using antacids that constant use of antacids can decrease calcium in the body. Antacids decrease acidity, thus decreasing calcium ionization.

- Check for prolonged bleeding or reduced clot formation. A low serum calcium level inhibits the production of prothrombin, which is needed in clot formation.

Hypercalcemia

- Monitor serum calcium levels, vital signs, and ECG strips, noting any changes.

- Promote active and passive exercises for bedridden clients. Immobilization promotes calcium loss from the bone.

- Identify symptoms of digitalis toxicity (bradycardia, nausea, vomiting, visual disturbances). An elevated serum calcium level while receiving a digitalis preparation enhances the action of digoxin.

- Teach the client with hypercalcemia to maintain hydration. Increased hydration increases calcium dilution and prevents renal calculi formation.

- Instruct clients with hypercalcemia to avoid foods rich in calcium.

- Monitor urinary output and urine pH. Calcium precipitates in alkaline urine and renal calculi can result. Acid-ash foods and juices such as cranberry and prune juices should be encouraged to increase the acidity of the urine. Acid urine increases the solubility of calcium. Orange juice will not change the urine pH.

- Instruct clients to increase fluid intake to dilute the serum and urine levels of calcium and to prevent the formation of renal calculi.

- Administer prescribed loop diuretics (Lasix) to enhance calcium excretion. Thiazide diuretics inhibit calcium excretion and are not indicated in hypercalcemia.

Evaluation/Outcome

- Evaluate the cause of calcium imbalance and document corrective measures taken.

- Evaluate the effects of the prescribed therapeutic regimen for hypocalcemia or hypercalcemia; serum calcium and ionized calcium levels within normal range.

- Remain free of signs and symptoms of hypocalcemia; absence of tetany symptoms, vital signs are within normal range.

- Include foods rich in calcium, such as dairy products; oral calcium supplements with vitamin D.

- Document compliance with the prescribed drug therapy and medical and dietary regimen.

Magnesium Imbalances

Joyce Lefever Kee, RN, MS

INTRODUCTION

Magnesium (Mg), the second most plentiful intracellular cation, has similar functions, causes of imbalances, and clinical manifestations as potassium. The normal serum magnesium level is 1.5–2.5 mEq/L or 1.8–3.0 mg/dl. A serum magnesium deficit is known as **hypomagnesemia,** and a serum magnesium excess is called **hypermagnesemia.**

One-third of magnesium is protein bound and approximately two-thirds is ionized, free magnesium that can be utilized by the body. Magnesium is absorbed from the small intestine. Table 8-1 provides the basic information related to magnesium balance.

Magnesium plays an important role in neuromuscular, cardiac, and enzyme activities. Magnesium acts as a coenzyme in the metabolism of carbohydrates and protein. Table 8-2 summarizes the various functions of magnesium.

PATHOPHYSIOLOGY

Excess magnesium can cause a sedative effect on the neuromuscular system by inhibiting neuromuscular responses. A magnesium deficit increases neuromuscular excitability. Table 8-3 describes the pathophysiologic factors related to hypomagnesemia and hypermagnesemia.

Table 8-1 Basic Information Related to Magnesium Balance

Categories	Magnesium Data
Distribution	Fifty percent of magnesium (Mg) is in bones; 49% of Mg is in intracellular fluid (ICF), and 1% is in extracellular fluid (ECF).
Functions	Influences neuromuscular activity, aids other electrolytes with cardiac contractions, activates many enzymes, and influences the utilization of K, Ca, and protein.
Normal serum values	Mg: 1.5–2.5 mEq/L; 1.8–3.0 mg/dl; 0.65–1.1 mmol/L.
Normal excretion (urine)	Mg: 120–140 mg daily.
Dietary daily requirement	For adults: 300–350 mg; for infants: 150 mg.
Food sources	Green vegetables, whole grains, fish and seafood, and nuts.
Excretion	Sixty percent is excreted in feces and 40% via kidneys.

Table 8-2 Magnesium and Its Functions

Body Involvement	Functions
Neuromuscular	Transmits neuromuscular activity. Important mediator of neural transmission in the CNS.
Cardiac	Contracts the heart muscle (myocardium).
Cellular	Activates many enzymes for proper carbohydrate and protein metabolism. Responsible for the transportation of sodium and potassium across cell membranes. Influences utilization of potassium, calcium, and protein. Magnesium deficits are frequently accompanied by a potassium and/or calcium deficit.

Table 8-3	Pathophysiology of Magnesium Imbalances
Magnesium Imbalance	**Explanation**
Hypomagnesemia	
Neuromuscular	Magnesium (Mg) deficit increases neuromuscular excitability. Mg deficit increases the release of acetylcholine from the presynaptic membrane of nerve fibers.
Cardiac	Can cause tachycardia, hypertension, cardiac dysrhythmias, ventricular fibrillation.
Gastrointestinal	GI dysfunction can inhibit Mg absorption from the small intestine.
Hormonal	Magnesium inhibits the release of the parathyroid hormone (PTH), which can cause a calcium deficit because of the decreased PTH.
Hypermagnesemia	
Neuromuscular	A serum Mg excess has a sedative effect on the neuromuscular system, resulting in a loss of deep tendon reflexes.
Cardiac	Hypermagnesemia can cause hypotension and heart block.
Respiratory	Can inhibit intercostal muscle action, thus decreasing respirations, which could result in respiratory paralysis.
Renal	Renal insufficiency can increase the magnesium level since 40% of magnesium is excreted by the kidneys.

● ETIOLOGY

Hypomagnesemia is probably the most frequently undiagnosed electrolyte deficiency. The total serum magnesium concentration is not representative of the cellular magnesium levels. Clients with hypomagnesemia are asymptomatic until the serum magnesium level approaches 1.0 mEq/L. Hence, many clients with hypomagnesemia are asymptomatic. Clients with hypokalemia or hypocalcemia who do not respond to potassium and/or calcium replacement may also have hypomagnesemia. Magnesium is important for potassium uptake and for maintaining cellular potassium. Correction of the magnesium deficit should be seriously considered when correcting serum potassium and serum calcium imbalances.

Hypermagnesemia occurs primarily because of magnesium intake, which occurs in laxatives, antacids, and many enema preparations. The elderly and those with renal insufficiency are at high risk for developing hypermagnesemia. The causes of hypomagnesemia and hypermagnesemia are presented in two tables. Table 8-4 lists the etiology and rationale for hypomagnesemia, and Table 8-5 lists the etiology and rationale for hypermagnesemia.

● CLINICAL MANIFESTATIONS

Magnesium influences the nervous system; too much or not enough magnesium affects the neuromuscular function. Severe hypomagnesemia may result in symptoms of tetany. Weakness, loss of deep tendon reflexes, and paralysis are signs and symptoms of hypermagnesemia. Central nervous system depression inhibits neuromuscular transmission, thus decreasing muscle tone and respiration. The serum magnesium level and the ECG changes determine the severity of the magnesium imbalance. Table 8-6 lists the clinical manifestations of hypomagnesemia and hypermagnesemia.

A **magnesium tolerance (load) test** may be prescribed to determine the presence of hypomagnesemia. With this test, a magnesium product is infused over 4–12 hours (check the procedure). Urine is collected over 24 hours starting with the beginning of the infusion. The normal magnesium excretion is 60–80% in 24 hours. Abnormal findings represent less than 50% of magnesium excretion.

● CLINICAL MANAGEMENT

Clinical management of hypomagnesemia includes a diet consisting of green vegetables, legumes, nuts (peanut butter), and fruits. Oral or intravenous magnesium salts may be prescribed when there is a marked to severe magnesium deficit. Table 8-7 lists the methods of clinical management for hypomagnesemia. Correction for magnesium deficit may take 3–4 days, depending upon the severity of the deficit. With asymptomatic hypomagnesemia, oral magnesium replacement is

Table 8-4 — Causes of Hypomagnesemia (Serum Magnesium Deficit)

Etiology	Rationale
Dietary Changes	
Inadequate intake, poor absorption, GI losses	Magnesium is found in various foods, e.g., green, leafy vegetables and whole grains.
Malnutrition, starvation	Inadequate nutrition can result in a magnesium deficit.
Total parenteral nutrition (TPN, hyperalimentation)	Continuous use of TPN without a magnesium supplement can cause a magnesium deficit.
Chronic alcoholism	Alcoholism promotes inadequate food intake and GI loss of magnesium.
Increased calcium intake	Calcium absorption promotes magnesium loss in feces.
Chronic diarrhea, intestinal fistulas, chronic use of laxatives	Chronic diarrhea impairs magnesium absorption. Prolonged use of laxatives can cause a magnesium deficit.
Renal Dysfunction	
Diuresis: diabetic ketoacidosis	Diuresis due to diabetic ketoacidosis causes magnesium loss via the kidneys.
Acute renal failure (ARF)	ARF in the diuretic phase promotes magnesium loss.
Cardiac Dysfunction	
Acute myocardial infarction (AMI)	Hypomagnesemia may occur from the first to the fifth day post-acute MI.
Heart failure (HF)	Prolonged diuretic therapy for HF can cause a magnesium deficit.
Electrolyte and Acid-Base Influence	
Hypokalemia	The cations potassium and calcium are interrelated with magnesium action.
Hypocalcemia Metabolic alkalosis	Hypomagnesemia can occur with hypokalemia, hypocalcemia, and metabolic alkalosis.
Drug Influence	
Aminoglycosides, potassium-wasting diuretics, cortisone, amphotericin B, digitalis	These drugs promote the loss of magnesium. Hypomagnesemia enhances the action of digitalis; digitalis toxicity may result.

Table 8-5 Causes of Hypermagnesemia (Serum Magnesium Excess)

Etiology	Rationale
Dietary Changes	
Excessive administration of magnesium products	Hypermagnesemia rarely occurs unless there is a prolonged excess use of
IV magnesium sulfate	magnesium-containing antacids (Maalox),
Antacids with magnesium	laxatives (milk of magnesia), and IV
Laxatives with magnesium	magnesium sulfate.
Renal Dysfunction	
Renal insufficiency	Renal insufficiency or failure inhibits the
Renal failure	excretion of magnesium.
Severe Dehydration	
Diabetic ketoacidosis	Loss of body fluids due to diuresis from diabetic ketoacidosis causes a hemoconcentration of magnesium, which can result in an increased magnesium level.

Table 8-6 Clinical Manifestations of Magnesium Imbalances

Body Involvement	Hypomagnesemia	Hypermagnesemia
Neuromuscular abnormalities	Hyperirritability	CNS depression
	Tetany-like symptoms	Lethargy, drowsiness, weakness, paralysis
	Tremors	
	Twitching of face	Loss of deep tendon reflexes
	Spasticity	
	Increased tendon reflexes	
Cardiac abnormalities	Hypertension	Hypotension (if severe, profound hypotension)
	Cardiac dysrhythmias	
	Premature ventricular contractions	Complete heart block
	Ventricular tachycardia	
	Ventricular fibrillation	
ECG/EKG	Flat or inverted T wave	Widened QRS complex
	Depressed ST segment	Prolonged QT interval
Others		Flushing
		Respiratory depression

Table 8-7	Suggested Clinical Management for Hypomagnesemia	
Drug Name	**Route for Administration**	**Rationale**
Magnesium gluconate (Magonate)	Orally	Used for mild hypomagnesemia
Magnesium-protein complex (Mg-PLUS)	Orally	Used for mild hypomagnesemia
Magnesium sulfate	Intramuscularly	Used for moderate hypomagnesemia: 1 gram or 2 mL of 50% $MgSO_4$ q8h
	Intravenously	Used for severe hypomagnesemia: 2 grams or 4 mL of 50% $MgSO_4$ diluted in 100 mL of D_5W, administer in 10–15 min

usually prescribed and with symptomatic hypomagnesemia, parenteral (IV, IM) magnesium sulfate is usually prescribed.

Correcting hypermagnesemia should include underlying causes and using intravenous saline or calcium salts to decrease the serum magnesium level. Intravenous calcium is an antagonist to magnesium; therefore, calcium decreases the symptoms of hypermagnesemia. If renal failure is the cause of severe hypermagnesemia, dialysis may be necessary.

Drugs and Their Effect on Magnesium Balance

Sodium inhibits tubular absorption of magnesium and calcium. Long-term administration of saline infusions may result in losses of magnesium and calcium. Diuretics, certain antibiotics, laxatives, and steroids are drug groups that promote magnesium loss. An excess intake of magnesium salts is the major cause of serum magnesium excess.

Hypomagnesemia (like hypokalemia) enhances the action of digitalis and causes digitalis toxicity. Magnesium sulfate corrects hypomagnesemia and symptoms of digitalis toxicity. Table 8-8 lists the drugs that affect magnesium balance.

Table 8-8	Drugs Affecting Magnesium Balance	
Magnesium Imbalance	**Drugs**	**Rationale**
Hypomagnesemia (serum magnesium deficit)	Diuretics Furosemide/Lasix Ethacrynic acid/ Edecrin Mannitol	Diuretics promote urinary loss of magnesium.
	Antibiotics Gentamicin Tobramycin Carbenicillin Capreomycin Neomycin Polymyxin B Amphotericin B	These agents can cause magnesium loss via kidney.
	Digitalis Calcium gluconate Insulin	
	Laxatives Cisplatin	Laxative abuse causes magnesium loss via GI.
	Corticosteroids Cortisone Prednisone	Steroids can decrease serum magnesium levels.
Hypermagnesemia (serum magnesium excess)	Magnesium salts: Oral and enema Magnesium hydroxide/MOM Magnesium sulfate/ Epsom salt Magnesium citrate	Excess use of magnesium salts can increase serum magnesium levels.
	Magnesium sulfate (maternity)	Use of excess $MgSO_4$ in treatment of toxemia can cause hypermagnesemia.
	Lithium	Hypermagnesemia can be associated with lithium therapy.

● CLINICAL CONSIDERATIONS: MAGNESIUM

1. Signs and symptoms of hypomagnesemia are similar to those of hypokalemia; see Table 8.4 on page 8.

2. Excess use of laxatives and antacids that contain magnesium can cause hypermagnesemia.

3. A magnesium deficit is often accompanied by a potassium and calcium deficit (40% of clients with hypomagnesemia also have hypokalemia). If a potassium deficit does not respond to potassium replacement, hypomagnesemia should be suspected.

4. Severe hypomagnesemia can cause symptoms of tetany.

5. IV magnesium sulfate diluted in intravenous solution should be administered at a slow rate. Rapid infusion can cause hot flashes.

6. In emergency situations, IV calcium gluconate is given to reverse hypermagnesemia.

7. Long-term administration of saline (NaCl) infusions can result in magnesium and calcium losses. Sodium inhibits renal absorption of magnesium and calcium.

8. A magnesium deficit enhances the action of digoxin.

9. Thiazides and loop (high-ceiling) diuretics decrease serum magnesium levels.

10. Mild to moderate hypermagnesemia is presently asymptomatic.

● CLIENT MANAGEMENT

Assessment

● Obtain a health history for possible causes of hypomagnesemia or hypermagnesemia; see Tables 8-4 and 8-5.

● Assess for signs and symptoms of hypomagnesemia [tetanylike symptoms (tremors, twitching of the face)] or hypermagnesemia (decreased neuromuscular activity, decreased respiration, and hypotension).

● Obtain a serum magnesium level that can be used as a baseline for comparison of future serum magnesium levels.

● Assess dietary intake and use of intravenous therapy without magnesium. Prolonged intravenous therapy including total parenteral nutrition (TPN) may be a cause of hypomagnesemia.

● Check the ECG/EKG strips for changes. Report abnormal findings.

Nursing Diagnoses

● *Imbalanced Nutrition, less than body requirements,* related to poor nutritional intake, chronic alcoholism, chronic laxative abuse, and chronic diarrhea

● *Imbalanced Nutrition, more than body requirements,* related to oral and intravenous magnesium supplements and chronic use of drugs containing magnesium

● *Decreased Cardiac Output,* related to a serum magnesium deficit

Interventions

Hypomagnesemia

● Instruct the client to eat foods rich in magnesium.

● Report when clients receive continuous magnesium-free IV fluids. TPN solutions should contain some magnesium.

● Administer IV magnesium sulfate diluted in IV solution, slowly unless the client has a very severe deficit. Rapid infusion can cause a hot or flushed feeling.

● Have IV calcium gluconate available for emergency to reverse hypermagnesemia from overcorrection.

● Monitor vital signs and ECG strips. Report abnormal findings.

● Report urine output <25 ml/h or 600 ml/day when the client is receiving magnesium supplements. Magnesium excess is excreted by the kidneys.

● Check for positive Trousseau's or Chvostek's signs, indicating severe hypomagnesemia. Tetany symptoms can occur in both magnesium and calcium deficits.

Hypermagnesemia

● Monitor vital signs, ECG strips, and urine output. Report abnormal findings.

● Monitor serum magnesium levels. A serum Mg <1.0 mEq/L or >10 mEq/L can cause a cardiac arrest.

● Instruct client to avoid prolonged use of antacids and laxatives that contain magnesium.

● Suggest that the client increase fluid intake for the purpose of diluting the serum magnesium level unless contraindicated for other health problems.

Evaluation/Outcome

● Evaluate that the cause of the magnesium imbalance has been corrected. Check that serum potassium level is within normal range. Because potassium and magnesium are cations and have similar functions, one electrolyte imbalance affects the other electrolyte balance.

● Evaluate the effect of the therapeutic regimen for the correction of magnesium imbalance; serum magnesium is within normal range.

● Remain free of signs and symptoms of hypomagnesemia or hypermagnesemia; ECG, vital signs, etc., return to the client's normal baseline patterns.

Phosphorus Imbalances

Joyce LeFever Kee, RN, MS

INTRODUCTION

Phosphorus (P) is a major anion that has its highest concentration in the intracellular fluid. Phosphorus and calcium have similar and opposite effects. Both electrolytes need vitamin D for intestinal absorption and are present in bones and teeth. The parathyroid hormone (PTH) acts on phosphorus and calcium differently. PTH decreases serum phosphorus levels by stimulating the renal tubules to excrete phosphorus and increases serum calcium levels by pulling calcium from the bone.

The normal serum phosphorus range is 1.7–2.6 mEq/L or 2.5–4.5 mg/dl. A phosphorus deficit is known as **hypophosphatemia,** and a phosphorus excess is called **hyperphosphatemia.** The ions phosphorus (P) and phosphate (PO_4) are used interchangeably. Phosphorus is measured in the serum, where it appears as the form of phosphate. Forty-five percent of phosphorus is protein bound and 55% is ionized (free) phosphorus, which is physiologically active. Table 9-1 summarizes the basic information related to phosphorus balance.

Phosphorus has many functions. It is a vital element needed in the formation of bones and teeth and for neuromuscular activity. As an essential component of the cell (nucleic acids and cell membrane), it is incorporated into the enzymes needed for metabolism, e.g., adenosine triphosphate (ATP), a transmission of hereditary traits, and acts as an acid-base buffer. Table 9-2 explains the functions of phosphorus.

Table 9-1	Basic Information Related to Phosphorus Balance
Categories	**Phosphorus Data**
Distribution	Approximately 85% of phosphorus is located in bones and teeth and 15% is located in the intracellular fluid (ICF).
Functions	For neuromuscular activity, durability of bones and teeth, formation of ATP, utilization of B vitamins, transmission of hereditary traits, metabolism of CHO, proteins, and fats, and as a contributing factor in acid-base balance.
Normal serum values	Phosphorus: 1.7–2.6 mEq/L; 2.5–4.5 mg/dl; 0.81–1.45 mmol/L.
Dietary requirements	Eight hundred to 1200 mg daily.
Food sources	Whole grain, cereal, cheese, milk, eggs, dry beans, beef, pork, fish, poultry, and most carbonated beverages.
Excretion	Ninety percent is excreted via kidneys and 10% is lost via GI secretions.

PATHOPHYSIOLOGY

Hypophosphatemia can occur within 3–4 days after an inadequate nutrient intake. Initially, the kidneys compensate by decreasing urinary phosphate excretion; however, a continuous inadequate intake of phosphorus results in extracellular fluid shift to the cells in order to replace phosphorus loss in the intracellular fluid.

PTH promotes renal excretion of phosphorus (phosphate) and calcium reabsorption. When there is a high serum concentration of phosphorus, aluminum-containing antacids decrease hyperphosphatemia and its symptoms. Hyperphosphatemia causes hypocalcemia.

ETIOLOGY

Dietary changes, gastrointestinal disturbances, hormonal influence, selected drugs, and cellular changes are all associated with hypophosphatemia. Respiratory alkalosis can result from hypophosphatemia. Any carbohydrate-loading diet can

Table 9-2	Phosphorus and Its Functions
Body Involvement	**Functions**
Neuromuscular	Normal nerve and muscle activity.
Bones and teeth	Bone and teeth formation, strength, and durability.
Cellular	Formation of high-energy compounds (ATP, ADP). Phosphorus is the backbone of nucleic acids and stores metabolic energy.
	Formation of the red-blood-cell enzyme 2,3-diphosphoglycerate (2,3-DPG) is responsible for delivering oxygen to tissues.
	Utilization of B vitamins.
	Transmission of hereditary traits.
	Metabolism of carbohydrates, proteins, and fats.
	Maintenance of acid-base balance in body fluids.

cause a phosphorus shift from the serum into the cell, resulting in a decreased serum phosphorus level. Tissue repair following trauma causes phosphorus to shift into the cells.

Excessive use of phosphate supplements and renal insufficiency are factors associated with hyperphosphatemia. Hyperphosphatemia causes hypocalcemia by decreasing the production of calcitriol. Calcitriol promotes calcium absorption from the intestines, so with a decrease of calcitriol, the serum calcium level would be decreased. The acid-base disorders, metabolic acidosis and acute respiratory acidosis, can be causes for the occurrence of hyperphosphatemia. Tables 9-3 and 9-4 list the causes of a phosphorus deficit and excess.

● CLINICAL MANIFESTATIONS

Clinical manifestations of hypophosphatemia and hyperphosphatemia are determined by the etiology of the phosphorus imbalance. Neuromuscular irregularities, hematologic and cardiopulmonary abnormalities, and abnormal serum phosphorus level are the most common manifestations. Because the symptoms of phosphorus imbalance are often

Table 9-3	Causes of Hypophosphatemia (Serum Phosphorus Deficit)
Etiology	**Rationale**
Dietary Changes	
Malnutrition	Poor nutrition results in a reduction of phosphorus intake.
Chronic alcoholism	Alcoholism contributes to dietary insufficiencies and increased diuresis.
Total parenteral nutrition (TPN, hyperalimentation)	TPN is usually a phosphorus-poor or -free solution. IV concentrated glucose and protein given rapidly shifts phosphorus into the cells, thus causing a serum phosphorus deficit.
Gastrointestinal Abnormalities	
Vomiting, anorexia	Loss of phosphorus through the GI tract decreases cellular ATP (energy) stores.
Chronic diarrhea	
Intestinal malabsorption	Vitamin D deficiencies inhibit phosphorus absorption. Phosphorus is absorbed in the jejunum in the presence of vitamin D.
Hormonal Influence	
Hyperparathyroidism (increased PTH)	Parathyroid hormone (PTH) production enhances renal phosphate excretion and calcium reabsorption.
Drug Influence	
Aluminum-containing antacids	Phosphate binds with aluminum to decrease the serum phosphorus level.
Diuretics	Most diuretics promote a decrease in the serum phosphorus level.
Cellular Changes	
Diabetic ketoacidosis	Glycosuria and polyuria increase phosphate excretion. A dextrose infusion with insulin causes a phosphorus shift into the cells; decreasing the serum phosphorus level.
Burns	Phosphorus is lost due to its increased utilization in tissue building.
Acid-Base Disorders	
Respiratory alkalosis Metabolic alkalosis	Respiratory alkalosis from prolonged hyperventilation decreases the serum phosphorus level by causing an intracellular shift of phosphorus. Metabolic alkalosis can also cause this shift.

Table 9-4	Causes of Hyperphosphatemia (Serum Phosphorus Excess)	
Etiology	**Rationale**	
Dietary Changes		
Oral phosphate supplements Intravenous phosphate	Excessive administration of phosphate-containing substances increases the serum phosphorus level.	
Hormonal Influence		
Hypoparathyroidism (lack of PTH)	Lack of PTH causes a calcium loss and a phosphorus excess.	
Renal Abnormalities		
Renal insufficiency	Renal insufficiency or shutdown decreases phosphorus excretion.	
Drug Influence		
Laxatives containing phosphate	Frequent use of phosphate laxatives increases the serum phosphorus level.	
Acid-Base Disorders		
Metabolic acidosis Respiratory acidosis	Acidosis is a cause of hyperphosphatemia. It prevents accumulation of cellular phosphates.	

vague, serum values are needed. Table 9-5 lists the clinical manifestations of phosphorus deficit and excess.

● CLINICAL MANAGEMENT

When the serum phosphorus level falls below 1.5 mEq/L or 2 mg/dl, oral and/or intravenous phosphate-containing solutions are usually prescribed. If the serum phosphorus level falls below 0.5 mEq/L or 1 mg/dl, severe hypophosphatemia occurs. Intravenous phosphate-containing solutions (sodium phosphate and potassium phosphate) are indicated. Sodium phosphate is the preferred solution if the client has oliguria.

Table 9-5	Clinical Manifestations of Phosphorus Imbalances	
Body Involvement	**Hypophosphatemia**	**Hyperphosphatemia**
Neuromuscular Abnormalities	Muscle weakness Tremors Paresthesia Bone pain Hyporeflexia Seizures	Tetany (with decreased calcium) Hyperreflexia Flaccid paralysis Muscular weakness
Hematologic Abnormalities	Tissue hypoxia (decreased oxygen-containing hemoglobin and hemolysis) Possible bleeding (platelet dysfunction) Possible infection (leukocyte dysfunction)	
Cardiopulmonary Abnormalities	Weak pulse (myocardial dysfunction) Hyperventilation	Tachycardia
GI Abnormalities	Anorexia Dysphagia	Nausea, diarrhea Abdominal cramps
Laboratory Values		
Milliequivalents per liter	<1.7 mEq/L	>2.6 mEq/L
Milligrams per deciliter	<2.5 mg/dl	>4.5 mg/dl

Suggested Phosphorus Replacement for Severe Hypophosphatemia

Uncomplicated P deficit:	IV phosphate salt: 0.6 mg/kg/h
Complicated P deficit:	IV phosphate salt: 0.9 mg/kg/h
Serum P level:	>1.5 mEq/L or 2 mg/dl oral phosphate salt

Check phosphorus level q6h.

Administration of insulin and glucose can lower the serum phosphorus level by shifting phosphorus from the extracellular fluid into the cells. The use of insulin and glucose is normally a temporary treatment to correct hyperphosphatemia.

Drugs and Their Effect on Phosphorus Balance

The major drug group that causes hypophosphatemia is the aluminum antacids. Other drug groups causing a phosphorus deficit include diuretics, steroids, and calcium salts. Excess use of phosphate laxatives, phosphate enemas, and oral and intravenous phosphates are often responsible for hyperphosphatemia. Table 9-6 lists the drugs that can cause a phosphorus deficit and excess.

Table 9-6	Drugs That Affect Phosphorus Balance	
Phosphorus Imbalance	**Drugs**	**Rationale**

Hypophosphatemia (serum phosphorus deficit)	Sucralfate
	Aluminum antacids
	  Amphojel
	  Basaljel
	Aluminum/magnesium
	  antacids
	  Di-Gel
	  Gelusil
	  Maalox
	  Maalox Plus
	  Mylanta
	  Mylanta II
	Calcium antacids
	  Calcium carbonate
		Aluminum-containing antacids bind with phosphorus; therefore the serum phosphorus level is decreased. Calcium promotes phosphate loss.

	Diuretics
	  Thiazide
	  Loop (high-ceiling)
	  Acetazolamide
		Phosphorus can be lost when diuretics are used.

(continues)

Table 9-6	**Drugs That Affect Phosphorus Balance—*continued***	
Phosphorus Imbalance	**Drugs**	**Rationale**

Hypophosphatemia (serum phosphorus deficit), *cont'd*	Androgens
	Corticosteroids
	  Cortisone
	  Prednisone
	Glucagon
	Gastrin
	Epinephrine
	Mannitol
	Salicylate overdose
	Insulin and glucose
		These agents have a mild to moderate effect on phosphorus loss.

Hyperphosphatemia (serum phosphorus excess)	Oral phosphates
	Sodium phosphate/
	  Phospho-Soda
	Potassium phosphate/
	  Neutra-Phos K
	Intravenous phosphates
	  Sodium phosphate
	  Potassium phosphate
		Excess oral ingestion and IV infusion can increase the serum phosphorus level.

	Phosphate laxatives
	  Sodium phosphate
	  Sodium biphosphate/
	  Phospho-Soda
	Phosphate enema
	Fleet sodium
	  phosphate
	Excessive vitamin D
	Antibiotics
	  Tetracyclines
	  Methicillin
		Continuous use of phosphate laxatives and enemas can increase the serum phosphorus level.

● CLINICAL CONSIDERATIONS: PHOSPHORUS

1. Phosphorus is needed for durable bones and teeth, formation of ATP (high-energy compound for cellular activity), metabolism of carbohydrates, proteins, and fats, utilization of B vitamins, transmission of hereditary traits, and others.

2. Phosphorus and calcium are similar and yet differ in action. Both need vitamin D for intestinal absorption. PTH promotes renal excretion of phosphorus (phosphate) and calcium reabsorption from the bones.

3. Vomiting and chronic diarrhea cause a loss of phosphorus.

4. Acute hypophosphatemia may result from an abrupt shift of phosphorus into the cells. Respiratory alkalosis and metabolic alkalosis can cause shifting of phosphorus into the cells.

5. Concentrated IV phosphates are hyperosmolar (hypertonic) and must be diluted. If IV potassium phosphate is given in intravenous solution, the IV rate should be no more than 10 mEq/h to avoid phlebitis and a potassium overload.

6. Aluminum-containing antacids decrease the serum phosphorus level; phosphate binds with the aluminum. Aluminum-containing antacids are useful for hyperphosphatemia.

7. Continuous use of phosphate laxatives can cause an elevated serum phosphorus level.

● CLIENT MANAGEMENT

Assessment

● Obtain a health history of clinical problems associated with hypophosphatemia (malnutrition, chronic alcoholism, chronic diarrhea, vitamin D deficiency, hyperparathyroidism, continuous use of aluminum-containing antacids, and respiratory alkalosis) and with hyperphosphatemia (continuous use of phosphate-containing laxatives, hypoparathyroidism, and renal insufficiency).

● Assess for signs and symptoms of a phosphorus deficit or phosphorus excess (refer to Table 9-5).

● Check the serum phosphorus level. The serum phosphorus level is needed as a baseline level for assessing future serum phosphorus levels.

● Check serum calcium level. An elevated calcium level causes a decreased phosphorus level and vice versa.

- Check vital signs. Report abnormal findings, such as weak pulse, tachypnea.
- Check urinary output. Report abnormal findings. A decrease in urine output, < 600 ml/day, increases the serum phosphorus level.

Nursing Diagnoses

- *Imbalanced Nutrition, less than body requirements,* related to inadequate nutritional intake, chronic alcoholism, vomiting, chronic diarrhea, lack of vitamin D intake, and intravenous fluids (including TPN), which lack a phosphate additive
- *Imbalanced Nutrition, more than body requirements,* related to excess intake of phosphate-containing compounds such as some laxatives, intravenous potassium phosphate, and others

Interventions

Hypophosphatemia

- Monitor serum phosphorus and calcium levels. Report abnormal results.
- Monitor oral and intravenous phosphate replacements. An oral phosphate salt, Neutrophos, which comes in capsules, may be indicated if nausea is present. Administer IV potassium phosphate slowly to prevent hyperphosphatemia and irritation of the blood vessel. Rapid intravenous potassium phosphate can cause phlebitis.
- Check for signs of infiltration at the IV site; KPO_4 is extremely irritating to the subcutaneous tissue and can cause sloughing of tissue and necrosis.
- Encourage the client to eat foods rich in phosphorus, such as meats, milk, whole grain cereal, and nuts. Most carbonated drinks are high in phosphates.
- Instruct the client to avoid taking antacids that contain aluminum hydroxide, such as Amphojel. Phosphorus binds with aluminum products; a low serum phosphorus level results.

Hyperphosphatemia

● Monitor vital signs. Report abnormal results.

● Monitor serum phosphorus and calcium levels. Report abnormal results.

● Observe the client for signs and symptoms of hypocalcemia (e.g., tetany). An increased serum phosphorus level decreases the calcium level.

● Monitor urine output. Report inadequate urine output. Phosphorus is excreted by the kidneys and poor renal function can cause hyperphosphatemia.

● Instruct the client to eat foods that are low in phosphorus and to avoid carbonated beverages, which are high in phosphorus.

Evaluation/Outcome

● Evaluate that the cause of phosphorus imbalance has been eliminated.

● Evaluate the effect of clinical management in the correction of hypophosphatemia or hyperphosphatemia; serum phosphorus levels are within normal range.

● Determine that the signs and symptoms of phosphorus imbalance are absent; client is free of neuromuscular abnormalities, such as muscle weakness and tetany symptoms.

● Document compliance with prescribed drug therapy and medical and dietary regimen.

ACID-BASE BALANCE AND IMBALANCE

INTRODUCTION

Our body fluid must maintain a balance between acidity and alkalinity in order for life to be maintained. The concentration of hydrogen ions (plus or minus) determine either the acidity or the alkalinity of a solution. The amount of ionized hydrogen in extracellular fluid is extremely small: around 0.0000001 g/L. The pH symbol stands for the negative logarithm of the hydrogen ion concentration. Mathematically, it is expressed as 10^{-7}. When the minus sign is dropped, the symbol is used to designate the hydrogen ion concentration as pH 7. As the hydrogen ion concentration rises in solution, the pH value falls, thus indicating increased acidity. As the hydrogen ion concentration falls, the pH rises, thus indicating increased alkalinity.

The hydroxyl ions (OH^-) are base ions and, when in excess, increase the alkalinity of the solution. A solution with a pH 7 is neutral because at this concentration the number of hydrogen ions is exactly balanced with the number of hydroxyl ions.

The pH of extracellular fluid in a healthy individual is maintained at a level between 7.35 and 7.45, resulting in a body fluid level that is slightly alkaline. If the pH value is below 7.35, acidosis is present, and if the pH value exceeds 7.45, alkalosis results. Within the body, the pH of the different body fluids varies. Table U3-1 lists the various body fluids and their pH ranges.

In health, there are $1\frac{1}{3}$ mEq/L of acid to each 27 mEq of alkali for each liter of extracellular fluid. This represents a ratio of 1 part acid to 20 parts alkali. Figure U3–1 demonstrates by the arrow that the body is in acid-base balance; a pH of 7.4 represents this balance. If the arrow tilts left due to an alkali deficit or acid excess, then acidosis occurs. If the arrow tilts right due to an alkali excess or acid deficit, then alkalosis occurs.

Table U3-1	The pH of Body Fluids
Body Fluid	**pH**
Extracellular fluid	7.35–7.45
Intracellular fluid	6.9–7.2
Urine	6.0
Gastric juice	1.0–2.0
Intestinal juice	6.6–7.6
Bile	5.0–6.0

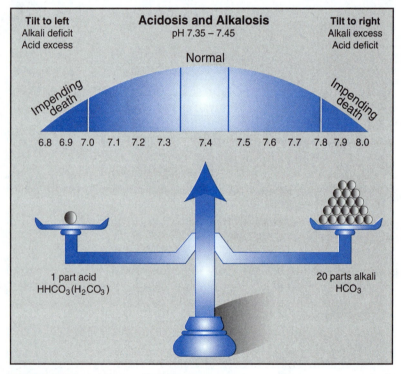

FIGURE U3-1 Acidosis and alkalosis.

REGULATORY MECHANISMS FOR PH CONTROL

The four major regulatory mechanisms for pH control are:

1. Buffer systems
2. Ion exchange

3. Respiratory regulation

4. Renal regulation

The buffer systems maintain the acid-base balance of body fluids by protecting the fluids against changes in pH. The most important buffer system in the body is the bicarbonate–carbonic acid buffer, which maintains the acid-base balance 55% of the time. Table U3-2 provides specific data related to the regulation of pH control for the four major regulatory mechanisms.

Table U3-2	Regulatory Mechanism for pH Control
Regulatory Mechanism	**Intervention**
Buffer Systems	
a. Bicarbonate–carbonic acid buffer system (principal buffer system of body)	Acids combine with bicarbonates in blood to form neutral salts (bicarbonate salt) and carbonic acid (weak acid). Carbonic acid (H_2CO_3) is weak and unstable acid, changing to water and carbon dioxide in fluid ($H_2CO_3 \rightleftharpoons H_2O + CO_2$). A strong base combines with weak acid, e.g., H_2CO_3.
b. Phosphate buffer system	The phosphate buffer system increases the amount of sodium bicarbonate ($NaHCO_3$) in extracellular fluids, making extracellular fluids more alkaline. The H^+ is excreted as NaH_2PO_4 and Na and bicarbonate ions combine.
c. Hemoglobin-oxyhemoglobin buffer system	Maintains same pH level in venous and arterial blood.
d. Protein buffer system	Proteins can exist in form of acids (H protein) or alkaline salts (B protein) and in this way are able to bind or release excess hydrogen as required.

(continues)

Table U3-2	Regulatory Mechanism for pH Control—*continued*
Regulatory Mechanism	**Intervention**
Ion exchange	Ion exchange of HCO_3 and Cl occurs in red blood cells (RBCs) as result of O_2 and CO_2 exchange. There is redistribution of anions in response to increase in CO_2. Chloride ion enters RBCs as bicarbonate ion and diffuses into plasma in order to restore ionic balance.
Respiratory regulation (acts quickly in case of emergency)	For regulation of acid balance, the lungs blow off more CO_2, and for regulation of alkaline balance, the respiratory center slows respirations in order to retain CO_2. It takes 1–3 minutes for the respiratory system to readjust H^+ concentration.
Renal Regulation a. Acidification of phosphate buffer salts	Exchange mechanism occurs between H^+ of renal tubular cells and disodium salt (Na_2HPO_4) in tubular urine.
b. Reabsorption of bicarbonate	Carbon dioxide is absorbed by tubular cells from blood and combines with water present in cells to form carbonic acid, which in turn ionizes, forming H^+ and HCO_3^-. Na^+ of tubular urine exchanges with H^+ of tubular cells and combines with HCO_3^- to form sodium bicarbonate and is reabsorbed into blood.
c. Secretion of ammonia	Ammonia (NH_3) unites with HCl in renal tubules and H^+ is excreted as NH_4Cl (ammonium chloride).

● SUMMARY OF ACID-BASE IMBALANCES

Table U3-3 gives a summary account of the four types of acid-base imbalances.

Table U3-3	Causes, Manifestations, and Laboratory Findings in Metabolic and Respiratory Acidosis and Alkalosis

Metabolic Acidosis	Metabolic Alkalosis
Clinical Manifestations	
Kussmaul breathing (rapid and vigorous)	Shallow breathing
Flushing of the skin (capillary dilation)	Tetany-like symptoms
Decrease in heart rate and cardiac output	Irritability, confusion
Nausea, vomiting, abdominal pain	Vomiting
Dehydration	
Laboratory Findings	
Bicarbonate deficit	*Bicarbonate excess*
pH<7.35, HCO$_3$ <24 mEq/L,	pH>7.45, HCO$_3$>28 mEq/L, BE>+2,
BE < − 2, plasma CO$_2$ <22 mEq/L	plasma CO$_2$ >32 mEq/L
Causes	
Diabetic acidosis, severe diarrhea or starvation, tissue trauma, renal and heart failure, shock, severe infection	Peptic ulcer, vomiting, gastric suction

Respiratory Acidosis	Respiratory Alkalosis
Clinical Manifestations	
Dyspnea, inadequate gas exchange	Rapid, shallow breathing
Flushing and warm skin	Tetany-like symptoms
Tachycardia	(numbness, tingling of
Weakness	fingers)
	Palpitations
	Vertigo
Laboratory Findings	
Carbonic acid excess (CO$_2$ retention)	*Carbonic acid deficit*
pH<7.35, PaCO$_2$ >45 mm Hg	pH>7.45, PaCO$_2$ <35 mm Hg
Causes	
COPD (emphysema, chronic bronchitis, severe asthma), narcotics, anesthetics, barbiturates, pneumonia, chest injuries	Anxiety, hysteria, drug toxicity, fever, pain, brain tumors, early salicylate poisoning, excessive exercise

Determination of Acid-Base Imbalances

Larry Dale Purnell, RN, PhD, FAAN

INTRODUCTION

Hydrogen ions circulate throughout the body fluids in two forms, *volatile acid* and *nonvolatile acid.* A volatile acid (carbonic acid [H_2CO_3]) circulates as CO_2 and H_2O and is excreted as a gas, CO_2. A nonvolatile acid (fixed acid, e.g., lactic, pyruvic, sulfuric, phosphoric acids) results from the various organic acids within the body. They are excreted from the body in urine. The lungs and the kidneys aid in the regulation of acid-base balance; the lungs excrete the volatile acid and the kidneys excrete nonvolatile acids. The formula that demonstrates respiratory and renal regulation for acid-base balance is shown in Figure 10-1.

Arterial blood gases are drawn to determine acid-base balance and/or imbalance. The three values (pH, $PaCO_2$, and HCO_3) are analyzed from the arterial blood specimen to indicate the type of acid-base imbalance. The pH indicates either that the extracellular fluid is neutral (7.35–7.45), acidotic (<7.35) or alkalotic (>7.45). $PaCO_2$ is the respiratory component for checking acid-base imbalance. If the $PaCO_2$ is >45 mm Hg, respiratory acidosis occurs; if $PaCO_2$ is <35 mm Hg, respiratory alkalosis is present. The metabolic or renal component is HCO_3. If the HCO_3 is <24 mEq/L, metabolic acidosis occurs; if it is >28 mEq/L, metabolic alkalosis is present. Other measurements to determine metabolic acidosis and alkalosis are base excess (BE) and serum CO_2, a serum bicarbonate determinant. The norm for base excess is -2 to $+2$. BE relates to the bicarbonate range of 24 to 28 mEq/L,

Table 10-1 Determination of Acid-Base Imbalance

Blood Tests	Normal Values	Imbalance
pH	Adult: 7.35–7.45 Newborn: 7.27–7.47 Child: 7.33–7.43	Adult: <7.35 = acidosis >7.45 = alkalosis
$PaCO_2$ (respiratory component)	Adult and child: 35–45 mm Hg Newborn 27–41 mm Hg	Adult and child: <35 mm Hg = respiratory alkalosis (hyperventilation) >45 mm Hg = respiratory acidosis (hypoventilation)
HCO_3^2 (metabolic and renal component)	Adult and child: 24–28 mEq/L Newborn: 22–30 mEq/L	Adult and child: <24 mEq/L = metabolic acidosis >28 mEq/L = metabolic alkalosis
Base excess (BE) (metabolic and renal component)	Adult and child +2 to −2	Adult and child < −2 = metabolic acidosis > +2 = metabolic alkalosis
CO_2^* (metabolic and renal component)	Adult and child: 22–32 mEq/L	Adult and child: <22 mEq/L = metabolic acidosis >32 mEq/L = metabolic alkalosis

*Serum CO_2 is a serum bicarbonate determinant and is frequently called *CO_2 combining power.* It refers to the amount of cations, e.g., H^+, Na^+, K^+, etc., available to combine with HCO_3^-. The level of HCO_3^- in the blood is determined by the amount of CO_2 dissolved in the blood.

Respiratory Regulation	Renal Regulation
$H_2 + CO_2 \leftrightarrows \quad (H_2CO_3) \quad \leftrightarrows H^+ + HCO_3$	
(excreted as volatile acid)	(excreted as nonvolatile acid)

FIGURE 10-1 Respiratory and renal regulation of acid-base balance.

with a BE norm of 26 mEq/L ($-2 = 24$ mEq/L and $+2 = 28$ mEq/L). Table 10-1 presents the normal values for these tests and the types of acid-base imbalances that occur.

To determine the type of acid-base imbalance:

1. pH should be checked first. If it is less than 7.35, acidosis is present. If it is greater than 7.45, alkalosis is present.

2. $PaCO_2$ is checked next. If it is within normal range, respiratory acidosis or alkalosis is *not* occurring. If the $PaCO_2$ is greater than 45 mm Hg and the pH is less than 7.35, respiratory acidosis occurs.

3. HCO_3 is checked. If the bicarbonate is less than 24 mEq/L and the pH is less than 7.35, metabolic acidosis is present.

Figure 10-2 outlines the method for determining acid-base imbalances.

● COMPENSATION FOR PH BALANCE

There are specific compensatory reactions in response to metabolic acidosis and alkalosis and to respiratory acidosis and alkalosis. The pH returns to normal or close to normal by changing the component ($PaCO_2$ or HCO_3) that originally was *not* affected.

The respiratory system can compensate for metabolic acidosis and alkalosis. In metabolic acidosis, the lungs (stimulated by the respiratory center) hyperventilate to decrease the CO_2 level; the $PaCO_2$ decreases due to "blowing off" of carbon dioxide and water, which decreases the body's carbonic acid (H_2CO_3) level. An example of respiratory compensation is pH 7.33, $PaCO_2$ 32 mm Hg, and HCO_3 18 mEq/L. The pH shows slight acidosis, and the HCO_3 is definitely low, confirming metabolic acidosis. The $PaCO_2$ should be normal (35 to 45 mm Hg); however, it is low because the respiratory center compensates for the acidotic state by "blowing off" CO_2 (hyperventilating); respiratory compensation occurs. Without this compensation, the pH would be extremely low; e.g., pH of 7.2.

The renal system can compensate for respiratory acidosis and alkalosis. With respiratory acidosis, the kidneys excrete more acid, H^+, and conserve HCO_3. With a pH of 7.34, $PaCO_2$ of 68, and HCO_3 of 35, the pH reveals a slight acidosis

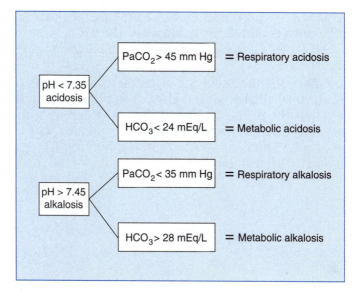

FIGURE 10-2 Types of acid-base imbalances.

and the $PaCO_2$ is highly elevated, indicating CO_2 retention (carbon dioxide and water = carbonic acid) and respiratory acidosis. The HCO_3 indicates renal or metabolic compensation. Without this compensation, the pH would be lower.

● CLINICAL CONSIDERATIONS: DETERMINATION OF ACID-BASE IMBALANCES

1. Hydrogen ions circulate in the body fluid in the form of a volatile acid (carbonic acid [H_2CO_3]). The volatile acid is excreted as a gas, CO_2, from the lungs, and the nonvolatile acid (fixed acid, e.g., lactic, pyruvic, ketones), which is excreted in the urine. The lungs and kidneys regulate the hydrogen ions; thus, lung and kidney disorders can cause an acid-base imbalance.

2. To determine acid-base imbalance, the pH should be checked first. The pH determines if the body fluids are within normal range (7.35–7.45), acidotic (<7.35) or alkalotic (>7.45).

3. To determine metabolic acidosis or metabolic alkalosis, first check the pH, then the bicarbonate (HCO_3). If the

pH is <7.35 and the HCO_3 is <24 mEq/L, the acid-base imbalance is metabolic acidosis. If the pH is >7.45 and the HCO_3 is >28 mEq/L, metabolic alkalosis is occurring.

4. To determine the presence of respiratory acidosis or respiratory alkalosis, first check the pH, and then the $PaCO_2$. If the pH is <7.35 and the $PaCO_2$ is >45 mm Hg, the acid-base imbalance is respiratory acidosis. If the pH is >7.45 and $PaCO_2$ <35 mm Hg, respiratory alkalosis is occurring.

Metabolic Acidosis and Metabolic Alkalosis

Larry Dale Purnell, RV, PhD

INTRODUCTION

The metabolic/renal components for metabolic acidosis and alkalosis include arterial bicarbonate (HCO_3), base excess (BE), and serum CO_2. In metabolic acidosis, the pH is decreased, or <7.35, the HCO_3 is <24 mEq/L, and the base excess (BE) is < -2. In metabolic alkalosis, the pH is increased or >7.45, the HCO_3 is >28 mEq/L, and the BE is $> +2$.

PATHOPHYSIOLOGY

Metabolic acidosis is characterized by a decrease in bicarbonate concentration or acid excess. With metabolic alkalosis, there is an increase in bicarbonate concentration or a loss of the hydrogen ion (strong acid) in the extracellular fluid.

Anion gap is a useful indicator for determining the presence or absence of metabolic acidosis. The anion gap can be obtained by using the following formula:

$$\text{Serum sodium (Na)} - (\text{Serum chloride} + \text{Serum } CO_2) = \text{Anion gap}$$

$$\text{Example: } 142 \text{ mEq/L} - (102 \text{ mEq/L} + 18 \text{ mEq/L}) =$$
$$142 - 120 = 22 \text{ mEq/L}$$

If the anion gap is >16 mEq/L, metabolic acidosis is suspected. According to the example, the anion gap is 22 mEq/L, so metabolic acidosis is present.

Conditions associated with an anion gap that is greater than 16 mEq/L are diabetic ketoacidosis, lactic acidosis, poisoning, and renal failure. If a client takes excessive amounts of baking soda or commercially prepared acid neutralizers to ease indigestion or stomach ulcer pain, the anion gap is much less than 16 mEq/L, so the imbalance results in metabolic alkalosis.

● ETIOLOGY

The causes of metabolic acidosis include starvation, severe malnutrition, chronic diarrhea, kidney failure, diabetic ketoacidosis, hyperthyroidism, thyrotoxicosis, trauma, shock, excessive exercise, severe infection, and prolonged fever. Table 11-1 describes the causes and rationale for each disorder. In metabolic alkalosis, typical etiologic factors include vomiting, gastric suction, peptic ulcers, and hypokalemia. Table 11-2 describes each cause and rationale.

● CLINICAL MANIFESTATIONS

When metabolic acidosis occurs, the central nervous system (CNS) is depressed. Symptoms can include apathy, disorientation, weakness, and stupor. Deep rapid breathing is a respiratory compensatory mechanism for decreasing the acid content in the blood.

In metabolic alkalosis, excitability of the CNS occurs. These symptoms may include irritability, mental confusion, tetanylike symptoms, and hyperactive reflexes. Hypoventilation may occur as a compensatory mechanism for metabolic alkalosis to conserve the hydrogen ions and carbonic acid. Table 11-3 lists the clinical manifestations related to metabolic acidosis and alkalosis.

In metabolic acidosis, the renal and respiratory mechanisms try to reestablish the pH balance. The H^+ exchanges with the Na^+, and thus H^+ is excreted in the urine. Kussmaul breathing (rapid deep breathing) causes CO_2 to be blown off through the lungs, decreasing carbonic acid (H_2CO_3) levels.

In metabolic alkalosis, the buffer, renal, and respiratory mechanisms try to reestablish balance. With the buffer mechanism, the excess bicarbonate reacts with buffer acid salts to

Table 11-1	Causes of Metabolic Acidosis
Etiology	**Rationale**
Gastrointestinal Abnormalities	
Starvation Severe malnutrition	Nonvolatile acids, i.e., lactic and pyruvic acids, occur as the result of an accumulation of acid products from cellular breakdown due to starvation and/or severe malnutrition.
Chronic diarrhea	Loss of bicarbonate ions in the small intestines is in excess. Also, the loss of sodium ions exceeds that of chloride ions. Cl^- combines with H^+, producing a strong acid (HCl).
Renal Abnormalities	
Kidney failure	Kidney mechanisms for conserving sodium and water and for excreting H^+ fail.
Hormonal Influence	
Diabetic ketoacidosis	Failure to metabolize adequate quantities of glucose causes the liver to increase metabolism of fatty acids. Oxidation of fatty acids produces ketone bodies, which cause the ECF to become more acid. Ketones require a base for excretion.
Hyperthyroidism, thyrotoxicosis	An overactive thyroid gland can cause cellular catabolism (breakdown) due to a severe increase in metabolism, which increases cellular needs.
Others	
Trauma, shock	Trauma and shock cause cellular breakdown and the release of nonvolatile acids.
Excess exercise, severe infection, fever	Excessive exercise, fever, and severe infection can cause cellular catabolism and acid accumulation.

decrease the number of bicarbonate ions in the extracellular fluid and increase the concentration of carbonic acid. The renal mechanism functions by conserving the hydrogen ions and excreting the sodium, potassium, and bicarbonate ions. The respiratory mechanism maintains balance through hypoventilation, retaining carbon dioxide and increasing the concentration of carbonic acid in the extracellular fluid.

Table 11-2	Causes of Metabolic Alkalosis
Etiology	**Rationale**
Gastrointestinal Abnormalities	
Vomiting, gastric suction	With vomiting and gastric suctioning, large amounts of chloride and hydrogen ions that are plentiful in the stomach are lost. Bicarbonate anions increase to compensate for chloride loss.
Peptic ulcers	Excess of alkali in ECF occurs when a client takes excessive amounts of acid neutralizers such as $NaHCO_3$ to ease ulcer pain.
Hypokalemia	Loss of potassium from the body is accompanied by loss of chloride.

Table 11-3	Clinical Manifestations of Metabolic Acidosis and Metabolic Alkalosis	
Body Involvement	**Metabolic Acidosis**	**Metabolic Alkalosis**
CNS Abnormalities	Restlessness, apathy, weakness, disorientation, stupor, coma	Irritability, confusion, tetanylike symptoms, hyperactive reflexes
Respiratory Abnormalities	Kussmaul breathing: deep, rapid, vigorous breathing	Shallow breathing
Skin Changes	Flushing and warm skin	
Cardiac Abnormalities	Cardiac dysrhythmias, decrease in heart rate and cardiac output	
Gastrointestinal Abnormalities	Nausea, vomiting, abdominal pain	Vomiting with loss of chloride and potassium
Laboratory Values		
pH	<7.35	>7.45
HCO_3, BE	<24 mEq/L; < −2	>28 mEq/L > +2
Serum CO_2	<22 mEq/L	>32 mEq/L

CLINICAL MANAGEMENT

The first line of treatment for metabolic acidosis and alkalosis is to determine the cause of the imbalance. Correcting the cause may completely alleviate the symptoms. Giving fluids intravenously and restoring electrolytes and nutrients assist by correcting metabolic acid-base imbalances. Figure 11-1 outlines the body's normal defense actions and various methods of treatment for restoring balance in metabolic acidosis and alkalosis.

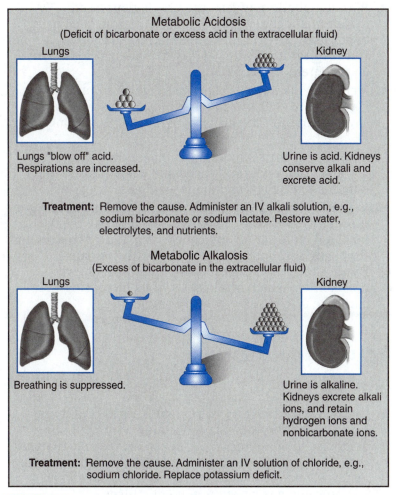

Metabolic Acidosis
(Deficit of bicarbonate or excess acid in the extracellular fluid)

Lungs   Kidney

Lungs "blow off" acid.   Urine is acid. Kidneys
Respirations are increased.   conserve alkali and
                                 excrete acid.

Treatment: Remove the cause. Administer an IV alkali solution, e.g., sodium bicarbonate or sodium lactate. Restore water, electrolytes, and nutrients.

Metabolic Alkalosis
(Excess of bicarbonate in the extracellular fluid)

Lungs   Kidney

Breathing is suppressed.   Urine is alkaline.
                                 Kidneys excrete alkali
                                 ions, and retain
                                 hydrogen ions and
                                 nonbicarbonate ions.

Treatment: Remove the cause. Administer an IV solution of chloride, e.g., sodium chloride. Replace potassium deficit.

FIGURE 11-1 Body's defense action and treatment for metabolic acidosis and alkalosis.

● CLINICAL CONSIDERATIONS: METABOLIC ACIDOSIS AND ALKALOSIS

1. Metabolic acidosis is characterized by a decrease in bicarbonate concentration or acid excess. The pH is <7.35, HCO_3 is <24 mEq/L, base excess (BE) is < -2.

2. The anion gap is a useful indicator for determining the presence or absence of metabolic acidosis. If the anion gap is >16 mEq/L, metabolic acidosis is suspected. The formula used is: Serum sodium $-$ (Serum chloride $+$ Serum CO_2) $=$ Anion gap

3. With metabolic acidosis, the CNS is depressed; symptoms include apathy, disorientation, weakness, and stupor. Deep, rapid breathing (Kussmaul breathing) is a respiratory compensatory mechanism to decrease acid content in the blood.

4. Metabolic alkalosis is characterized by an increase in bicarbonate concentration or a loss of a strong acid (hydrogen ion). The pH is >7.45, HCO_3 is >28 mEq/L, BE $> +2$.

5. Vomiting, gastric suction, and ingestion of large amounts of a sodium bicarbonate preparation are common causes of metabolic alkalosis.

6. In metabolic alkalosis, the buffer, renal, and respiratory mechanisms try to reestablish balance. The renal mechanism functions by conserving hydrogen ions, and excreting sodium, potassium, and bicarbonate. Hypoventilation is a respiratory compensatory mechanism, which retains CO_2, thus increasing the carbonic acid (H_2CO_3) concentration.

● CLIENT MANAGEMENT

Assessment

● Obtain a client history of current clinical problems. Identify health problems associated with metabolic acidosis, such as starvation, severe or chronic diarrhea, diabetic ketoacidosis, trauma and shock, kidney failure, and problems associated with metabolic alkalosis, such as vomiting, gastric suction, peptic ulcer.

● Check the arterial bicarbonate, base excess, and serum CO_2 levels for metabolic acid-base imbalances. Compare with the norms for arterial blood gases.

● Obtain baseline vital signs for comparison with future vital signs.

● Check laboratory results, especially blood sugar and electrolytes.

Nursing Diagnoses

● *Imbalanced Nutrition, less than body requirements,* related to the body's inability to use nutrition

● *Decreased Cardiac Output,* related to severe metabolic acidotic state

● *Deficient Fluid Volume,* related to nausea, vomiting, and increased urine output

Interventions

Metabolic Acidosis

● Monitor dietary intake and report inadequate nutrient and fluid intake.

● Report abnormal laboratory results regarding electrolytes, blood sugar, and arterial blood gases (ABGs). A pH <7.35 and HCO_3 <24 mEq/L indicate metabolic acidosis.

● Monitor vital signs. Report the presence of Kussmaul respirations that relate to diabetic ketoacidosis or severe shock.

● Monitor signs and symptoms related to metabolic acidosis (refer to Table 11-3).

● Monitor fluid intake and output. Report the amount of fluid loss via vomiting and gastric suctioning.

● Administer adequate fluid replacement with sodium bicarbonate as prescribed by the health care provider to correct acidotic state.

Metabolic Alkalosis

● Monitor serum electrolytes and ABG values. A pH >7.45 and HCO_3 >28 mEq/L indicate metabolic alkalosis.

● Monitor vital signs. Note if the respirations remain shallow and slow.

● Monitor signs and symptoms of metabolic alkalosis (refer to Table 11-3).

● Report the consumption of large quantities of acid neutralizers that contain bicarbonate compounds such as Bromo-Seltzer.

● Record the amount of fluid loss via vomiting and gastric suctioning. Hydrogen and chloride are lost with the gastric secretions, thus the pH is increased and metabolic alkalosis results.

● Provide comfort and alleviate anxiety when possible.

Evaluation/Outcome

● Evaluate that the cause of metabolic acidosis or metabolic alkalosis has been corrected or controlled.

● Evaluate the therapeutic effect on the correction of metabolic acidosis or metabolic alkalosis; ABGs are returning to or have returned to normal range.

● Remain free of signs and symptoms of metabolic acidosis or metabolic alkalosis; vital signs returned to normal range, especially respiration.

● Client is able to perform activities of daily living.

Respiratory Acidosis and Respiratory Alkalosis

Larry Dale Purnell, RN, PhD, FAAN

INTRODUCTION

The $PaCO_2$ is the respiratory component that determines respiratory acidosis and alkalosis. In respiratory acidosis, the CO_2 is conserved by mixing it with water to form carbonic acid (H_2CO_3). In respiratory acidosis, the pH is decreased (<7.35) and the $PaCO_2$ is increased (>45 mm Hg). In respiratory alkalosis, the pH is increased (>7.45) and the $PaCO_2$ is decreased (<35 mm Hg).

PATHOPHYSIOLOGY

Respiratory acidosis is characterized by an increase in carbon dioxide and carbonic acid concentration in the extracellular fluid. Respiratory alkalosis is characterized by a decrease in carbon dioxide and carbonic acid in the extracellular fluid. Figure 12-1 demonstrates the relationship of the pH to the $PaCO_2$. When the pH is decreased and the $PaCO_2$ is increased, respiratory acidosis occurs. Likewise, if the pH is increased and the $PaCO_2$ is decreased, respiratory alkalosis occurs.

Very often, inadequate ventilation is the cause of respiratory acidosis. The characteristic breathing pattern associated with respiratory acidosis is dyspnea or shortness of breath because hypoventilation usually causes a decrease in the $PaCO_2$. In respiratory alkalosis, breathing is rapid and shallow (hyperventilation). In respiratory acidosis, the

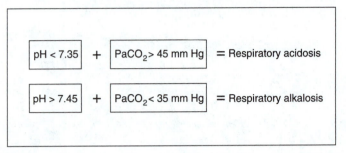

FIGURE 12-1 Relationship of pH and PaCO$_2$ in respiratory acid-base imbalances.

buffer, renal, and respiratory mechanisms try to reestablish balance. As a result of a chloride shift, bicarbonate ions are released to neutralize carbonic acid excess. In respiratory alkalosis, the buffer mechanism produces more organic acids which react with the excess bicarbonate ions. There is an increase in bicarbonate excretion and a retention of the hydrogen ion.

● ETIOLOGY

Inadequate exchange of gases in the lungs causes a retention of CO_2 and carbonic acid in the blood ($CO_2 + H_2O = H_2CO_3$), resulting in respiratory acidosis. Respiratory alkalosis results from a CO_2 loss, lungs blowing off carbon dioxide. Tables 12-1 and 12-2 list the causes of respiratory acidosis and alkalosis.

Narcotics, sedatives, chest injuries, respiratory distress syndrome, pneumonia, and pulmonary edema can cause acute respiratory acidosis (ARA). ARA results from rapidly increasing CO_2 levels and retention of CO_2 in the blood. With chronic obstructive pulmonary disease (COPD), the PaCO$_2$ gradually increases over a prolonged period of time (days to months). The body can compensate for CO_2 accumulation by excreting excess hydrogen ions and conserving the bicarbonate ion. The client's PaCO$_2$ can be extremely elevated and the HCO$_3$ also elevated, indicating metabolic/renal compensation. An example of compensated ABG for a client with COPD is pH 7.22, PaCO$_2$ 98 mm Hg, HCO$_3$ 40. Refer to Chapter 10 for a discussion of acid-base compensation mechanisms.

Table 12-1	Causes of Respiratory Acidosis
Etiology	**Rationale**
CNS Depressants Drugs: narcotics [morphine, meperidine (Demerol)], anesthetics, barbiturates	These drugs depress the respiratory center in the medulla, causing retention of CO_2 (carbon dioxide), which results in hypercapnia (increased partial pressure of CO_2 in the blood).
Pulmonary Abnormalities Chronic obstructive pulmonary disease (COPD: emphysema, severe asthma)	Inadequate exchange of gases in the lungs due to a decreased surface area for aeration causes retention of CO_2 in the blood.
Pneumonia, pulmonary edema	Airway obstruction inhibits effective gas exchanges, resulting in a retention of CO_2.
Poliomyelitis, Guillain-Barré syndrome, chest injuries	Weakness of the respiratory muscles decreases the excretion of CO_2, thus increasing carbonic acid concentration.

Table 12-2	Causes of Respiratory Alkalosis
Etiology	**Rationale**
Hyperventilation Psychologic effects: anxiety, hysteria, overbreathing	Excessive "blowing off" of CO_2 through the lungs results in hypocapnia (decreased partial pressure of CO_2 in the blood).
Pain	Overstimulation of the respiratory center in the medulla results in hyperventilation.
Fever	
Brain tumors, meningitis, encephalitis	
Early salicylate poisoning	
Hyperthyroidism	

Those in respiratory alkalosis are often very apprehensive and anxious. They hyperventilate to overcome their anxiety. This causes them to blow off excessive quantities of carbon dioxide, which results in a respiratory alkalotic state.

CLINICAL MANIFESTATIONS

In respiratory acidosis, an increase in hypercapnia causes dyspnea (difficulty in breathing), an increased pulse rate, and an elevated blood pressure. The skin may be warm and flushed due to vasodilation from the increased CO_2 concentration.

When respiratory alkalosis occurs, there is CNS hyperexcitability and a decrease in cerebral blood flow. Tetany-like symptoms and dizziness frequently result. Table 12-3 lists the signs and symptoms of respiratory acidosis and alkalosis.

CLINICAL MANAGEMENT

The three treatment modalities for respiratory acidosis are: remove the cause; have the client perform deep breathing exercises; use a ventilator. In respiratory acidosis, the kidneys conserve alkali and excrete hydrogen or acid in the urine. Ex-

Table 12-3 Clinical Manifestations of Respiratory Acidosis and Respiratory Alkalosis		
Body Involvement	**Respiratory Acidosis**	**Respiratory Alkalosis**
Cardiopulmonary Abnormalities	Dyspnea Tachycardia Blood pressure	Rapid, shallow breathing Palpitations
CNS Abnormalities	Disorientation Depression, paranoia Weakness Stupor (later)	Tetany symptoms: numbness and tingling of fingers and toes, positive Chvostek's and Trousseau's signs Hyperactive reflexes Vertigo (dizziness) Unconsciousness (later)
Skin	Flushed and warm	Sweating may occur
Laboratory Values		
pH	<7.35 (when compensatory mechanisms fail)	>7.45 (when compensatory mechanisms fail)
$PaCO_2$	>45 mm Hg	<35 mm Hg

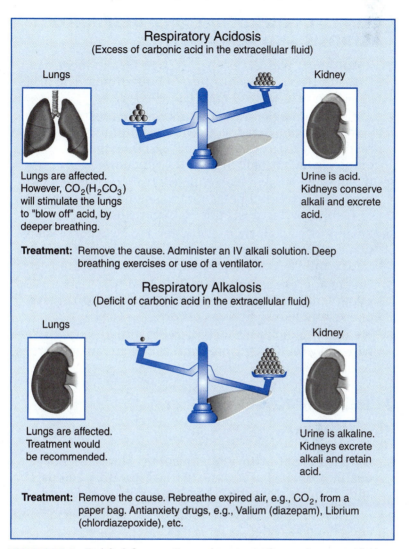

FIGURE 12-2 Body's defense action and treatment for respiratory acidosis and alkalosis.

cess CO_2 accumulation stimulates the lungs to blow off carbon dioxide or acid to compensate for the respiratory acidotic state.

With respiratory alkalosis, the three treatment modalities include: remove the cause; have the client rebreathe expired air to obtain CO_2; use antianxiety drugs. The kidneys excrete alkaline ions (HCO_3) and retain acid or hydrogen ions. Figure 12-2 demonstrates the body's defense action and treatment for respiratory acidosis and alkalosis.

CLINICAL CONSIDERATIONS: RESPIRATORY ACIDOSIS AND ALKALOSIS

1. Respiratory acidosis is characterized by an increase in CO_2 and H_2CO_3 concentration in body fluids. The pH is <7.35 and $PaCO_2$ >45 mm Hg.

2. ABGs should be closely monitored when respiratory acidosis is suspected; e.g., with chest injuries, respiratory distress syndrome, COPD (asthma, emphysema, chronic bronchitis), pneumonia.

3. Warm, flushed skin (vasodilation from increased CO_2), dyspnea, increased pulse rate are signs and symptoms of respiratory acidosis due to hypercapnia.

4. Respiratory alkalosis is characterized by a decrease in CO_2 and H_2CO_3 concentration in body fluids. The pH is >7.45 and $PaCO_2$<35 mm Hg.

5. Severe apprehension and anxiety lead to hyperventilation and respiratory alkalosis. Dizziness and tetany-like symptoms occur.

6. Treatment modalities include rebreathing expired air via paper bag (not plastic bag) and use of antianxiety drugs.

CLIENT MANAGEMENT

Assessment

- Obtain a client history of clinical problems. Identify health problems associated with respiratory acidosis and alkalosis (refer to Tables 12-1 and 12-2).

- Check for signs and symptoms of respiratory acidosis and alkalosis (refer to Table 12-3).

- Obtain vital signs for a baseline record to compare with future vital signs.

- Check arterial blood gases (ABGs), particularly the pH and $PaCO_2$. A pH <7.35 and $PaCO_2$ >45 mm Hg are indicative of respiratory acidosis; a pH >7.45 and $PaCO_2$ <35 mm Hg are indicative of respiratory alkalosis.

Nursing Diagnoses

- *Impaired Gas Exchange,* related to alveolar hypoventilation secondary to COPD
- *Ineffective Airway Clearance,* related to thick bronchial secretions and/or bronchial spasms
- *Risk for Injury,* related to hypoxemia and hypercapnia
- *Ineffective Breathing Pattern,* related to inadequate ventilation
- *Ineffective Breathing Pattern,* related to hyperventilation and anxiety
- *Risk for Injury,* related to dizziness, lightheadedness, and syncope secondary to respiratory alkalosis (hyperventilating)

Interventions

Respiratory Acidosis

- Monitor the client's respiratory status for changes in respiratory rate, distress, and breathing pattern.
- Monitor arterial blood gases.
- Auscultate breath sounds periodically to determine wheezing, rhonchi, or crackles that indicate poor gas exchange.
- Monitor vital signs for tachycardia or cardiac dysrhythmias associated with hypercapnia and hypoxemia (oxygen deficit in the blood).
- Encourage the client to breathe slowly, deeply, and cough to eliminate bronchial secretions and improve gas exchange.
- Assist the client with use of an inhaler containing a bronchodilator drug.
- Administer chest clapping on COPD clients to break up mucous plugs and secretions in the alveoli.
- Teach breathing exercises and postural drainage to clients with COPD to remove secretions that are trapped in overextended alveoli.

● Encourage the client to increase fluid intake in order to decrease tenacity of secretions.

● Monitor the client's state of sensorium for signs of disorientation due to a lack of oxygen to the brain.

● Encourage the client to participate in a pulmonary rehabilitation program.

Respiratory Alkalosis

● Encourage the client who is overanxious and hyperventilating to take deep breaths and breathe slowly to prevent respiratory alkalosis.

● Listen to the client who is emotionally distressed. Encourage the client to seek professional help.

● Demonstrate a slow, relaxed breathing pattern to decrease overbreathing, which causes respiratory alkalosis.

● Administer a sedative as prescribed to relax the client and restore a normal breathing pattern.

● Monitor ABGs and vital signs.

Evaluation/Outcome

● Evaluate that the cause of respiratory acidosis or respiratory alkalosis is corrected or controlled; ABGs are returning to or have returned to normal range.

● The client remains free of signs and symptoms of respiratory acidosis or respiratory alkalosis.

● The client exhibits a patent airway and the breath sounds have improved.

● The client ambulates with little or no assistance and without breathlessness.

● Document compliance with prescribed drug therapy and medical regimen.

INTRAVENOUS THERAPY

INTRODUCTION

This unit discusses the basic classifications of intravenous solutions in terms of their osmolality and the various types of fluids for intravenous administration. The two chapters in this unit are Intravenous Solutions and their Administration and Total Parenteral Nutrition (TPN). Purposes for IV therapy include: (1) hydration to restore fluid loss (rehydrate) and improve renal output; (2) maintenance to meet daily fluid needs; (3) replacement for ongoing fluid losses; and (4) replacement of electrolyte losses.

Many of the solutions used for IV therapy are produced commercially to meet clients' needs associated with specific types of fluid, electrolyte, and acid-base imbalances. IV solutions are classified as being hypotonic, isotonic, or hypertonic. IV osmolality of a solution is determined by the concentration or the number of particles (osmols) suspended in the solution. The greater the number of particles in the solution, the higher the osmolality of the solution. Hypotonic (hypo-osmolar) solutions have less than 240 mOsm/L; isotonic (iso-osmolar) solutions have approximately 240–340 mOsm/L; and hypertonic (hyperosmolar) solutions have more than 340 mOsm/L. Table U4-1 lists IV solutions according to their osmolality and uses; e.g., hydrating solutions, replacement solutions, protein solutions, and plasma expanders.

CRYSTALLOIDS

Commonly used crystalloid solutions include dextrose and water (D_5W), saline (NSS), and lactated Ringer's solutions. Isotonic solutions such as 5% dextrose and water (D_5W) have approximately 250 mOsm/ L. A normal saline solution (0.9% NaCl or NSS) has 310 mOsm/L, and lactated Ringer's solution has approximately the same number of milliosmols. Hypotonic solutions include 0.33% NaCl (one-third normal saline) with

Table U4-1	Selected Solutions Used in IV Therapy		
Categories and Solutions	**Tonicity (Osmolality)**	**Electrolytes (mEq/L)**	**Rationale**
Hydrating Solutions			
0.45% NaCl [$^1/_2$ normal saline solution (NSS)]	Hypotonic	Na 77; Cl: 77	Useful for establishing renal function. Not for replacement therapy.
Dextrose 2.5% in 0.45% saline	Isotonic	Calories: 85, Na: 77, Cl: 77	Helpful in establishing renal function.
Dextrose 5% in 0.2% saline	Isotonic	Calories: 170, Na: 38, Cl: 38	Useful for daily maintenance of body fluids when less Na and Cl are required.
Dextrose 5% in 0.33% saline	Hypertonic	Calories: 170, Na: 51, Cl: 51	Useful for daily maintenance of body fluids.
Dextrose 5% in 0.45% saline	Hypertonic	Calories: 170, Na: 77, Cl: 77	Calories: 170, maintenance of body fluids and for treating fluid volume deficits.
Dextrose 5% in water (Dextrose 10% in water is occasionally used)	Isotonic	Calories: 170	Helpful in rehydration and elimination. May cause urinary, sodium loss. Good vehicle for IV potassium.
Replacement Solutions			
Dextrose 5% in 0.9% NaCl [normal saline solution (NSS)]	Hypertonic	Calories: 170, Na: 154, Cl: 154	Replacement of fluid, sodium, chloride; and calories.
Lactated Ringer's	Isotonic	Na: 130, K: 4, Ca: 3, Cl: 109; lactate: 28	Resembles the electrolyte composition of normal blood serum/plasma. Potassium amount does not meet body's daily K-requirement.
Dextrose 5% in lactated Ringer's	Hypertonic	Calories: 170, Na: 130, K: 4, Ca: 3, Cl: 109, lactate: 28	Same contents as lactated Ringer's plus calories.
Ringer's solution	Isotonic	Na: 147, K: 4, Ca: 3, Cl: 154	Does not contain lactate which may be harmful to clients who lack enzymes essential to metabolize lactic acid.

(continues)

Table U4-1		Selected Solutions Used in IV Therapy—*continued*	
Categories and Solutions	**Tonicity (Osmolality)**	**Electrolytes (mEq/L)**	**Rationale**
Normal saline solution (NSS)	Isotonic	Na: 154, Cl: 154	Restores ECF volume and replaces sodium and chloride deficits.
Hypertonic saline 3% NaCl	Hypertonic	Na: 513, Cl: 513	Helpful in hyponatremia. Helpful in eliminating intra-cellular fluid excess.
Protein Solutions			
Aminosyn RF 5.2%	Hypertonic	Calories: 175, K: 5.4, amino acids	Provides protein and fluid for the body, and promotes wound healing.
Aminosyn II 3.5% with dextrose 5%	Hypertonic	Calories: 345, Na: 18, amino acids	Provides protein, calories, and fluids. Helpful for the malnourished and for clients with hypoproteinemia. Not to be used in severe liver damage.
Plasma Expander			
Dextran 40 in normal saline or 5% dextrose in water	Isotonic		Colloidal solution used to increase plasma volume. Dextran 40 is a short-lived plasma volume expander (4 to 6 hours). Useful in early shock to correct hypovolemia, increase arterial blood pressure, improve pulse pressure and cardiac output. It improves micro-circulation and increases small vessel perfusion. *Caution.* NOT to be used in severely dehydrated clients in renal disease, thrombocytopenia, or clients who are actively hemorrhaging.

103 mOsm/L, and 0.45% NaCl (one-half normal saline) with 154 mOsm/L. *Although 5% dextrose and water is isotonic, it becomes a hypotonic solution as soon as the dextrose is metabolized in the body.* When 5% dextrose and water without sodium chloride is used consistently over a period of time, the client is actually receiving a hypotonic solution, which can cause ICFVE or water intoxication. Hypertonic solutions include 5% dextrose with 0.9% NaCl (NSS), which contains 560 mOsm/L, 5% dextrose in lactated Ringer's solution (525 mOsm/L), and 3% saline solution (810 mOsm/L).

Dextrose solutions for intravenous therapy are prepared in two strengths, 5% and 10%. Five percent dextrose means that there are 5 grams of dextrose in 100 ml of solution. Therefore, 1 L or 1000 ml of 5% dextrose contains 50 grams (50 g) of dextrose. One gram of dextrose is equivalent to 4 calories, thus 50 grams is equivalent to 200 calories. One liter of 5% dextrose and water does not supply many calories. Potassium that is administered intravenously must be diluted in a solution such as 5% dextrose and water. Potassium should *never* be given as a bolus injection because lethal cardiac dysrhythmias will result.

Normal saline solution (NSS or 0.9% NaCl) is isotonic and similar to plasma; however, it contains a slightly higher concentration of sodium chloride (Na = 154 mEq/L and Cl = 154 mEq/L). NSS is useful in replacing fluid and ECF electrolyte losses. It is considered a plasma volume expander. A hypertonic saline solution (3% NaCl) may be used in treating a client with severe hyponatremia; the serum sodium level is usually <115 mEq/L.

Lactated Ringer's solution is similar to plasma. It contains sodium, potassium, calcium chloride, and lactate (lactate is metabolized to bicarbonate). It is isotonic and frequently called a balanced electrolyte solution (BES). This solution is usually prescribed following trauma or surgery to replace "plasma-like" fluid. Lactated Ringer's and normal saline solutions can be used interchangeably for acute fluid replacement.

There are numerous commercially-prepared, balanced electrolyte solutions. Most of these IV solutions contain sodium, potassium, magnesium, chloride, and either acetate, lactate, or gluconate; some also contain calcium and phosphate. These solutions are prescribed for either maintenance needs or for replacement losses such as severe vom-

Table U4-2 Commercially Prepared, Balanced Electrolyte Solutions (BES)

Solution	mEq/L Concentration
Abbott Solutions	
Normosol R	Na: 140; K: 5; Mg: 3; Cl: 98; Acetate: 27; Gluconate: 23
Normosol M	Na: 40; K: 13; Mg: 3, Cl: 40; Acetate: 16
Ionosol B (also in 5% dextrose)	Na: 57; K: 25; Mg: 5; Cl: 49; HPO$_4$: 7; lactate: 25
Ionosol MB (also in 5% dextrose)	Na: 25; K: 20; Mg: 3; Cl: 22; HPO$_4$: 3; lactate: 23
Baxter Solutions	
Plasma-Lyte 148	Na: 140; K: 5; Mg: 3; Cl: 98; Acetate: 27; Gluconate: 23
Plasma-Lyte R	Na: 140; K: 10 Ca: 5; Mg: 3; Cl: 103; Acetate: 47; lactate: 8
Plasma-Lyte M	Na: 40; K: 16; Ca: 5; Mg: 3; Cl: 40; Acetate: 12; lactate: 12
McGaw Solutions	
Isolyte E	Na: 140; K: 10; Ca: 5; Mg: 3; Cl: 103; Acetate: 49; Citrate: 8
Isolyte S	Na: 140; K: 5; Mg: 3; Cl: 98; Acetate: 27; Gluconate: 23
Isolyte R	Na: 40; K: 16; Ca: 5; Mg: 3; Cl: 40; Acetate: 24
Isolyte M	Na: 38; K: 35; Cl: 40; HPO$_4$: 15; Acetate: 20

iting, burns, diabetic acidosis, or postoperative dehydration. Table U4-2 lists commercially produced, balanced electrolyte solutions according to the companies that manufacture these products.

COLLOIDS

Colloids are frequently called volume expanders or plasma expanders; they physiologically function like plasma proteins in the blood by maintaining oncotic pressure. Commonly used colloids include albumin, dextran, Plasmanate, and hetastarch (artificial blood substitute). Hypotension and allergic reactions can occur with their use.

Dextran is a colloidal solution that is used to expand the plasma volume. Dextran can affect clotting by coating the platelets and reducing their ability to clot. Dextran comes in two concentrations, dextran 40 and dextran 70. Dextran 40 remains in the circulatory system for 6 hours and dextran 70 remains in circulation for 20 hours. Dextran 70 is infrequently used because it can cause severe dehydration and can affect blood typing and crossmatching. Dextran 40 is useful in correcting hypovolemia in early shock by increasing arterial blood pressure and increasing cardiac output; it also increases pulse pressure. Another purpose for dextran 40 is to improve microcirculation by reducing red blood cell aggregation in the capillaries.

The use of dextran 40 is contraindicated for clients having severe dehydration, renal disease, thrombocytopenia, or active hemorrhaging. In severe dehydration, dextran 40 increases dehydration by pulling more fluid from the cells and tissue spaces into the vascular space. If urine output is good, the vascular fluid is excreted. Both cellular and extracellular dehydration occur. However, if renal function is decreased, fluid hypervolemia might occur. If oliguria is due to hypovolemia, dextran 40 may improve urine output, but if renal damage is present, dextran 40 may cause renal failure. Dextran 40 tends to clot platelets and prolong bleeding time, so this solution is not indicated for a client with thrombocytopenia. Dextran 40 improves microcirculation, and during active bleeding, additional blood loss can occur from the capillaries if hemorrhage is prolonged.

Albumin concentrate is useful in restoring body protein. It is considered to be a plasma volume expander. Too much albumin or albumin administered too rapidly can cause fluid to be retained in the pulmonary vasculature. Plasmanate is a commercially prepared protein product that is used instead of plasma and albumin to replace body protein.

● BLOOD AND BLOOD COMPONENTS

Blood and blood components are another type of intravenous therapy. Whole blood, packed red cells (whole blood minus the plasma), plasma, and platelets can be administered intravenously. Fifty-five percent of whole blood is plasma. Various components of whole blood can be fractionated and transfused separately. These components include red blood cells (RBC or packed cells), plasma, platelets, white blood cells (WBC), albumin, and blood factors II, VII, VIII, IX, and X. Red blood cells, also known as packed cells, are composed of whole blood minus the plasma. A unit of RBC or packed cells is 250 ml. When RBC replacement is needed without an increase in fluid volume, a unit of RBC is often prescribed instead of whole blood.

The shelf life of refrigerated whole blood is 42 days. Red blood cells and plasma can be frozen to extend their shelf life to 10 years for red blood cells and 1 year for plasma. Platelets must be administered within 5 days after they have been extracted from whole blood. As whole blood ages, potassium leaves the red blood cells, thus increasing the serum potassium level. After 3 weeks of shelf life, serum potassium in the whole blood can increase to 20 mEq/L or greater. A client who has an elevated or a slightly elevated serum potassium level should not receive whole blood that has a long shelf life. This "old blood" could dangerously increase the client's serum potassium level.

The hematocrit measures the volume of red blood cells in proportion to the extracellular fluid. A rise or drop in the hematocrit can indicate a gain or loss of intravascular extracellular fluid. An increased concentration of red blood cells is known as hemoconcentration. A transfusion of whole blood or plasma decreases the hemoconcentration, thus lowering the hematocrit, increasing the blood pressure, and establishing renal flow. The treatment of choice to decrease osmolality is a transfusion of plasma or the administration of crystalloids.

CHAPTER 13

Intravenous Solutions and Their Administration

Sheila G. Cushing, MS, RN

INTRODUCTION

Concepts related to intravenous administration and therapy are presented in this chapter through the use of six sub-headings: (1) basic purposes of IV therapy, (2) IV flow rate and calculation for IV infusion, (3) types of IV infusion devices for short-term IV therapy, (4) central venous catheters for long-term IV therapy, (5) assessment factors in IV therapy, and (6) possible complications resulting from IV therapy. Client Management, including assessment, diagnoses, interventions, and evaluation/outcome, summarizes the important functions for the health professional.

BASIC PURPOSES OF INTRAVENOUS THERAPY

Healthy people normally do not require fluid and electrolyte therapy; however, certain illnesses and conditions compromise the body's ability to adapt to fluid changes. When a client cannot maintain this balance, IV therapy may be indicated. People requiring intravenous therapy may depend on intravenous therapy to meet daily maintenance needs for water, electrolytes, calories, vitamins, and other nutritional substances.

The five purposes of IV therapy are to: (1) provide maintenance requirements for fluids and electrolytes, (2) replace previous losses, (3) replace concurrent losses, (4) provide nutrition, and (5) provide a mechanism for the administration of medications and/or the transfusion of blood and blood components. Multiple electrolyte solutions are helpful in replacing previous and concurrent fluid losses. Fluid and electrolyte losses that occur from diarrhea, vomiting, and/or gastric suction are an example of concurrent losses. When a client is unable to meet his or her nutritional needs through oral intake, total parenteral nutrition (TPN) may be prescribed; TPN is discussed in Chapter 14. IV therapy is also used for administering medications and blood products. Sufficient kidney function is necessary while the client is receiving IV fluids and electrolyte therapy. Renal dysfunction may result in fluid overload and electrolyte imbalances.

Fluids and electrolytes for maintenance therapy should be ordered on a daily basis and administered over a period of 24 hours. If a client receives his or her full 24-hour maintenance parenteral therapy in 8 hours, two-thirds of the water and electrolytes are in excess of the body's current needs, and a large portion of the excess maintenance fluids is excreted.

Tolerance for sudden changes in water and electrolytes is limited for extremely ill clients following major surgery, older adults, small children, and infants. Rapid administration of replacement fluids that exceed a person's physiologic tolerance can cause hyponatremia, pulmonary edema, and other complications.

● IV FLOW RATE AND CALCULATIONS FOR INTRAVENOUS INFUSIONS

The desired amount of solution (ml) per day and the IV flow rate are generally calculated in relation to the type of therapy needed; e.g., maintenance, replacement with maintenance, or hydration. Urinary output needs to be reestablished before maintenance therapy is started. Table 13-1 outlines the three types of IV therapy, the amount of suggested IV solutions, and the suggested IV flow rate. The IV flow rate may need to be adjusted if the client is very ill, an older adult, a small child, or infant. Today, many institutions use IV controllers or pumps to deliver IV fluids. The health professional needs to know how to calculate the flow rate and regulate the various types of infusion devices.

Table 13-1 Types of IV Therapy

Type of Therapy	Amount of Solution Desired (ml)	Rate of Flow
Maintenance therapy	1500–2000	62–83 ml/h or 1–1.5 ml/min if given over 24 h
Replacement with maintenance therapy	2000–3000	83–125 ml/h or 1.5–2 ml/min (depends on individual)
Hydration therapy	1000–3000	60–120 ml/h or 1–2 ml/min

Note: These guidelines may be adapted to individual circumstances. The health care provider orders the 24-h requirements and the health professional computes 1-h requirements from this. The amount of solution to be administered and the rate of flow can vary greatly with the very sick; the older adult, the small child, the infant, and the postsurgical client.

The prescribed order for IV therapy includes the type of fluid for infusion and the amount to be administered in a specified period of time. The health professional must compute the number of milliliters per hour (ml/h) and then calculate the drops per minute for the infusion. Electronic infusion pumps are frequently used to administer IV solutions and are usually regulated to deliver milliliters per hour.

When using IV infusion sets for IV therapy administration, first check the drop factor or drip rate that is printed on the manufacturer's box or package. The number of drops per milliliter (gtt/ml) varies with each manufacturer. Drop factors range from 10–20 gtt/ml for the macrodrip chambers and 60 gtt/ml for microdrip chambers. Table 13-2 lists the drop factors according to macrodrip sets and microdrip sets.

Table 13-2 Intravenous Sets

Drops (gtt) Per Milliliter

Macrodrip Sets	Microdrip Sets
10 gtt/ml	60 gtt/ml
15 gtt/ml	
20 gtt/ml	

There are two methods used to calculate IV flow rate (gtt/minute):

Two-Step Method:

a. Amount of fluid ÷ hours to administer = ml/h

b. $\dfrac{\text{mlh} \times \text{gtt/ml (IV set)}}{60 \text{ min}} = \text{gtt/min}$

One-Step Method:

$\dfrac{\text{Amount of fluid} \times \text{gtt/ml (IV set)}}{\text{Hours to administer} \times \text{Minutes per hour (60)}} = \text{gtt/min}$

Example:
Order: 2000 ml of 5% dextrose in 0.45% NaCl (one-half normal saline solution) and 1000 ml of D_5W to run over 24 hours. The drop factor on the manufacturer's box is 10 gtt/ml. Using the two-step method, the client should receive 125 ml/h and 21 gtt/min.

Using the two-step method:
a. 3000 ml ÷ 24 h = 125 ml/h

b. $\dfrac{125 \text{ ml/h} \times 10 \text{ gtt/ml (IV-set)}}{60 \text{ min (1 hr)}} = \dfrac{1250}{60} = 21 \text{ gtt/min}$

Using the one-step method:

$\dfrac{3000 \text{ ml} \times 10 \text{ gtt/ml}}{24 \text{ h} \times 60 \text{ min}} = \dfrac{30000}{1440} = 20.8 \text{ (21 gtt/min)}$

If the health professional uses an electronic IV infusion pump or controller, the volume per hour must be calculated (in this case 125 ml/h) and entered on the pump.

● TYPES OF IV INFUSION DEVICES FOR SHORT-TERM IV THERAPY

There are three common types of infusion devices for routine short-term IV therapy: the butterfly (steel needle), the over-needle catheter, and the inside-needle catheter. The winged-tip, or butterfly, set consists of a wing-tip needle with a steel cannula, plastic or rubber wings, and a plastic catheter or hub. The needle is $\frac{1}{2}$ to $1\frac{1}{2}$ inches long with needle gauges of 16 to 26. The infusion needle and clear tubing are bonded into a single unit.

Advantages of the butterfly infusion set are that it is a one-piece apparatus, has a short beveled needle, and is easy to tape securely. The butterfly reduces the risk of secondary puncture and infiltration on puncture. Disadvantages of this IV apparatus are that the butterfly should be used only for very short-term IV therapy (in many cases, less than 2 hours). The butterfly method is commonly used in children and older adults whose veins are likely to be small or fragile.

The second type of commonly used IV device is the over-needle catheter (ONC). The bevel of the needle extends beyond the catheter, which is $1\frac{1}{4}$ to 8 inches in length. Twelve to 24 gauge needles are available. With its short, large cannula, the ONC is preferable for rapid IV infusion and is more comfortable for the client. Catheters used in ONCs and INCs are constructed of silicone, Teflon, polyvinyl chloride, or polyethylene.

The third type of IV device is the inside-needle catheter (INC), which is constructed exactly the opposite of the ONC. Needle length is $1\frac{1}{2}$ to 3 inches with a catheter length of 8 to 25 inches. Catheter gauges from 2 to 24 are available. The INC set comes with a catheter sleeve guard that must be secured over the needle bevel to prevent severing the catheter. With its longer, narrower catheter, the INC is preferred when vein catheterization is necessary for prolonged infusions.

● CENTRAL VENOUS CATHETERS AND LONG-TERM IV THERAPY

Central venous catheters are another type of IV device. These catheters are radiopaque and may have a single, double, or triple lumen. Since the insertion of a central venous catheter presents critical risks, its insertion is followed by an x-ray to confirm the position and tip placement of the catheter.

Four common reasons for using a central venous catheter are: (1) to measure the central venous pressure, (2) for infusion of TPN, (3) for infusion of multiple IV fluids and/or medications, and (4) to infuse chemotherapeutic or irritating medications. Hickman, Groshong, and Cook are examples of central venous catheters that must be inserted in the operating room. The implantable vascular access device (IVAD) is another example of a central venous line that must be surgically inserted.

For clients without adequate peripheral sites and for those requiring long-term IV therapy, a central venous site is the optimal choice. Central venous sites are the superior vena cava and the inferior vena cava. The superior vena cava is accessed from the internal jugular vein and the right or left subclavian vein, whereas the inferior vena cava is accessed from the femoral vein. Figure 13-1 presents the central venous access sites. The catheter may be a single or multilumen. A peripherally inserted central catheter (PICC) line is used for long-term IV therapy (2 weeks to 1 year) and is frequently used in home care settings for clients who require IV therapy. The PICC line is inserted into the antecubital vein. A specifically trained or certified PICC insertion health professional inserts the catheter and an x-ray is taken to confirm accurate placement. Guidelines for flushing solutions and volume are presented in Table 13-3.

Complications that may occur with insertion of a central venous line into the subclavian and jugular veins are pneumothorax, hemorrhage, air embolism, thrombus dislodgement, and cardiac dysrhythmias. Long-term complications such as hemorrhage, phlebitis, air embolism, thrombus formation, infection, dislodgement, cardiac dysrhythmias, and circulatory impairment might occur with central venous lines.

● ASSESSMENT FACTORS IN INTRAVENOUS THERAPY

The IV solutions and devices are selected by the health professional. He or she must know and understand the various solutions, needles, catheters, tubings, IV sites, flow rate, positioning, and taping IV tubing in order to accurately assess, initiate, and monitor infusions. Table 13-4 provides the assessment factors, interventions, and rationale related to IV therapy.

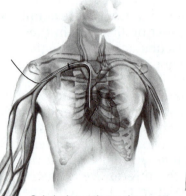

Subclavian catheter site

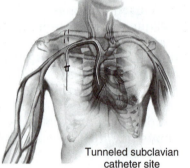

Peripherally inserted
central catheter (PICC)

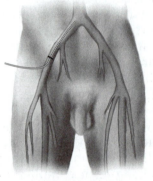

Femoral catheter site

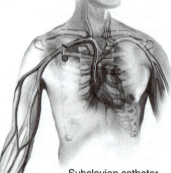

Tunneled subclavian
catheter site

Septum   Reservoir   Catheter

Vascular access port

Subclavian catheter
with vascular access port

FIGURE 13-1 Examples of central venous access sites.

Table 13-3	Venous Access Devices: Flushing Guidelines (Always follow institutional procedure)			
Type	**Length (inches)**	**Flush Solution**	**Volume (ml)**	**Frequency**
Peripheral Venous	1–2	Normal saline	1–3	After each use or q8h
Single lumen(central)	8	Heparinized saline	1–3*	After each use or q24h
Multilumen	8	Heparinized saline	1–3* per port	After each use or q24h
External-tunneled Hickman or Cook	35	Heparinized saline	2–5* per port	After each use or q24h
Groshong	35	Normal saline	2–5*	After each use or q8h
Peripherally inserted central catheter (PICC)	20	Heparinized saline	3–5*	After each use or q12h
Implanted vascular access device	35	Heparinized saline	3–5*	After each use, q5–7d when not in use

*Use 10cc syringe to decrease pressure on the catheter.

Intravenous solutions with <240 mOsm are considered hypotonic. If a hypotonic solution is used continuously, ICFVE or water intoxication results. Five percent dextrose and water is an example of an isotonic solution that converts to a hypotonic solution when used continuously. Constant use of hyperosmolar solutions may cause dehydration.

If IV fluids are to run at less than 50 ml per hour for 12 hours, IV and/or infusion control device with a microdrip chamber is the best choice. IV tubing should be changed every 72 hours, and the IV container (bag) should not hang for longer than 24 hours according to agency policy. Needles and IV catheters should be changed at least every 3 days. The body areas preferred for the insertion of peripheral IV devices are hand veins and distal arm veins. The problem with the use of ONCs is severing of the catheter with the needle tip, and the problem with INCs is that a leak can occur at the infusion insertion site. IV fluids running too fast can cause overhydration.

Table 13-4 Assessment Factors in IV Therapy

Assessment	Interventions	Rationale
Types of IV Solutions	Note the types of IV fluid ordered: hypotonic, isotonic, or hypertonic solutions.	An excessive use of hypotonic solutions can cause a fluid volume excess. Excessive use of hypertonic solutions may cause a fluid volume deficit. An isotonic solution has 240–340 mOsm/L; less than 240 is hypo-osmolar, and greater than 340 is hyperosmolar.
	Report extended use of continuous IVs of dextrose in water.	Dextrose 5% in water administered continuously becomes a hypotonic solution. Dextrose is metabolized rapidly and the remaining water decreases the serum osmolality. Alternate use of D/W with D/NSS (saline) to prevent this complication.
	Observe for signs and symptoms of fluid volume deficit, i.e., dry mucous membranes, poor skin turgor, and increased pulse and respiration rates, when using hyperosmolar solutions. Creatinine/ BUN ratio, 1:10/20; hemoconcentration, 1:20 or greater.	Continuous use of hyperosmolar solutions pulls fluid from intra-cellular compartments to the extracellular compartments. The fluid is excreted by the kidneys. Poor kidney function causes fluid retention, increasing the risk for a fluid volume excess.
Intravenous Tubing and Bag	Inspect IV bags for leaks by gently squeezing.	Microorganisms can enter IV bags through small leak sites contaminating the fluid.
	Check drop size on the equipment box. Use IV tubing with macrodrip chamber (10–20 gtt/ml) for administering IV fluids at a rate of 50 ml/h or greater.	Use of a microdrip chamber (IV tubing) for fluids that are ordered to run at a rate greater than 50 ml/h is inaccurate.

(continues)

Table 13-4	Assessment Factors in IV Therapy—*continued*	
Assessment	**Interventions**	**Rationale**
	Use microdrip chamber (60 gtt/ml) for administering IV fluids at a rate under 50 ml/h.	Infusion pumps increase the accuracy and decrease the risks associated with IV fluids that are to run for 12–24 h and meet specific client fluid needs.
	Change IV tubing every 72 h at time of new hanging.	Studies have shown that IV tubing left hanging for 72 h is free of bacteria when proper aseptic technique is used.
	New IV containers are hung according to agency policy.	An IV bag should not be used for longer than 24 h. If the order is for KVO (keep vein open), a 250–500-ml container with a microdrip chamber set is suggested.
Needles and IV Catheters (cannulas)	Recognize the types of IV needles and catheters used for IV fluids: Straight needles Scalp vein needles/ butterfly (steel) needles Heparin lock Over-needle catheter (ONC) Inside-needle catheter (INC)	Needles (straight and scalp vein) are used for short-term IV therapy and for clients with autoimmune problems. Catheters made of silicone and Teflon are less irritating than polyvinyl chloride and polyethylene catheters.
	Change IV site every 2–3 days according to agency policy.	Needles and catheters in longer than 72 h increase the risk of phlebitis.
	Check the ONC for placement and function.	There are many types of ONCs, i.e., Angiocath, A-Cath, Vicra Quik-Cath, etc. Catheter length can be 1–3 inches. Care should be taken to avoid severing the catheter with the needle tip.

(continues)

Table 13-4	Assessment Factors in IV Therapy—*continued*	
Assessment	**Interventions**	**Rationale**
	Check for fluid leaks at the insertion site after the insertion of an INC.	An INC is used for central venous pressure monitoring, TPN (hyperalimentation), etc. It is frequently inserted in large veins, i.e., subclavian vein, internal jugular, or femoral vein. Leaks result from needle punctures that are larger than the catheter.
Injection Site	Insert needle or catheter in the hand or the distal veins of the arm. Use the antecubital fossa (elbow) site last.	The upper extremity is preferred for the infusion site, since the occurrence of phlebitis and thrombosis in the upper extremities is not as prevalent as it is in the lower extremities.
	Avoid using the leg veins if possible.	Circulation in the leg veins is reduced and thrombus formation can occur.
	Avoid using limbs affected by a stroke or mastectomy for IV sites.	Circulation is usually decreased in affected extremities.
	Apply arm board and/or soft restraints to the extremity with the IV when the client is restless or confused.	Prevention of extremity movement with an IV decreases the chance of dislodging the needle and phlebitis.
Flow Rate and Irrigation	Check types of solutions clients are receiving.	Knowledge of tonicity (osmolality) of fluids aids in determining rate of flow. Rate of hypertonic solutions should be slower than isotonic solutions.
	Observe drip chamber and regulate accordingly.	Regulation of IV fluids is important to prevent overhydration, i.e., cough, dyspnea, neck vein engorgement, and chest crackles. Do not play "catch-up" with IV fluids.

(continues)

Table 13-4	Assessment Factors in IV Therapy—*continued*	
Assessment	**Interventions**	**Rationale**
	Regulate KVO (keep vein open) rate to run 10–20 ml/h or according to agency policy, or use an infusion pump.	KVO IVs should run approximately 10–20 ml/h.
	Label IV bag for milliliters (ml) to be received per hour. Check rate of flow every 30 min to 1 h with hypertonic and toxic solutions and every hour with isotonic solutions.	Hypertonic solutions administered rapidly can cause cellular dehydration and, if the kidneys are properly functioning, vascular dehydration. Hypertonic fluids act as an osmotic diuretic and can cause diuresis; when administered rapidly, speed shock can occur; and if extravasation occurs, necrotic tissue can result.
	Restore IV flow if stopped by opening flow clamp, milking the tubing, raising the height of IV bag, or repositioning the extremity.	If IV flow has stopped and does not start by opening clamp, milking tubing, raising the bag, or repositioning extremity, then the IV catheter should be removed. Irrigating IV catheters is prohibited in some institutions and should never be attempted with clotted lines. Forceful irrigation can dislodge clot(s) and cause the movement of an embolus to the lungs.
Position of IV Line	Position and tape IV tubing to prevent kinking.	Kinking of the tubing may cause the IV to be discontinued and to be restarted at a different site.
	Hang IV bag $21\frac{1}{2}$–3 feet above client's infusion site.	The higher the IV bag, the faster the gravity flow rate. If the IV bag is too low, IV fluids may stop due to an insufficient gravity pull.

● POSSIBLE COMPLICATIONS RESULTING FROM IV THERAPY

Numerous complications may result from the use of intravenous therapy. Infiltration, phlebitis, hematoma, and infections are common problems associated with IV infusions. Other serious problems include speed shock, air embolus, pulmonary embolus, and pulmonary edema. Speed shock occurs when drugs in solution are given too rapidly. It increases the drug concentration in the body and produces shocklike symptoms. An air embolus can be fatal when more than 50 ml of air is injected into the vein. Pulmonary embolus results when a thrombus in the peripheral veins becomes an embolus and travels to the lungs. This may occur when a clotted IV needle or catheter is irrigated forcefully, or when the lower extremities are used for administering IV fluids. Restlessness, chest pain, cough, dyspnea, and tachycardia are clinical signs and symptoms of a pulmonary embolus. Table 13-5 lists problems and complications that may occur from IV administration of fluids and medications.

Table 13-5	Possible Complications Resulting from IV Administration	
Complications	**Interventions**	**Rationale**
1. Infiltration	Observe insertion site for infiltration, i.e., swelling, coolness, and soreness.	Infiltration is accumulation of nonmedicated fluid in the subcutaneous tissue. When infiltration or extravasation occurs, the IV should be discontinued and restarted at a different site. Notify the health care provider if extravasation is observed.
2. Phlebitis	Observe insertion site for phlebitis, i.e., red, swollen, hard, painful, and warm to touch. Apply warm, moist heat to area as ordered.	Phlebitis is an inflammation of the vein that can be caused by irritating substances. Drugs and hyperosmolar solutions may cause phlebitis. Application of moist heat decreases inflammation.
		(continues)

Table 13-5	Possible Complications Resulting from IV Administration—*continued*	
Complications	**Interventions**	**Rationale**
3. Systemic infection	Observe for pyrogenic reactions (septicemia), i.e., chills, fever, headache, fast pulse rate. Check vital signs q4h for shocklike symptoms. Utilize aseptic technique when inserting IV catheters and changing IV tubing and IV bag.	Aseptic technique should be used at all times with IV therapy. Prevention of systemic infections is of primary importance.
4. Speed shock	Observe for signs and symptoms of speed shock, i.e., tachycardia, syncope, decreased blood pressure.	Speed shock occurs when solutions with potent drugs are given rapidly. High drug concentration accumulates rapidly in the body and can cause shocklike symptoms.
5. Air embolism	Remove air from tubing to prevent air embolism.	Air can be removed from tubing by (1) inserting a needle with syringe into side arm of tubing set and withdrawing the air and (2) using a pen or pencil on tubing, distal to the air, and rolling tubing until air is displaced into the drip chamber.
	Observe for signs and symptoms of air embolism. These include pallor, dyspnea, cough, syncope, tachycardia, decreased blood pressure.	Air embolism occurs when air inadvertently enters the vascular system. Injection of more than 50 ml of air can be fatal. It occurs more frequently in the central veins, and symptoms usually appear within 5 min.
	Immediately place client on left side in Trendelenburg position.	Air is trapped in the right atrium, which prevents it from going to the lungs.

(continues)

Table 13-5	Possible Complications Resulting from IV Administration—*continued*	
Complications	**Interventions**	**Rationale**
6. Pulmonary embolism	Report signs and symptoms of pulmonary embolism, i.e., restlessness, chest pain, cough, dyspnea, tachycardia.	Thrombus originating in the peripheral vein becomes an embolus and can lodge in a pulmonary vessel.
	Administer oxygen, analgesics, anticoagulants, and IV fluids as ordered.	Preventive measures should be taken, such as *never* forcefully irrigating an IV catheter to reestablish flow and avoiding the use of veins in the lower extremities.
7. Pulmonary edema	Auscultate lungs for crackles. Check neck veins for engorgement. Decrease IV flow rate.	IV fluids administered too rapidly or in large amounts can cause over-hydration. Excess fluids accumulate in the lungs.
8. "Runaway" IV fluids	Monitor IV fluid every hour even if on an electronic infusion pump (EIP).	Control clamp on IV tubing is opened.
	Check EIP flow rate and alarm set.	Alarm was not set properly on EIP.
9. Hematoma	Observe for hematoma with unsuccessful attempts to start IV therapy.	Hematoma (blood tumor) is a raised ecchymosed area.
	Apply ice pack immediately, then warm compresses after 1 hour.	Ice stops bleeding into tissue. Warm compresses cause vasodilation and improve blood flow and healing.
Additives to IV Fluids	Recognize the untoward reactions of drugs in IV fluids: potassium, Levophed, low-pH drugs, vitamins, antibiotics, antineoplastic drugs.	Potassium, antineoplastic drugs, and Levophed irritate the blood vessels and body tissue. Phlebitis is common with these drugs; and if infiltration occurs, sloughing of tissues may result. Vitamins and antibiotics should not be mixed together. They are incompatible. Always check

(continues)

Table 13-5	Possible Complications Resulting from IV Administration—*continued*	
Complications	**Interventions**	**Rationale**
		compatibility charts before adding medications to IV fluids.
	Stay with the client 10–15 min when the client is receiving drugs that are classified as a possible cause of anaphylaxis.	Allergic reactions often occur within the first 15 min when drugs are administered by IV.
	Inject drugs into IV container and invert several times before administering.	Equal drug distribution throughout the solution ensures proper dilution. *Do not* add drugs, i.e., potassium, into the IV bag while it is being administered unless the IV is temporarily stopped and the bag is inverted several times to promote equal distribution.
Intake and Output	Check urine output every 4–8 h. If a critically ill client is receiving potassium, urine output should be checked every hour.	If renal function is poor, overhydration can occur when excessive or continuous IV fluids are given. Potassium is excreted by the kidneys; thus, a decreased urine output can result in hyperkalemia.

● CLIENT MANAGEMENT

Assessment

● Check the prescribed IV solutions to ensure that the prescribed solutions are not all hypotonic or hypertonic. When 3000 ml of 5% dextrose in water is administered daily, this solution becomes hypotonic, and the dextrose is metabolized in the body, leaving water.

- Determine which IV tubing with drip chamber should be used. This is generally determined according to how long the IV fluids are to run. If the 1000 ml is to run 8 hours or more, the macrodrip chamber tubing should be selected.

- Select and observe infusion sites carefully. To reduce the risk of phlebitis and dislodged thrombus, the upper extremities are preferred infusion sites.

- Calculate flow rates and regulate the IV solutions. Patency of the IV system and regulation of the flow rate are essential.

- Assess for problems and complications of IV infusion.

Nursing Diagnoses

- *Excess Fluid Volume,* related to runaway IV or volume infusion too great for client's physical condition
- *Deficient Risk for Fluid Volume,* related to inadequate fluid intake
- *Risk for Infection,* related to contaminated IV fluid, contaminated equipment, or a break in aseptic technique
- *Deficient Knowledge,* related to a lack of familiarity with IV therapy or infusion devices

Interventions

- Monitor the rate of IV flow. Avoid fluid overload from IV solutions that run too fast. Pulmonary edema can result. IV solutions that run too slowly can cause an inadequate fluid intake.

- Monitor vital signs and chest sounds for signs of fluid overload; these include tachycardia, dyspnea, chest crackles, and vein engorgements.

- Use aseptic technique when inserting an infusion device, changing IV tubing, changing IV bags, and changing site dressings. A break in the system provides the potential for bacterial invasion.

- Change peripheral IV site, IV tubing, and dressing sites according to the agency's policy.

- Check frequently for fluid leaks from IV site and tubing, and for pain, redness, and swelling at the site.

- Monitor urine output. Decreased urinary output may be an indication of fluid overload or dehydration.

- Monitor laboratory results, particularly serum electrolytes, BUN, serum creatinine, hematocrit, and hemoglobin. These results can indicate overhydration, dehydration, and/or electrolyte imbalances.

Evaluation/Outcome

- Evaluate the effects of intravenous therapy to replace fluid and electrolyte losses, to meet concurrent fluid losses, and maintain fluid balance.

- Evaluate the tonicity of the prescribed daily IV fluids to avoid constant use of either hypotonic or hypertonic solutions.

- The client remains free of problems and complications, such as phlebitis, infiltration, fluid overload, air embolus, and pulmonary embolus, related to IV therapy.

CHAPTER 14

Total Parenteral Nutrition (TPN)

Sheila G. Cushing, MS, RN

INTRODUCTION

Total parenteral nutrition (TPN), sometimes referred to as hyperalimentation, is the infusion of amino acids, hypertonic glucose, fat emulsions, and additives such as vitamins, electrolytes, minerals, and trace elements. TPN can meet a client's total nutritional needs and is commonly used for clients whose caloric intake is insufficient. This method of nutrition is recommended for those who need nutritional support for a long period of time and cannot tolerate enteral feedings. Administering a high concentration of glucose solutions in peripheral veins can cause phlebitis at the infusion site; therefore, central vein administration is used for TPN. Central veins such as the right subclavian vein and the internal jugular vein can accommodate a high volume of hypertonic solutions because of their size and ability to dilute the infused fluid.

ETIOLOGY

Candidates for TPN include clients with severe burns who are in negative nitrogen balance; who cannot take enteral feedings; with severe debilitating diseases (cancer, AIDS); with gastrointestinal disorders such as ulcerative colitis, gastrointestinal fistulas, and other GI conditions in which the GI tract cannot consume enteral feedings.

For clients who are unable to tolerate oral or gastric feeding and suffer from severe malnutrition, TPN helps to restore a positive nitrogen balance. Following a major bowel resection, the absorptive area of the intestines is reduced; TPN aids in providing adequate nutrients. The benefit TPN provides clients with a gastrointestinal fistula is to allow the intestine to rest while providing nutrients. Table 14-1 lists indications for TPN.

Table 14-1	Indications for TPN (Hyperalimentation)
Indications	**Rationale**
Oral or nasogastric feedings are contraindicated or not tolerated	Long-term use of IV glucose solutions can cause protein wasting. TPN maintains a positive nitrogen balance.
Severe malnutrition	Malnutrition can cause severe protein loss and wasting syndrome. Negative nitrogen (protein) balance occurs. TPN restores positive nitrogen balance.
Malabsorption syndrome	The inability to absorb nutrients in the small intestine requires nutrients to be offered intravenously.
Dysphagia	Difficulty in masticating and swallowing due to pharyngeal radiation treatment prevents clients from breaking down food sufficiently for digestion.
Gastrointestinal fistula	Fistulas promote protein losses. TPN allows the intestine to rest and decreases gallbladder, pancreas, and small intestine secretions.
Major bowel resection and ulcerative colitis	These disorders reduce the absorptive area of the small intestine. TPN increases the intestine's ability to absorb nutrients more quickly than oral feedings and it permits the bowel to rest.
Extensive surgical trauma and stress	Extensive surgery requires 3500–5000 calories a day to maintain protein balance. TPN lowers the chance for infection and provides a positive nitrogen balance to aid in wound healing. TPN before surgery improves the nutritional status so that the client can withstand surgery and its stresses.
Extensive burns	Extensive burns require 7500–10,000 calories daily. TPN improves wound healing and formation of granulation tissue and promotes successful skin grafting.
Metastatic cancer or AIDS with anorexia and weight loss	Clients with wasting syndrome and debilitating diseases, such as cancer or AIDS, frequently are in negative nitrogen balance. TPN restores protein balance and tissue synthesis.

● TPN SOLUTIONS

The typical TPN solution for 1 L or 1000 ml contains 25% dextrose mixed in a commercially prepared protein (amino acid) source. Vitamins and electrolytes are added prior to administration. Electrolytes are frequently added immediately before the infusion according to the client's serum electrolyte levels. Frequently, the pharmacy department prepares these solutions using aseptic technique under a laminar airflow hood according to the prescribed order. Dextrose (glucose) is the choice carbohydrate for TPN because it can be metabolized by all tissues. The protein source for TPN is crystalline amino acids. Intravenous fat emulsions are added to the solution to increase the number of calories and prevent hyperglycemia or they may also be given through an extra line. Clients with diabetes mellitus may need a higher percentage of fat emulsion to prevent hyperglycemia. Standard TPN solutions contain dextrose, amino acids, sodium, potassium (added later), magnesium, calcium, chloride, phosphate, acetate, vitamins (added later), and trace elements. Other additives may be included according to individual needs.

Daily TPN solutions can be administered through a central venous access device such as a PICC line or a Hickman catheter as a continuous infusion or intermittent infusion that runs for approximately 12 hours. By having a 12-hour TPN infusion time, the client is free the remaining 12 hours for normal activities, such as work, school, or play. Today, many clients receive the 12-hour method of infusion in the home. A support system is usually available for client's needs and questions.

Usually 1 L of solution is ordered for the first 24 hours when initiating TPN therapy. This allows the pancreas to accommodate the increased glucose concentration of the solution. Additional daily increases of 500 to 1000 ml per day are ordered until the desired daily volume is reached. A usual maintenance volume of $2\frac{1}{2}$ to 3 liters of the hypertonic TPN solution is administered over 24 hours. A continuous infusion rate prevents fluctuations in blood glucose levels. If blood sugar levels are under control, a 12-hour TPN method may be used.

Generally medications are not administered in TPN solutions, but there are a few exceptions. For example, regular insulin can be added to TPN to control hyperglycemia.

Some medications are compatible with TPN and can be administered at the same site, but most often a multilumen central venous catheter or additional peripheral site is used if the client requires IV fluids, blood product, and/or IV medications.

● ELECTROLYTE AND GLUCOSE IMBALANCES ASSOCIATED WITH TPN

Because of high glucose concentration potassium shifts from the extracellular fluid sites to the cells (ICF). Increased potassium is needed in the TPN solutions, otherwise the client's potassium level begins to fall after 8–12 hours of TPN therapy. Hypokalemia may result from clients receiving insulin to manage hyperglycemia. Insulin moves potassium back into the cells. The client should generally receive 60 to 90 mEq of potassium per day in the TPN solutions (in some cases, more potassium per day is added to the solutions). Hyperkalemia may result from decreased renal function, systemic sepsis, or tissue necrosis. Serum potassium levels and urine output need to be closely monitored while the client is receiving potassium.

Hypophosphatemia (decreased serum phosphorus level) is a common problem associated with TPN. Increased glucose concentration in TPN solutions moves phosphate back into the cells. During TPN therapy, protein synthesis promotes the shift of phosphates back into the cells.

Hypomagnesemia does not occur as frequently as hypokalemia and hypophosphatemia; however, it can occur in clients who are severely malnourished, have excessive loss of intestinal secretions, have a long-term alcoholic problem, or are receiving daily magnesium-wasting diuretics.

Hyponatremia and hypocalcemia are not as common as hypokalemia and hypophosphatemia. A decreased serum sodium level may result from the Syndrome of Inappropriate Antidiuretic Hormone (SIADH) or from excessive fluid intake. Hypocalcemia usually results from a decrease in albumin levels associated with malnutrition. Hypercalcemia may occur during long-term TPN therapy. This results when calcium is lost from the bone. Table 14-2 lists the types of electrolyte and glucose imbalances, daily electrolyte requirements, and causes of the imbalance.

Table 14-2 Electrolyte and Glucose Imbalances Related to TPN

Imbalances	Suggested Replacement	Causes
Electrolytes		
Hypokalemia	60–90 mEq/d	High blood glucose levels Insulin
Hyperkalemia		Decreased renal function
		Systemic sepsis
		Tissue necrosis
Hypophosphatemia	15–45 mEq/d	High blood glucose levels
		Protein synthesis
Hypomagnesemia	4–40 mEq/d	Severe malnutrition
		Excessive loss of intestinal secretions
		Chronic alcohol problem
Hyponatremia	30–50 mEq/L	SIADH
		Excessive fluid intake
Hypocalcemia	5–10 mEq/L	Decreased albumin levels
		Malnourishment
Glucose		
Hyperglycemia	25% dextrose/L	Rapidly administered TPN solutions
		Stress
		Illness

Hyperglycemia is a problem related to the high glucose concentration of TPN solutions. Excess blood glucose levels occur more frequently during early TPN therapy. Other causes include rapidly infused glucose solutions, stress, and illness. TPN is primarily started with one liter of solution for the first day and then the volume of solution is increased to meet the client's nutritional needs.

● COMPLICATIONS RELATED TO TPN

Major complications that can result from TPN therapy are air embolus, phlebitis, thrombus, infection, hyperglycemia or hypoglycemia, and fluid overload. TPN is an excellent medium for the growth of organisms, bacteria, and yeast. Strict asepsis is necessary when IV tubing and dressings are changed. Most hospitals have a procedure for changing dressings in which strict aseptic technique, i.e., gloves, masks, and antibiotic ointment, are mandated.

When IV tubing is changed at the central venous catheter site, all lines must be clamped before they are disconnected to prevent air from entering the circulation. As a further safeguard the tubing is generally changed during the expiratory phase of the respiratory cycle. When changing the catheter, all clients with a central line should carry a readily available plastic clamp to prevent an air embolism in case there is inadvertent damage to the catheter. The client must lie flat and perform the Valsalva maneuver (take a breath, hold it, and bear down) to prevent air from being sucked into the circulation. The Valsalva maneuver increases intrathoracic pressure.

Increased blood glucose (hyperglycemia) occurs as a result of rapid infusion of the hypertonic dextrose solution used in TPN. An elevated blood glucose level may occur during early TPN until the pancreas adjusts to the hyperglycemic load. Regular insulin, either in the IV solution or by subcutaneous injection, may be required to prevent or control hyperglycemia. Other complications that can occur include hypoglycemia from abruptly discontinuing hyperosmolar dextrose solutions, fluid volume excess from the infusion of an excessive volume of fluid, or a fluid shift from intracellular to extracellular compartments. Table 14-3 lists the five major complications associated with TPN therapy (hyperalimentation), their related causes, symptoms, and corresponding interventions.

Hypertonic dextrose in a protein hydrolysate solution promotes yeast and bacteria growth. It has been reported that these organisms do not grow as rapidly in a crystalline amino acid solution as they do in protein hydrolysate solution. Many of the TPN solutions contain a crystalline amino acid solution, not a protein hydrolysate solution.

Table 14-3 Complications of TPN

Complications	Causes	Symptoms	Interventions
Air embolism	IV tubing disconnected Catheter not clamped Injection port fell off Improper changing of IV tubing Catheter damage (leak or tear)	Coughing Shortness of breath Chest pain Cyanosis	Clamp catheter Client must lie on left side with head down Check vital signs (VS) Notify health care provider
Infection	Poor aseptic technique when catheter inserted Contamination when changing tubing Contamination when solution mixed Contamination when dressing changed	Temperature above 100° (37.7°C) Pulse increased Chills Sweating Redness, swelling, drainage at insertion site Pain in neck, arm, or shoulder Lethargy Urine: glycosuria Bacteria Yeast growth	Notify health care provider Change dressing every 24–48 h according to agency policy Change solution every 24 h Change tubing every 24 h according to agency policy Check VS every 4 h
Hyperglycemia	Fluids rapidly infused Insufficient insulin coverage Infection	Nausea Weakness Thirst Headache Blood glucose elevated	Monitor blood glucose Notify health care provider Decrease infusion rate Regular insulin as required Monitor blood glucose every 4 h and prn

(continues)

Table 14-3 Complications of TPN—*continued*

Complications	Causes	Symptoms	Interventions
Hypoglycemia	Fluids abruptly discontinued Too much insulin infused	Nausea Pallor Cold, clammy Increased pulse rate Shaky feeling Headache Blurred vision	Notify health care provider Increase infusion rate with NO insulin, as per order or hospital policy *or* Orange juice with 2 teaspoons of sugar if client can tolerate fluids *or* Glucose IV, as per order or hospital policy *or* Glucagon, as per order or hospital policy
Fluid overload (hypervolemia)	Increased rate of IV infusions Fluid shift from cellular to vascular due to hyperosmolar solutions	Cough Dyspnea Neck vein engorgement Chest crackles Weight gain	Check VS every 4 h Weigh daily Monitor intake and output Check neck veins for engorgement Check chest sounds Monitor electrolytes Monitor BUN and creatinine

● CLIENT MANAGEMENT

Assessment

- Check TPN solutions, infusion site, and IV line. TPN lines are not to be interrupted except for lipids that may be piggybacked into the TPN line. It is highly recommended that flow rates be maintained by an electronic infusion pump (EIP).
- Check vital signs. Use vital signs measurements as a baseline for future comparison of vital signs.
- Check laboratory results, especially serum electrolyte and blood glucose levels. These values will be used for comparison with future laboratory results.
- Assess nutritional status, weight, energy level, and skin changes.

Nursing Diagnoses

- *Risk for Infection,* related to TPN therapy, concentrated glucose solutions, and invasive lines requiring dressing and tubing changes
- *Risk for Deficient Fluid Volume,* related to inadequate fluid intake and osmotic diuresis
- *Excess Fluid Volume,* related to excess fluid infusion or a health condition that is unable to tolerate a high concentration solution administered at an increased rate
- *Ineffective Breathing Pattern,* related to complications of central venous lines and fluid volume excess
- *Deficient Knowledge,* related to unfamiliarity with TPN therapy and procedures specific to IV therapy equipment

Interventions

- Change IV tubing according to agency policy (every 72 hours). To prevent an air embolus when changing the IV tubing always clamp the central venous line (use plastic or padded clamps only). If an air embolus is suspected, immediately place the client in a Trendelenburg position on his or her left side.

● Never use an existing TPN line for blood samples.

● Place prepared solutions not in use in the refrigerator (remove the solution 2 hours before hanging). TPN is usually started at 1000 ml for the first 24 hours and is increased at a rate of 500 to 1000 ml daily until the desired volume is reached. When discontinuing TPN, decrease the daily rate gradually over 12 to 72 hours according to the order.

● Change central venous line dressings according to hospital policy, usually every 24 to 72 hours using strict sterile technique.

● Monitor the central venous line infusion site for signs of infection or thrombus. Complaints of pain, numbness, or tingling in the fingers, neck, or arm on the same side as the catheter may indicate a thrombus formation. Elevated temperature and labored or rapid breathing, pain, redness, swelling, and drainage at the infusion site are indicators of infection and/or phlebitis.

● Check for signs of pulmonary edema such as dyspnea.

● Observe for signs and symptoms of reactions to lipid solutions; e.g., elevated temperature, flushing, sweating, pressure sensation over eyes, nausea or vomiting, headache, chest or back pain, and dyspnea.

Evaluation/Outcome

● Evaluate the effects of total parenteral nutrition on providing adequate or increased nutrition, i.e., weight increase, fluid and electrolyte balance, and osmolality levels within normal range.

● Client remains free of complications, i.e., infection, air embolism, pulmonary embolism, pulmonary edema.

● Maintain a support system.

FLUID, ELECTROLYTE, AND ACID-BASE IMBALANCES AND CLINICAL SITUATIONS

INTRODUCTION

In the clinical and chronic care settings, health professionals provide care for persons experiencing a variety of problems related to fluid, electrolyte, and acid-base imbalances. This unit addresses two developmental situations that focus on infants and children, and the older adult. The remaining six chapters focus on clinical problems and acute disorders related to trauma and shock, burns and burn shock, gastrointestinal surgical interventions, increased intracranial pressure, and chronic disorders related to cancer, heart failure, diabetic ketoacidosis, and chronic obstructive pulmonary disease. To assess clients' needs and provide the appropriate care needed for persons with selected health problems, the health professional must have a working knowledge and understanding of concepts related to fluid and electrolyte balance. Knowledge of these concepts allows the health professional to assess physiologic changes that occur with fluid, electrolyte, and acid-base imbalances and to plan appropriate interventions to assist clients as they adapt to these changes.

In each of these chapters, the pathophysiology (physiologic changes), etiology, clinical manifestations, clinical management, clinical considerations, and client management (assessment, diagnoses, interventions, and evaluations/outcome) are included. Clinical considerations summarize important facts related to the fluid, electrolyte, and acid-base problems for the specific health disorder. These considerations should be useful to health care providers when providing care for clients.

CHAPTER 15

Fluid Problems in Infants and Children

Gail Wade, RN, DNSc

INTRODUCTION

The health professional's understanding of the physiologic differences in infants and children that have implications for fluid and electrolyte balance is essential to providing optimal health care. Since these physiologic differences vary significantly throughout infancy and childhood, important regulatory factors must be viewed in terms of the maturity of the infant or child when addressing fluid balance problems that can be life-threatening in this vulnerable age group.

PATHOPHYSIOLOGY

Neonates, infants, and young children exhibit major physiologic differences from adults in their total body surface area, immature renal structures, endocrine system, and high rate of metabolism affecting hemostatic control. Each of these factors predisposes them to developmental variations in fluid and electrolyte balance. Water distribution in the newborn or infant is not the same as in an adult. Infants' proportionately higher ECF volume to ICF volume predisposes them to rapid fluid losses, increasing their vulnerability to dehydration. Table 15-1 compares the percent of an individual's fluid volume to body weight over the life span.

Table 15-1	Comparison of Fluid Volumes to Body Weight Over the Life Span		
	Low Birth Weight Infants	**Infants to 1 Year**	**Children Over 1 Year through Adulthood**
Total Fluid Volume to Body Weight	80–90%	70–80%	60%
ECF Volume		50%	20%

Table 15-2 outlines important physiologic differences in infants and children that predispose them to fluid balance problems. The combination of these differences stimulates the metabolic processes of infants and young children to respond to even small changes in fluid volume, resulting in electrolyte imbalances. Untreated imbalances may have major health consequences that are developmental in nature.

Table 15-2	Physiological Differences in Infants that Predispose Them to Fluid Imbalances
Developmental Physiologic Differences	**Pathophysiologic Implications**
1. Increased body surface area	Excess water loss via skin (the smaller the infant, the greater the loss)
2. Immature kidneys (can take up to 2 years for kidneys to mature)	Limited ability to retain water Increased water loss (limited ability to retain water)
3. Proportionately higher ratio of ECF volume (50%/wt. compared to 20% in adults)	Predisposes infant to rapid losses of fluid, resulting in dehydration
4. Higher metabolic rate	Predisposes infant to more rapid use of water
5. Immature endocrine system	Limits rapid response of appropriate regulatory system
6. Increased pH in newborns (lasts a few days to a few weeks or may persist in low birth weight infants)	Indicative of metabolic acidosis

As the child grows, fluid shifts from the ECF to the ICF compartment. At 1 year, the percentage of the child's total body water is similar to the percentage of the adult's (60%) total body water; however, the proportion of ECF and ICF is still different. Generally, serum electrolyte levels in infants and children are similar to adult levels.

ETIOLOGY

Infants' and children's increased risk for fluid balance problems is often complicated by their small size, the immaturity of various body regulatory systems, their overall health status, and the extent of their fluid reserve. A summary of the etiological factors associated with fluid balance problems in infants and children is listed in Table 15-3. The most common fluid balance problem in infants and children is dehydration (deficient fluid volume). Electrolyte imbalances are associated with fluid volume problems. Etiological factors associated with common fluid and electrolyte balance problems in infants and children are listed in Table 15-4.

Table 15-3	Common Etiological Factors Associated with Fluid Balance Problems in Infants and Children
Type of Problem	**Etiological Factors**
Dehydration (deficient fluid volume)	Diarrhea
	Vomiting
	Inadequate fluid intake
Overhydration (excess fluid volume)	Excessive insensible water loss
	Radiant warmers/phototherapy
	Intravenous overloading
	Large intake of fluids (especially in infants with underdeveloped thirst mechanism)
	Administration of inappropriately prepared formulas
	Tap-water enemas
	Rapid reduction of glucose levels in diabetic ketoacidosis

Table 15-4	Common Electrolyte Balance Problems with Related Etiological Factors
Problems	**Etiological Factors**
Hyponatremia (sodium depletion)	Vomiting/diarrhea Overhydration with 5% dextrose in water (D_5W) Diuretics Low sodium intake Excessive insensible water loss Water intoxication related to excessive intake of electrolyte-free solutions (tap water) Irrigation of body cavities with water Disease states (nephrotic syndrome, HF, acute renal failure, cirrhosis, burns, SIADH)
Hypernatremia (sodium excess)	Vomiting/diarrhea High salt intake (oral or intravenous) High solute intake without water replacement (tube feedings) Excessive insensible water loss Disease states (diabetes insipidus, nephropathy)
Hypokalemia (potassium depletion)	Vomiting/diarrhea Laxative and enema abuse Medications (steriods, antibiotics, diuretics) High carbohydrate intake Disease states (diabetic ketoacidosis, Cushing's syndrome, anorexia nervosa)
Hyperkalemia (potassium excess)	Intravenous potassium overload Blood transfusions with aged blood Medications (potassium-sparing diuretics, chemotherapy) Disease states (renal failure, hypoaldosteronism, metabolic acidosis, crush injuries, burns, sickle cell crisis)
Hypocalcemia (calcium depletion)	Inadequate diet (deficient in vitamin D and calcium) Cow's milk formula Medications (diuretics, anticonvulsants, antacids, laxatives, phosphate-containing preparations, antineoplastics) Disease states (renal insufficiency, hypoparthyroidism, alkalosis, pancreatitis, GI disorders)

(continues)

Table 15-4	Common Electrolyte Balance Problems with Related Etiological Factors—*continued*
Problems	**Etiological Factors**
Hypercalcemia (Calcium excess)	Prolonged immobilization Excessive IV or oral intake Medications (vitamin D intoxication, diuretics-thiazides) Disease states associated with bone catabolism (hyperparathyroidism, hyperthyroidism, leukemia and other malignancies, kidney disease)

● CLINICAL MANIFESTATIONS

Signs and symptoms of fluid imbalance vary with the infant's or child's level of maturity, state of hydration, and the source of the problem.

Fluid intoxication from overhydration occurs when excessive fluid ingestion results in low serum sodium levels and central nervous system irritation. Infants are especially vulnerable since their thirst mechanism and kidneys are not well-developed. The typical signs, symptoms, and laboratory findings in overhydration are displayed in Table 15-5.

Dehydration is the most common type of fluid balance problem in infants and children. It occurs when the total amount of fluid output exceeds the total fluid intake. Dehydration associated with diarrhea is the number one cause of fluid and electrolyte imbalance in infants and children. When vomiting occurs with diarrhea, fluid and electrolyte losses are more severe.

Losses in body weight can be used to determine the degree of body fluid loss. For every 1% of weight loss, 10 ml/kg of body fluid is lost. Dehydration is classified as mild, moderate, or severe based on body loss measurements. Table 15-6 provides guidelines to assess the degree of dehydration in infants and children. Table 15-7 outlines the types, clinical manifestations, and suggested interventions for dehydration.

Table 15-5	Overhydration: Possible Signs, Symptoms, and Laboratory Findings	
Signs and Symptoms		**Laboratory Findings**
Rapid weight gain (> 10% of body weight) Generalized edema Adventitious lung sounds Slow, bounding pulse CNS disturbances (irritability, headache, seizures, lethargy) Blurring of vision Nausea and vomiting Cramps and muscle twitching		Low urine specific gravity Decreased levels of serum electrolytes Decreased hematocrit

Table 15-6	Clinical Assessment of Degree of Dehydration in Infants and Children		
% Deyhydration (ml/kg body weight)			
	Infants	**Children**	**Clinical Assessment**
Mild	5% (50 ml/kg)	3% (30 ml/kg)	Thirst Slightly dry mucous membranes Decreased skin elasticity Skin color pale Tears present Fontanel flat Heart rate normal to slightly increased Urine output normal to slightly decreased Alert, restless

(continues)

Table 15-6	Clinical Assessment of Degree of Dehydration in Infants and Children—*continued*		
% Deyhydration (ml/kg body weight)			
	Infants	**Children**	**Clinical Assessment**
Moderate	10% (100 ml/kg)	60% (60 ml/kg)	Increased severity of symptoms Skin and mucous membranes dry Tenting Capillary filling 2–3 seconds Skin color gray Tears reduced Fontanel soft and depressed Deep set eyes Heart rate increased Urine output decreased
Severe	15% (150 ml/kg)	9% (90 ml/kg)	Restless to lethargic Marked severity of symptoms Skin clammy Mucous membranes parched/cracked Skin turgor absent Capillary filling > 3 seconds Skin color mottled Tears absent Fontanel and eyes sunken Heart rate significantly increased Urine output low Lethargic to comatose

Source: Adapted from *The Harriet Lane Handbook: A Manual for Pediatric House Officers* (15th ed., p. 231). St. Louis: Mosby, 2000.

Table 15-7	Types of Dehydration: Isonatremic, Hypernatremic, and Hyponatremic				
Types of Dehydration	**Water and Sodium Loss**	**Serum Sodium Level**	**ECF and ICF Loss**	**Causes**	**Symptoms**	**Treatment**
Isonatremic dehydration (iso-osmolar or isotonic dehydration)	Proportionately equal loss of water and sodium	130–150 mEq/L	Extracellular fluid volume is markedly decreased (severe hypovolemia). Since sodium and water loss are approximately the same, there is no osmotic pull from ICF to ECF. The plasma volume is significantly reduced and shock occurs from decreased circulating blood volume. ICF volume remains virtually constant.	Diarrhea, vomiting, and malnutrition (decreases in fluid and food intake) are the most common causes.	With severe fluid loss, symptoms are characteristic of hypovolemic shock: rapid pulse rate, rapid respiration; later, a decreasing systolic blood pressure. Other symptoms are weight loss, irritability, lethargy, pale or gray skin color, dry mucous membranes, reduced skin turgor, sunken eyeballs, sunken fontanels, absence of tearing and salivation, and decreased urine output.	Fluid should be restored rapidly to correct hypovolemic shock. Iso-osmolar solutions, i.e., Ringer's lactate and 5% dextrose in 0.2% NaCl or 0.3% NaCl, are some of the choices. Replacement should be calculated over 24 h; if dehydration is severe, half of the amount of solution should be given the first 8 h and the remaining half over the next 16 h.

(continues)

Table 15-7 | **Types of Dehydration: Isonatremic, Hypernatremic, and Hyponatremic—*continued***

Types of Dehydration	Water and Sodium Loss	Serum Sodium Level	ECF and ICF Loss	Causes	Symptoms	Treatment
Hypernatremic dehydration (hyperosmolar or hypertonic dehydration) (second leading type of dehydration in children)	Water loss is greater than sodium loss; sodium excess	↑ 150 mEq/L	ECF and ICF volumes are both decreased. Increased ECF osmolality (solutes) results in a shift of fluid from the ICF to the ECF, causing severe cellular dehydration. ECF depletion may not be as severe as ICF depletion. Loss of hypo-osmolar fluid raises the osmolality of ECF.	Severe diarrhea (water is lost in excess to solutes) and high solute intake with decreased water intake are the two most common causes. Others include fever, poor renal function, rapid breathing, or any combination of these conditions.	Shock is less apparent since ECF loss is not as severe. Symptoms include weight loss, avid thirst, confusion, convulsions, tremors, thickened and firm skin turgor, sunken eyeballs and fontanels, absence of tearing, moderately rapid pulse, moderately rapid respirations, frequently normal blood pressure, normal to decreased urine output, and intracranial hemorrhage.	The goal is to increase the ICF and ECF volumes without causing water intoxication. Giving excessive hypo-osmolar solutions or only 5% dextrose in water dilutes ECF, causing water to shift to the ICF and water intoxication (ICF volume excess) to occur. A gradual reduction over 48 h of solution is safest. Dextrose 5% with 0.2% NaCl may be ordered, and later, lactated Ringer's solution. With normal urinary flow, potassium can be added to the solution (2–3 mEq/kg).

| Hyponatremic dehydration (hypo-osmolar or hypotonic dehydration) | Sodium loss is greater than water loss; excess water | ↓ 130 mEq/L | ECF is severely decreased, and ICF is increased. The osmolality of ECF is lower than the osmolality of ICF. Water shifts from the ECF to the ICF (lesser to the greater concentration). The cerebral cells are frequently affected first as the excess water interferes with brain cell activity. | Severe diarrhea (sodium is lost in excess of water), excessive water intake, electrolyte-free fluid infusions (5% dextrose in water), sodium-losing nephropathy, and diuretic therapy. | Thirst, weight loss, lethargy, comatose, poor skin turgor, clammy skin, sunken and soft eyeballs, absence of tearing, shock symptoms (rapid pulse rate, rapid respirations, and low systolic blood pressure), and decreased urine output. | Ringer's lactate or 5% dextrose in 0.45% NaCl (1/2 NSS) can help to correct the serum sodium level (125–135 mEq/L). For serum sodium of 115 mEq/L, normal saline can be used. When the serum sodium is less than 115, 3% saline may be indicated. Rapid fluid correction with electrolytes can cause an excessive shift of cellular fluid into the plasma. The result can be overhydration and heart failure. |

● CLINICAL MANAGEMENT

Regardless of the type of fluid volume problem, immediate treatment of infants and children is needed to prevent hypovolemic shock and serious complications such as central nervous system disturbances. Oral rehydration is the treatment of choice for children with mild to moderate dehydration.

For mild dehydration, parents should be urged to give the child any kind of oral fluid that the child tolerates and to continue feedings as tolerated. Formula can be given to infants. If these approaches are unsuccessful, then oral electrolyte solutions should be given.

Table 15-8 contains a list of oral electrolyte solutions that are used for rehydration and maintenance. Generic brands are also available. When purchasing generic brands, however, it is important to select the appropriate solution for the type of rehydration or maintenance therapy needed.

Once rehydration is accomplished, the child should be encouraged to resume a normal diet. Some physicians prescribe diluted or lactose-free formulas for infants while others believe full-strength formula can be given. Feedings for breast-fed infants may be supplemented with an electrolyte solution (usually 100 ml/kg is recommended). Any ongoing losses (through stool or emesis) should also be replaced. For each loss through diarrhea stools, 10 ml/kg of the child's body weight should be replaced with an electrolyte solution.

With the resumption of a normal diet, physicians may prescribe 100 ml/kg of an oral electrolyte solution to sup-

Table 15-8 Oral Electrolyte Solution					
Product	**Na (mEq/L)**	**K (mEq/L)**	**Cl (mEq/L)**	**Base (mEq/L)**	**Glucose (g/L)**
Infalyte	50	25	45	30	30
Naturalyte	45	20	35	48	25
Pedialyte	45	20	35	30	25
Cerealyte	70	20	60	30	4.0
Rehydralyte	75	20	65	30	25
ORS (WHO)	90	20	80	30	20

Source: Adapted from J. Snyder (1994). *Seminars in Pediatric Infectious Disease* (Vol. 5, p. 231)

plement the diet. Diets that are low in simple carbohydrates and contain easily digestible foods such as cereal, yogurt, cooked vegetables, and soups can be given to older children. Toddlers may tolerate soft or pureed foods. The BRAT diet (bananas, rice, apples, and toast or tea) is no longer recommended because of its limited nutritional value and high carbohydrate, low electrolyte composition. Foods to avoid are fried foods, soda, and jello water.

Oral rehydration therapy is replaced with parenteral therapy in infants and children with severe vomiting, gastric distention, and severe dehydration. Emergency treatment of unstable children with severe dehydration is needed to prevent or correct hypovolemic shock. In emergency situations, fluids should be restored rapidly.

Careful consideration of the parameters for rehydrating children is essential. Overhydration can lead to cerebral edema with neurological symptoms such as seizures. Initial expansion of ECF volume is usually accomplished with a bolus of an isotonic solution such as 0.9% sodium chloride or lactated Ringer's solution. Recommended amount is 20 to 30 ml/kg. The bolus may be repeated if needed.

Initial expansion is to prevent shock by improving circulatory and renal function. Requirements for continued rehydration vary with the child's clinical status and the nature of the electrolyte imbalance. The amount of fluid replaced is based on the calculated loss as well as the fluid maintenance requirements.

The type of intravenous fluid administered is determined by the type of dehydration. For isonatremic dehydration, fluids are usually replaced and maintained with a solution of either Ringer's lactate or 5% dextrose in 0.2% or 0.3% NaCl. The concentration of NaCl for treatment of hyponatremic dehydration is dependent on the serum sodium level. Ringer's lactate or a 5% dextrose solution with 0.45% NaCl is often effective in treating small sodium deficits. Deficits between 115 mEq/L and 125 mEq/L may be treated with normal saline. Severe sodium deficits may require a 3% saline solution.

Assessment and treatment of hypernatremic dehydration is complicated because fluid shifts between the intracellular and extracellular space to preserve the circulating volume. Therefore, the potential of overhydrating the child and causing water intoxication is present. Generally a hypotonic solution (5% dextrose in 0.2% NaCl) is used to correct the osmolality. Isotonic fluids (Ringer's lactate) may be used to correct the fluid volume problem. Serum sodium correction in hypernatremia should not occur any more rapidly than 0.5–1.0 mEq/L/h. To ensure that serum sodium levels do not decrease too rapidly, levels should be monitored every 2 to 4 hours and the fluid level adjusted accordingly. The goal for correcting hypernatremic dehydration is to prevent water intoxication.

Infants and children are maintained on intravenous fluid only until their condition has stablized. Once the fluid and electrolyte imbalances have stabilized, oral rehydration should be initiated.

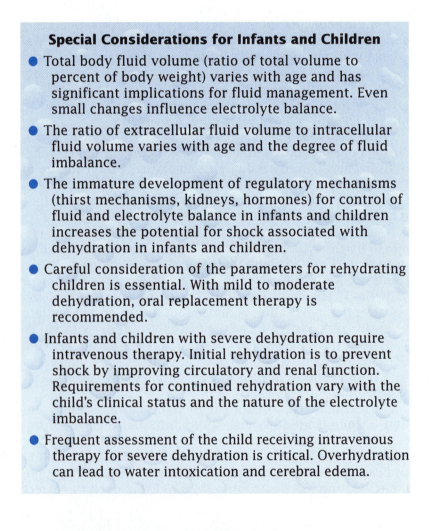

Special Considerations for Infants and Children

● Total body fluid volume (ratio of total volume to percent of body weight) varies with age and has significant implications for fluid management. Even small changes influence electrolyte balance.

● The ratio of extracellular fluid volume to intracellular fluid volume varies with age and the degree of fluid imbalance.

● The immature development of regulatory mechanisms (thirst mechanisms, kidneys, hormones) for control of fluid and electrolyte balance in infants and children increases the potential for shock associated with dehydration in infants and children.

● Careful consideration of the parameters for rehydrating children is essential. With mild to moderate dehydration, oral replacement therapy is recommended.

● Infants and children with severe dehydration require intravenous therapy. Initial rehydration is to prevent shock by improving circulatory and renal function. Requirements for continued rehydration vary with the child's clinical status and the nature of the electrolyte imbalance.

● Frequent assessment of the child receiving intravenous therapy for severe dehydration is critical. Overhydration can lead to water intoxication and cerebral edema.

● CLIENT MANAGEMENT

Assessment

● Complete a health history of the current problem.

● Complete a head-to-toe assessment of the infant or child to compare your findings with those of the health history and note symptoms of fluid overload or deficit. Refer to Table 15-9 for a complete head-to-toe assessment outline.

● Identify potential health problems related to factors associated with fluid and electrolyte balance, such as changes in weight, eating/drinking patterns, urine output, insensible perspiration, respiratory rate, vomiting, diarrhea, irritability, listlessness, skin (turgor, color, temperature), membranes, eyes, tears, fontanels, vital signs, neurological signs, neurovascular measurements, and stool frequency/consistency.

● Review studies (electrolytes, hemoglobin/hematocrit, urine specific gravity) to determine fluid and electrolyte balance problems.

● Obtain a baseline of vital signs, weight, and so on for comparison with future measurements.

Nursing Diagnoses

● *Deficient Fluid Volume,* related to decreased fluid reserve or excessive vomiting and diarrhea

● *Excess Fluid Volume,* related to inadequate fluid excretion and/or alternative fluid volume regulation

● *Imbalanced Nutrition, less than body requirements,* related to starvation, diabetic ketoacidosis

● *Deficient Knowledge (parents),* related to the fluid needs of infants and children

Interventions

Deficient Fluid Volume

● Monitor lab values (creatinine ratio, electrolyte, hemoglobin, hematocrit, urine specific gravity).

Table 15-9	Head-to-Toe Assessment of Fluid and Electrolyte Imbalance in Infants and Children	
Observation	**Assessment**	**Rationale**
Behavior and Appearance	Irritable/restless Anorexia Purposeless movement Unusual cry Lethargic Lethargy with hyperirritability on stimulation Unresponsive (comatose)	Early symptoms of fluid volume deficit are irritability, purposeless movements, and an unusual or high-pitched cry in infants. Young children may experience thirst with restlessness. As dehydration continues, lethargy and unconsciousness may occur.
Skin	Color ____ Temperature ____ Feel ____ Turgor ____	Skin color may be pale (mild), gray (moderate), or mottled (severe) depending on the degree of dehydration. Temperature is usually cold except with hypertonic dehydration where the temperature may be hot or cold. Skin feels dry with isotonic dehydration; clammy with hypotonic dehydration; and thickened and doughy with hypertonic dehydration. Turgor is measured by pinching the skin on the abdomen, chest wall, or medial aspect of the thigh and assessing the rate of skin retraction (elasticity). As dehydration progresses, elasticity decreases from fair to very poor. With hypertonic dehydration, turgor may remain fair. Skin turgor of obese infants or children may appear normal even with a deficit. Undernourishment can cause poor tissue turgor with fluid balance.
Mucous Membranes	Dryness in oral cavity (cheeks and gums) ____ Dry tongue with longitudinal wrinkles ____	The mucous membranes and tongue are dry with a fluid deficit. Sodium deficit causes the tongue to appear sticky, rough, and red. A dry tongue may also indicate mouth breathing. Some medications and vitamin deficiencies cause dryness of mucous membranes. Dryness in the oral cavity membranes (cheeks and gums) is a better indicator of fluid loss.

(continues)

Table 15-9	Head-to-Toe Assessment of Fluid and Electrolyte Imbalance in Infants and Children—*continued*	
Observation	**Assessment**	**Rationale**
	Thirst Mild ____ Avid ____	Thirst is an indicator of dehydration (fluid loss). Thirst may be difficult to determine when vomiting is present. Avid thirst may indicate serum hyperosmolality and cellular dehydration.
Eyes	Sunken ____ Tears ____ Soft eyeballs ____	Sunken eyes and dark skin around them may indicate a severe fluid volume deficit. Tears are absent with moderate to severe dehydration. (Tearing is not present until approximately 4 months of age.) Soft eyeballs may indicate isonatremic or hyponatremic dehydration.
Fontanel	Sunken ____ Bulging ____	Depression of the anterior fontanel is often an indicator of fluid volume deficit. A fluid excess results in bulging fontanel.
Vital Signs Temperature	Admission Temperature ____ Time ____ (1) ____ Time ____ (2) ____	Body temperature can be subnormal or elevated. Fever increases insensible water loss. The child's extremities may feel cold because of hypovolemia (fluid volume deficit), which decreases peripheral circulation. A subnormal temperature may be due to reduced energy output.
Pulse	Admission pulse ____ Pulse rate Time ____ (1) ____ Time ____ (2) ____ Pattern____	A weak and rapid pulse rate (over 160 for infant and over 120 for child) may indicate a fluid volume deficit (hypovolemia) and the possibility of shock. A full, bounding, not easily obliterated pulse may indicate a fluid volume excess. An irregular pulse can be due to hypokalemia. A weak, irregular, rapid pulse may indicate hypokalemia, while a weak, slow pulse may indicate hypernatremia.
Respiration	Admission rate ____ Respiration Time ____ (1) ____ Time ____ (2) ____	Note the rate depth and pattern of the infant's breathing. Dyspnea and moist crackles usually indicate fluid volume excess. Rapid breathing increases insensible fluid loss from the lungs. Rapid, deep, vigorous breathing (Kussmaul breathing) frequently

(continues)

Table 15-9	Head-to-Toe Assessment of Fluid and Electrolyte Imbalance in Infants and Children—*continued*

Observation	Assessment	Rationale
	Pattern _____	indicates metabolic acidosis. Acidosis can be due to poor hydrogen excretion by the kidneys, diarrhea, salicylate poisoning, or diabetes mellitus. Shallow, irregular breathing can be due to respiratory alkalosis.
Blood Pressure	Admission BP _____ Blood pressure Time _____ (1) _____ Time _____ (2) _____	Elasticity of young blood vessels may keep blood pressure stable even when a fluid volume deficit is present. Increased blood pressure may indicate fluid volume excess. Decreased blood pressure may indicate severe fluid volume deficit, extracellular shift from the plasma to the interstitial space, or sodium deficit.
Neurological Signs	Abdominal distention _____ Diminished reflexes (hypotonia) _____ Weakness/ paralysis _____ Tetany tremors (hypertonia) _____ Twitching, cramps _____ Sensorium Confusion _____ Comatose _____ Other _____	Abdominal distention and weakness may indicate a potassium deficit. Tetany symptoms can indicate a calcium and/or magnesium deficit. Serum calcium deficits occur easily in children, since their bones do not readily replace calcium to the blood. Confusion can be due to a potassium deficit and/or fluid volume imbalance.
Neurovascular Signs	Capillary filling time _____	A measure of systemic perfusion. Moderate to severe dehydration is often accompanied by delayed capillary filling time of > 2–3 seconds.
Weight	Preillness weight _____ Current weight _____	Weight loss can indicate the degree of dehydration (fluid loss): *Mild*—2–5% in infants and young children *Moderate*—5–10% in infants and young children; 3–6% in older children *Severe*—10–15% in infants and young children; 6–9% in older children Fluid loss can also be estimated by

(continues)

Table 15-9	Head-to-Toe Assessment of Fluid and Electrolyte Imbalance in Infants and Children—*continued*	
Observation	**Assessment**	**Rationale**
		considering that 1 g of weight loss equals 1 mL of fluid loss. Edema and ascites can occur with fluid imbalances. Fluid overloads can result in hepatomegaly (enlarged liver). Weights should be taken on the same scale, at the same time each day, and with the same covering.
Urine	Number of voidings in 8 h _____ Amt ml/8 h _____ Amt ml/h _____ Urine color _____ Specific gravity _____ Urine pH _____	Accurate measurements of intake and output from all sources is essential. Normal output ranges are: Infants: 2–3 ml/kg/h Young children: 2 ml/kg/h Older children: 1–2 ml/kg/h By subtracting the weight of a saturated urine diaper from a dry diaper, output in infants and toddlers can be determined (1 g wet diaper = 1 ml urine). Because of evaporative losses, diapers must be weighed within 30 min of the void to be accurate. Specific gravity can be obtained by refractometer or dipstick. Accurate assessment can be made within 2 h of the void. Oliguria (decrease in urine output) with very concentrated urine (dark yellow color) and increased specific gravity (>1.020 for infants and 1.030 for children) can indicate a moderate to severe fluid volume deficit, plasma to interstitial fluid shift, sodium deficit or severe sodium excess, potassium excess, or renal insufficiency. An elevated specific gravity is also indicative of glycosuria and proteinuria. With severe fluid deficit the infant may not void for 16–24 h and not show evidence of abdominal distention. Polyuria (increased urine output) with low specific gravity (<1.010) can indicate fluid excess, renal disease, a sodium deficit, or extracellular shift from interstitial fluid to plasma or decreased

(continues)

Table 15-9	Head-to-Toe Assessment of Fluid and Electrolyte Imbalance in Infants and Children—*continued*

Observation	Assessment	Rationale
		antidiuretic hormone (ADH). An acidic pH may indicate metabolic or respiratory acidosis, alkalosis with severe potassium deficit, or a fluid deficit. Alkaline urine may result from metabolic or respiratory alkalosis, hyperaldosteronism, acidosis with chronic kidney infection and tubular dysfunction, or diuretic therapy.
Stools	Number ＿＿＿＿ Consistency＿＿＿＿ Color ＿＿＿＿ Amount ＿＿＿＿	The consistency, color, and amount of each stool should be noted. If the stool is liquid, it should be measured. Frequent liquid stools can lead to fluid volume deficit, potassium and sodium deficit, and bicarbonate deficit (acidosis).
Vomitus	Number ＿＿＿＿ Consistency＿＿＿＿ Color ＿＿＿＿ Amount ＿＿＿＿	Vomitus needs to be described according to consistency, color, and amount. Frequent vomiting of large quantity leads to fluid loss, potassium and sodium loss, as well as hydrogen and chloride loss (alkalosis).
Other Fluid Loss	GI suction ＿＿Amount ＿＿＿＿ Drainage tube ＿＿Amount ＿＿＿＿ Fistula ＿＿Color ＿＿＿＿ ＿＿Amount ＿＿＿＿ Other ＿＿Amount ＿＿＿＿	Fluid loss from all sources should be measured. Fluid loss from GI suctioning, drainage tubes, and fistula can contribute to severe fluid and electrolyte imbalance.
Blood Chemistry and Hematology	Electrolytes Time ＿＿ Time ＿＿ K ＿＿ ＿＿ Na ＿＿ ＿＿ Cl ＿＿ ＿＿ Ca ＿＿ ＿＿ Mg ＿＿ ＿＿ BUN ＿＿ ＿＿ Creatinine ＿＿ ＿＿ ＿＿ Hgb ＿＿ ＿＿ Hct ＿＿ ＿＿	One set of blood chemistry is not sufficient for assessment. Electrolytes should be frequently monitored when they are not in normal range. Norms are: K: ＿＿Newborn 3.0–6.0 mEq/L ＿＿Infant & older 3.5–5.0 mEq/L Na: ＿＿Newborn 136–146 mEq/L ＿＿Infant 139–146 mEq/L ＿＿Child 135–148 mEq/L

(continues)

Table 15-9	Head-to-Toe Assessment of Fluid and Electrolyte Imbalance in Infants and Children—*continued*	
Observation	**Assessment**	**Rationale**
		Cl:
		Newborn 97–110 mEq/L
		Child 98–111 mEq/L
		Ca:
		Newborn 7–12 mg/dL
		Child 8–10.8 mg/dL
		Mg:
		All ages 1.3–2.0 mEq/L
		BUN:
		Newborn 4–18 mg/dL
		Child 5–18 mg/dL
		Creatinine:
		Newborn 0.3–1.0 mg/dL
		Infant 0.2–0.4 mg/dL
		Child 0.3–0.7 mg/dL
		Hgb:
		Newborn 14.5–22.5 g/dL
		Infant 9–14 g/dL
		Child 11.5–15.5 g/dL
		Hct:
		Newborn 44–72%
		Infant 28–42%
		Child 35–45%
		An elevated BUN can indicate fluid volume deficit or kidney insufficiency. Elevated creatinine frequently indicates kidney damage. Elevated hemoglobin and hematocrit may indicate hemoconcentration caused by fluid volume deficit. If anemia is present, the hemoglobin and hematocrit may appear falsely normal.

	Blood gases
	  pH _____
	  $PaCO_2$ _____
	  PaO_2 _____
	  HCO_3 _____
	  BE _____
		After the first day of life, normal range for pH is 7.35–7.45. A pH of 7.35 or less indicates acidosis. A pH of 7.45 or higher indicates alkalosis.
		Newborns and infants have $PaCO_2$ levels that range between 27 and 41 mm Hg. After infancy, $PaCO_2$ levels range from 35 to 48 mm Hg in males and from 32 to 45 mm Hg in females. Lower values indicate respiratory alkalosis or compensation (overbreathing, hyperventilating).

(continues)

	Head-to-Toe Assessment of Fluid and Electrolyte Imbalance in Infants and Children—*continued*
Table 15-9	

Observation	Assessment	Rationale
		Higher values mean respiratory acidosis.
		Normal range for HCO_3 in all ages is 21–28 mEq/L. BE (base excess) varies with age.
		Normal BE ranges are:
		Newborn $(-10)-(-2)$ mEq/L
		Infant $(-7)-(-1)$ mEq/L
		Child $(-4)-(+2)$ mEq/L
		HCO_3 below 21 and BE less than the normal value for age indicates metabolic alkalosis.
		HCO_3 above 28 and BE higher than the normal value for age indicates metabolic acidosis.

● Closely monitor for changes in general appearance, behaviors, and neurologic status.

● Monitor weight daily.

● Monitor vital signs in accordance with severity of health problems.

● Integrate observations to determine the type and degree (mild, moderate, severe) of dehydration.

● Monitor effects of fluid replacement on behavior and laboratory findings.

● Monitor balance in intake and output.

Excess Fluid Volume

● Attempt to identify the source of the fluid overload.

● Closely monitor intake and output for imbalance.

● Monitor laboratory values (electrolytes, hemoglobin, hematocrit, urine specific gravity, and creatinine ratio), and report even small changes.

● Monitor vital signs in accordance with severity of the imbalance.

- Monitor weight daily.
- Observe closely for CNS signs and symptoms that may result in seizures or coma.
- Monitor extremities, face, perineum, and torso for signs of edema.
- Provide a quiet, controlled environment.
- Record and report even small changes in findings.

Imbalanced Nutrition: Less Than Body Requirements

- Ask the parent or child to identify the child's food preferences. Whenever possible, these preferences should be respected.
- Diets that are low in simple carbohydrates and contain easily digestible foods such as cereal, yogurt, cooked vegetables, and soups are appropriate for older children. Toddlers may tolerate soft or pureed foods. The BRAT (bananas, rice, apples, and toast or tea) diet is no longer recommended because it is high in carbohydrates and low in electrolytes. Parents should also be advised to avoid giving their child fried foods, soda, or jello water.
- For mild dehydration, urge parents to give any kind of fluid that the child will tolerate and continue normal feeding. Formula can be given to the infant.
- Advise parents that ½ strength juices are a better choice than colas if the child is anorexic. Colas are high in glucose, potentially increasing serum osmolality.
- If the dehydration progresses and the child does not tolerate fluids, parents should be told to give an appropriate oral rehydration solution. Rehydration therapy for mild dehydration is 50 ml/kg given over 4 hours. For moderate dehydration, 100 ml/kg should be given over 4 hours. The solution can be given via an oral syringe or a teaspoon.
- Once the child's condition has stabilized and the child is interested in eating, advise the parents to provide foods that are low in simple carbohydrates and easily digestible. In the early stages of recovery, an oral rehydration solution may be prescribed.

Deficient Knowledge (Parents)

● Assess the parents' knowledge level about their child's condition.

● Encourage parents to continue using approaches that are successful.

● Answer parents' questions as necessary.

● Provide needed information about the child's condition and the treatment plan.

● Provide support and encouragement to the parents.

Evaluation/Outcome

● Evaluate that the cause of the fluid volume problem has been eliminated or controlled (disease state identified, vomiting and/or diarrhea controlled, hemorrhage) and the electrolyte imbalance and/or fluid intake has been adjusted appropriately.

● Evaluate the effectiveness of interventions through selected electrolyte studies (Na, Cl, K, Ca) to verify that they have returned to normal range.

● Document daily weight (in kilograms for infants and young children) for return to stable baseline weight (consult parents if necessary).

● Assess general appearance for a decrease in signs and symptoms of fluid imbalance (lethargy, hyperirritability, sunken or bulging fontanels in infants, edema, weak/shrill cry, limited tears, seizures, and so on).

● Assess hydration status (return of moist, pink mucous membranes, good skin turgor, and so on) of infant or child.

● Monitor fluid balance through intake and output measures.

● Document parental understanding of teaching related to the signs and symptoms of dehydration in children.

● Evaluate whether the child's nutritional status has returned to the preillness state.

Older Adults with Fluid and Electrolyte Imbalances

Ingrid Aboff, MSN RN

🔵 INTRODUCTION

The health professional's understanding of the normal age-related physiological changes of older adults is essential to providing optimal health care for this rapidly growing sector of the population. These age-related changes are often compounded by chronic health problems, thus, the older adult is more vulnerable to life-threatening complications from fluid and electrolyte imbalances. Health interventions must include careful attention to these imbalances.

🔵 PATHOPHYSIOLOGY

During the normal aging process the pulmonary, renal, cardiac, gastrointestinal, and integumentary systems undergo structural changes that will ultimately decrease their functional efficiency. While these changes do not intrinsically imply that a body system is impaired, it does explain why, in older adults, the ability to compensate for fluid and electrolyte imbalances may be decreased. In addition, risk factors such as chronic diseases increase the debilitating effects of normal functional changes in all of the body's systems and further inhibit the older adult's ability to maintain fluid and electrolyte balance.

Assessments provide information about age-related changes and factors that may place older adults at risk for fluid and electrolyte imbalances that can be manifested as functional consequences. Appropriate interventions are needed to foster positive functional consequences and decrease the debilitating effects of these risk factors and age-related changes.

Table 16-1 lists (a) age-related structural changes in five major body systems; (b) health risk factors for fluid and electrolyte imbalance; (c) functional changes resulting from age-related changes and potential risk factors; and (d) interventions to foster positive functional outcome

● ETIOLOGY

The older adult's ability to adapt to changes in fluid and electrolyte balance is often complicated by chronic disease, and/or medications. Refer to Table 16-2 for a summary of fluid problems commonly found in the older adult.

● CLINICAL MANIFESTATIONS

The severity of fluid and electrolyte imbalances in the older adult vary with the individual's ability to maintain a fluid reserve, the efficiency of the individual's regulatory systems, and any complicating disease factors. Since structural changes and underlying disease influence the manifestation of clinical symptoms, it is important to view health problems in terms of each system affected. Table 16-3 outlines typical symptoms of an older adult experiencing excess fluid volume. Table 16-4 outlines some presenting symptoms for an older adult experiencing a deficient fluid volume.

● CLINICAL MANAGEMENT

Effective management of fluid and electrolyte imbalances requires the health professional to integrate findings from their structural and functional assessments with health data related to individual risk factors and chronic diseases. Once this data is put into perspective, fluid balance can be managed by targeting outcomes appropriate to the client's age-related changes and current health problems. Table 16-5 lists actions to be taken in the clinical management of fluid balance in the older adult.

Table 16-1	Major Structural Changes, Risk Factors, and Functional Outcomes in Older Adults			
Organ System	**Structural Changes**	**Risk Factors**	**Functional Outcomes**	**Nursing Interventions**
Pulmonary function decreased	Loss of elasticity of parenchymal lung tissue with 20% decrease in weight	Chronic diseases	Defective alveolar ventilation	Increase breathing capacity to enhance the elimination of CO_2 by:
	Increased rigidity of chest wall, decreased recoil of lungs	Emphysema	Decreased gas exchange	1. Breathing exercises with prolonged expiration
	Fewer alveoli	Asthma	Increased work of breathing	2. Coughing after a few deep breaths
	Decreased strength of expiratory muscles	Chronic bronchitis	Respiratory rate may increase	3. Frequent position changes
	Decrease in internal surface area	Bronchiectasis	Baseline arterial oxygenation is lower	
	Decreased mucociliary transport system	Injuries from smoking	Decreased ability to clear mucus and foreign bodies (bacteria)	
		Longer sleeping hours	Decline in response to supplemental oxygen	
		Exposure to air pollutants	Decreased cough reflex	
		Occupational exposure to toxic substances	Accumulation of bronchial secretions	
		Infection	Increased CO_2 retention	
		Decreased immune system response	Increased difficulty in regulating pH	
			Decreased response to hypoxia and hypercapnia	

(continues)

Table 16-1	Major Structural Changes, Risk Factors, and Functional Outcomes in Older Adults—*continued*			
Organ System	**Structural Changes**	**Risk Factors**	**Functional Outcomes**	**Nursing Interventions**
Pulmonary function decreased (*continued*)			Decreased tolerance for exercise Decreased vital capacity response Increased residual volume	
Renal function decreased	Arteriosclerotic changes in large renal vessels Decrease in number of functioning cortical nephrons (begins by age 40) 30–50% less by age 70 Decrease in size and weight of the kidneys Increased interstitial tissue Reduced medullary nephron's ability to concentrate urine Decrease in number glomeruli Thickening of glomeruli and tubular membranes	Medications (e.g., nephrotoxic drugs, diuretics) Genitourinary diseases (e.g., infections, obstructions) Chronic renal insufficiency Hypertension Atherosclerotic vascular disease	Reduced glomerular filtration Decreased renal blood flow Impaired ability to excrete water and solutes causing: 1. A decrease in H^+ excretion; thus, metabolic acidosis can occur 2. Reduced ability to concentrate urine 3. Increased accumulation of waste products in body 4. Decreased ability to excrete drugs Decline in urine creatinine clearance of about 10% per decade after age 40	Assess adaptive capacity and maintain optimal renal function by: 1. Checking fluid intake and output balance 2. Encouraging fluid intake as appropriate 3. Checking acid-base balance according to serum CO_2 or HCO_3 4. Testing specific gravity to determine kidneys' ability to concentrate urine 5. Track renal function by monitoring serum creatinine, blood urea nitrogen (BUN), and urine creatinine clearance

Renal function decreased (continued)		(Note: Serum creatinine will remain within normal limits) Overall decrease in adaptive capacity of the kidneys to stress Decreased thirst perception (hypodipsia) Impaired responsiveness to sodium balance	6. Noting drugs that may be toxic to renal function 7. Observing for side effects from drug accumulation
Circulation and cardiac function decreased	Increased rigidity and decreased elasticity of arterial walls (arteriosclerosis) Decreased elasticity of blood vessels Thickening of cardiac vessels and valves Decrease in number of conductive cells	Myocardial infarction Cardiomyopathy Obesity Smoking Dietary habits that contribute to risk factors: Hyperlipidemia, excess salt and calories Inactivity Low potassium intake Diuretic therapy Excessive alcohol consumption Stress Air pollution Hormone changes	Potential increase in blood pressure Stasis of blood causing back pressure on capillaries, which in turn causes fluid to move into tissue areas causing edema Decreased cardiac reserve (capacity of heart to respond to increased burden) slows the adaptive functions as evidenced by: 1. Heart rate same as young adults except under stress takes longer to return to normal 2. Increased incidence of edema and congestive heart failure

Assess adaptive capacity of heart and maintain circulation and cardiac function by:

1. Checking blood pressure for elevations resulting from arteriosclerotic changes
2. Determining blood flow by checking peripheral pulses
3. Checking dependent extremities for edema from increased capillary pressure
4. Checking pulse rates (apical and radial)
5. Noting changes in heart rate following activity

(continues)

Table 16-1	Major Structural Changes, Risk Factors, and Functional Outcomes in Older Adults—*continued*			
Organ System	**Structural Changes**	**Risk Factors**	**Functional Outcomes**	**Nursing Interventions**
Circulation and cardiac function decreased *(continued)*			Diminished strength of cardiac contractions Decreased cardiac output and stroke volume Decreased compensatory responses to blood pressure changes Decreased maximum heart rate and aerobic capacity Decrease in maximum oxygen consumption Approximately 50% of older adults have abnormal resting electrocardiographs (EKGs)	6. Assessing lung sounds for crackles 7. Monitoring intake and output balance 8. Assessing for unexplained weight gain of 4.5 kg (10 lb), pitting edema 9. Administering diuretics as prescribed, assessing effectiveness 10. Observing for signs and symptoms of hypovolemia and electrolyte depletion (namely hypokalemia) as a result of diuretic therapy 11. Monitoring serum electrolytes 12. Encouraging regular exercise, longer cooling down periods

Gastrointestinal function decreased	Atrophy of gastric mucosa Muscular atrophy and loss of supportive structures in small intestines	Alcohol or medications Psychosocial factors (e.g., isolation, depression) Factors that interfere with ability to obtain, prepare, consume, or enjoy food and fluids (e.g., immobility, mental impairment) Extraintestinal disorders (diabetes, vascular disorders, and neurologic changes)	Decrease in gastric secretions, especially HCl Metabolic alkalosis related to decreased HCl Atrophic gastritis due to decreased HCl Weakened intestinal wall causing diverticuli Decreased motility (peristalsis) of gastrointestinal tract (may cause constipation) Decreased calcium and nutrient absorption Decreased solubility and absorption of some drugs	Assess for adaptive changes and maintain gastrointestinal function by: 1. Discussing client preferences for foods 2. Suggesting dietary alterations according to physiologic changes, individual preferences, and nutritional needs; may need increased calcium and vitamin D 3. Encouraging fluid intake 4. Checking frequency, consistency, and stool color in bowel elimination 5. Assessing bowel sounds and level of peristalsis
Liver function and endocrine gland function decreased	Liver decreases in mass of approximately 40% by age 80 Hormonal cells decrease in size and character, and outputs dwindle	Liver or endocrine diseases Medications (e.g., steroids, cardiac medications, antibiotics) Alcohol consumption	Liver: 1. Decreased hepatic capacity to detoxify drugs 2. Decreased synthesis of cholesterol and enzyme activity	Assess adaptive liver and endocrine gland functioning by: 1. Noting drugs client is taking that may be toxic to liver

(continues)

Table 16-1 Major Structural Changes, Risk Factors, and Functional Outcomes in Older Adults—*continued*

Organ System	Structural Changes	Risk Factors	Functional Outcomes	Nursing Interventions
Liver function and endocrine gland function decreased *(continued)*			Hormonal: 1. Decreased overall metabolic capacity 2. Decreased endocrine gland function to react to adverse drug action	2. Observing for toxic effects of drug buildup 3. Observing for desired effects of drugs 4. Assessing alcohol consumption and teaching accordingly 5. Assessing for jaundice 6. Assessing for fluid shift (e.g., ascites)
Skin function decreased	All three layers of the skin (epidermis, dermis, and subcutaneous) become thinner, lose elasticity and strength Blood flow—decreased Sebaceous glands—decreased production Sweat glands—decreased production Decrease in number of nerve endings	Exposure to ultraviolet rays (sunlight) Adverse medication effects Personal hygiene habits (e.g., too frequent bathing) Immobility Friction Chemical Mechanical injury Temperature—too high or low Pressure Gene influence	Drier, coarser skin Increased threshold level to pain and temperature sensitivity Decreased ability to produce sweat Impaired ability to maintain body temperature Decreased skin elasticity (making it difficult to assess skin turgor)	Maintain skin integrity and function by: 1. Maintaining hydration, monitoring fluid status 2. Maintaining optimal skin temperature 3. Maintaining and encouraging mobility to enhance circulation 4. Turning patient and elevating extremities when necessary to minimize edema and skin breakdown

Skin function
decreased
(continued)

Diabetes
Peripheral vascular
disease

5. Educating about
decreased sensitivity to
pain and temperature
6. Providing special
mattress for those at
risk
7. Padding, protecting
boney prominences
and pressure sites as
needed

Table 16-2 Body Fluid Problems in the Older Adult

Problems	Etiology	Interventions
Deficient Fluid Volume: Dehydration	1. Insufficient water intake 2. Increased urinary output 3. Decreased thirst mechanism 4. Diminished response to ADH (antidiuretic hormone) 5. Reduced ability to concentrate urine	1. Measure fluid intake and output to assess fluid balance 2. Encourage adequate oral fluid intake 3. Assess osmolality of IV fluid intake 4. Assess for clinical signs and symptoms of hypovolemia (dehydration) 5. Monitor other types of fluid therapy, e.g., IV clysis and tube feeding. Adjust rate of IV fluid according to age and physiologic state 6. Monitor levels of serum electrolytes, BUN, serum creatinine, hematocrit, and hemoglobin
Excess Fluid Volume Edema	1. Slightly elevated ECF 2. Overhydration from IV therapy 3. Increased capillary pressure 4. Cardiac insufficiency	1. Measure fluid intake and output to assess fluid balance. 2. Monitor daily weights 3. Adjust IV flow rate to prevent overhydration 4. Assess for peripheral edema in morning 5. Protect edematous skin from injury 6. Observe for signs and symptoms of hypervolemia—overhydration, which can lead to pulmonary edema such as headache, anxiety, shortness of breath, tachypnea, coughing, pulmonary crackles, and chest pain

(continues)

Table 16-2	Body Fluid Problems in the Older Adult—*continued*	
Problems	**Etiology**	**Interventions**
Constipation	1. Decrease in water intake	1. Encourage fluid intake
	2. Muscular atrophy of small and large intestines with decrease in GI motility	2. Assess bowel sounds for peristalsis
	3. Perceptual loss of bowel stimulation	3. Administer mild laxative and teach dangers of abuse
	4. Medications that influence gastric motility and hydration	4. Have patient eat at regular times
		5. Offer bedside commode
		6. Increase roughage in diet as tolerated
		7. Observe color, consistency, and frequency of stools
	1. Tube feedings with high carbohydrate content	1. Assess for problem causing diarrhea (infectious, impaction, medications)
	2. Constipation—with small amount of liquid stools	2. Administer drug(s), e.g., Lomotil, Kaopectate, Immodium, to decrease motility of bowel
	3. Partially digested nutrients	
	4. Viral or bacterial infection	3. Observe color, frequency, and consistency of stool
		4. Monitor closely for hypovolemia and electrolyte imbalance (potassium, sodium)
		5. Encourage clear liquids

Table 16-3 — Characteristics of an Older Adult with Excess Fluid Volume

Organ System Affected	Structural Changes	Risk Factors	Functional Changes	Diagnoses	Interventions	Rationale
Cardiac	Arteriosclerosis Increased capillary pressure Decreased effectiveness of cardiac contractions	Recent weight gain of 10 pounds Low protein intake HF HTN	High blood pressure Edema Decreased cardiac output Increased heart rate	Excess fluid volume: edema, related to decreased cardiac output as evidenced by weight gain of 10 pounds, lower extremity edema, and pulmonary crackles	1. Monitor intake and output, body weight, vital signs, and neck veins for distension 2. Monitor hemoglobin, hematocrit, serum creatinine, BUN, and electrolytes 3. Administer diuretics as ordered by physician	Checking for overhydration is important to measure the effectiveness for medical treatment and interventions Hemoglobin, hematocrit, serum creatinine, BUN, and electrolytes concentration are important to assess fluid balance changes A↓ Hgb and Hct levels can indicate fluid overload

System	Age-Related Change	Risk Factors	Nursing Diagnosis	Interventions	Rationale
Cardiac *(continued)*				4. If on diuretics, monitor K^+	Diuretics increase fluid loss and decrease edema. Many diuretics cause potassium loss
Respiratory	Loss of elasticity of the parenchymal lung tissue Increased rigidity of the chest wall	Immobility Hypoventilation	CO_2 retention Respiratory acidosis *and* Reduced breathing capacity	Impaired gas exchange Ineffective breathing patterns	
				1. Monitor chest for adventitious sounds	To assess for fluid overload
				2. Observe for cough, which may indicate pulmonary edema	Cough is an early sign of fluid overload
				3. Breathing exercises—prolonged expiration	Assists in removing excess CO_2
				4. Coughing after a few deep breaths	To enhance gas exchange (O_2 + CO_2)
				5. Change position frequently	Assists in lung expansion
Renal	Persistent renal vasoconstriction from arteriosclerotic changes and decreased numbers of functioning nephrons	Medications Genitourinary obstructions ↑ HTN	Reduced glomerular filtration rate and ability to excrete water and solute	Excess fluid volume related to renal insufficiency as evidenced by decreased urine output,	
				1. Assess intake and output	To determine amount of excess fluid volume
				2. Weigh daily, assess for edema	Daily weight is the best monitor of fluid status
				3. Auscultate lung and heart sounds	

(continues)

Table 16-3 Characteristics of an Older Adult with Excess Fluid Volume—*continued*

Organ System Affected	Structural Changes	Risk Factors	Functional Changes	Diagnoses	Interventions	Rationale
Renal *(continued)*				increased serum creatinine, and BUN	4. Assess urine specific gravity (SG) 5. Monitor serum creatinine and BUN 6. Monitor serum sodium, hemoglobin, and hematocrit 7. Monitor potassium 8. Administer diuretics as indicated	Fluid overload may lead to pulmonary edema and heart failure Increased urine SG indicates inadequate fluid intake or decreased renal function Assess progression and management of renal dysfunction May decrease in values as a result of hemodilution Lack of renal secretion may lead to hyperkalemia

Gastrointestinal				
Liver*				
Integumentary	Loss of elasticity and strength of skin Decreased blood flow, sebaceous and sweat gland production	Edema Immobility	Pitting edema noted in lower extremities, reducing protective function of skin and increasing risk of skin injury	Impaired skin integrity related to edema and immobility	1. Avoid friction, prolonged pressure, chemical irritation, mechanical injury, excessive temperature variations 2. Encourage mobility to enhance circulation 3. Elevate extremities 4. Implement interventions for excess fluid volume	To promote diuresis To reduce possible skin breakdown due to edema and/or immobility Good circulation improves skin repair To improve circulation and reduce edema Fluid balance reduces risks to integumentary system

*Not applicable

Table 16-4 **Characteristics of an Older Adult with Deficient Fluid Volume**

Organ System Affected	Structural Changes	Risk Factors	Functional Changes	Diagnoses	Interventions	Rationale
Cardiac Respiratory*	Increased rigidity and decreased elasticity of arterial walls (arteriosclerosis) Decreased elasticity of blood vessels Thickening of cardiac vessels and valves Decrease in number of conductive cells	Decreased fluid intake Diuretic therapy Excessive alcohol consumption	Potential decrease in blood pressure Diminished strength of cardiac contractions Decreased cardiac output and stroke volume Decreased compensatory responses to blood pressure changes Decreased maximum heart rate and aerobic capacity	Decreased cardiac output related to decreased desire to drink fluids, diuretic therapy as evidenced by decreased blood pressure; thready, rapid pulse; and fatigability	Assess adaptive capacity of heart and maintain circulation and cardiac function by: 1. Checking blood pressure and pulse for orthostatic changes 2. Determining blood flow by checking peripheral pulses 3. Assessing for increased fatigue in client	Orthostatic blood pressure and pulse changes may indicate dehydration Weak, thready pulse may be a sign of dehydration Fatigue may be a result of decreased cardiac output related to dehydration
Renal	Persistent renal vasoconstriction Decreased number of functioning nephrons	Obstructions Disease Medications	Decreased thirst mechanism	Deficient fluid volume related to decreased desire to drink fluids, high alcohol intake,	1. Observe for decreased urine output	Decreased skin turgor is a sign of dehydration. Decreased urine output may be due to

	Risk Factors	Physiological Changes	Nursing Diagnosis	Interventions	Rationale
		Reduced glomerular filtration rate. Decreased ability to excrete water and solute	and social isolation, as evidenced by dry lips, furrowed tongue, and decreased skin turgor	2. Measure intake and output. 3. Check specific gravity of urine. 4. Observe lab results for increased red blood cell count, hematocrit, hemoglobin, creatinine clearance, serum creatinine, and BUN	dehydration or renal dysfunction. To determine fluid balance. To assess renal function. Provide clues to extent of fluid deficit. Provide clues in regard to renal function
Gastrointestinal	Alcohol intake. Poor diet. Immobility. Decreased motivation to drink fluids other than alcohol. Social isolation	Decreased GI secretions. Decreased motility. Constipation. Decreased sensation of thirst	Constipation related to inadequate intake of food and fluids and lack of exercise, as evidenced by infrequent bowel movements, small, hard stools	1. Increase fluid intake of water and fluids. 2. Assess fluid balance. 3. Encourage a balanced diet with increased roughage. 4. Assess bowel sounds. 5. Observe color and consistency of stools	To enhance bowel elimination and soften stools. Fluid balance reduces risk for constipation. Balanced diet with fiber stimulates bowel elimination

(continues)

Table 16-4 Characteristics of an Older Adult with Deficient Fluid Volume—*continued*

Organ System Affected	Structural Changes	Risk Factors	Functional Changes	Diagnoses	Interventions	Rationale
Liver* Integumentary	All three layers of the skin (epidermis, dermis, and subcutaneous) become thinner, lose elasticity and strength Decreased blood flow Decreased number of nerve endings	Temperature—too high or too low Immobility Pressure Friction	Decreased skin integrity	Risk for impaired skin integrity	1. Observe for decreased skin turgor and dry mucous membranes 2. Maintain and encourage sufficient fluid intake	Decreased skin turgor and dry mucous membranes are signs of dehydration Adequate hydration will improve skin condition

*Not applicable

Table 16-5	Clinical Management of Fluid Balance in the Older Adult

- Adjust fluid and electrolyte replacement therapy to match the older adult's reduced functional efficiency and slower response rate (renal, cardiac, pulmonary, GI, integumentary, and regulatory systems).
- Alert client to side effects of diuretics and other medications and his or her increased risk for fluid and electrolyte imbalances (especially sodium and potassium).
- Recognize client's increased risk for fluid and electrolyte complications in acute illness or surgical interventions.
- Encourage client to select appropriate foods and fluids in balanced quantities to meet individual hydration needs.

CLINICAL CONSIDERATIONS: OLDER ADULTS

1. Efficiency of body systems decreases with age and chronic health problems reducing both the effectiveness and speed of bodily responses to stressors.
2. Hypernatremia associated with fluid imbalance is a common problem for the older adult. It is usually related to poor fluid consumption.
3. Potassium-depleting diuretics tend to induce hypokalemia in the older adult; potassium-sparing diuretics are more likely to produce hyperkalemia.
4. Fluid deficits are often associated with orthostatic hypotension.
5. Prolonged use of strong laxatives and enema dependency can cause hypokalemia and deficient fluid volume.
6. Standard colon-cleansing procedures can cause fluid and electrolyte complications in the marginally hydrated older adult.
7. Calcium deficiencies are often associated with osteoporosis. Risks increase with age and postmenopausal osteoporosis.
8. Heat stroke is more common in the older adult than in other age groups (age-related mortality rates increase after the age of 70).

9. The older adult is at an increased risk for postsurgical complications (cardiac, pneumonia, and fluid and electrolyte imbalance).

CLIENT MANAGEMENT

Assessment

- Complete an extensive health history with careful attention to fluid and electrolyte balance factors (dehydration, fluid overload, edema, mental clarity, cardiac, and renal function).
- Complete a head-to-toe physical assessment with specific attention to changes associated with aging.
- Identify risk factors and potential fluid and electrolyte health problems.
- Obtain complete list of medications and herbal supplements.
- Complete laboratory studies on electrolytes, hemoglobin/hematocrit ratio, BUN creatinine ratio, and urine specific gravity to identify fluid and electrolyte problems.
- Obtain baseline measurements of vital signs and weight for future reference.

Nursing Diagnoses

- *Deficient Fluid Volume,* related to severe imbalance between intake and output
- *Excess Fluid Volume,* related to inadequate fluid excretion associated with poorly functioning regulatory systems (heart, kidneys, endocrine, and lungs)
- *Imbalanced Nutrition,* less than body requirements, related to inadequate diet

Interventions

Deficient Fluid Volume

- Monitor lab values (BUN/creatinine ratio, electrolyte, hemoglobin, hematocrit, urine specific gravity).

- Closely monitor for changes in general appearance, behaviors, and neurologic activity.
- Monitor weight daily.
- Monitor vital signs in accordance with severity of health problems.
- Integrate observations to determine the degree (mild, moderate, severe) of dehydration.
- Monitor effects of fluid replacement with physical assessment and laboratory findings.
- Monitor balance in intake and output measures.

Excess Fluid Volume

- Attempt to identify the source of the fluid overload.
- Closely monitor intake and output for imbalance.
- Monitor laboratory values (serum electrolytes, hemoglobin, hematocrit, urine specific gravity, and serum creatinine).
- Monitor weight daily.
- Observe closely for signs and symptoms of pulmonary edema.
- Monitor extremities and torso for signs of edema.

Evaluation/Outcome

- Evaluate intake and output for fluid balance.
- Evaluate effectiveness of medications and fluid replacement in treatment.
- Monitor nutritional intake to ensure fluid balance.
- Evaluate body weight and vital signs for return to normal client values.
- Evaluate skin turgor, circulation, temperature, and moisture to reduce effects of risk factors.
- Monitor lab results for Hgb, Hct, Na, Cl, K, BUN, and creatinine until findings are within normal range.
- Maintain a support system.

Acute Disorders: Trauma and Shock

Linda Laskowski-Jones, MS, RN

INTRODUCTION

Numerous physiologic changes in fluid and electrolyte imbalances occur as a result of traumatic injuries and shock. Swift and accurate assessment and interventions are necessary to protect the life of the injured client. Chapter 17 is divided into two sections related to fluid, electrolyte, and acid-base changes: trauma and shock.

TRAUMA

Fluid, electrolyte, and acid-base changes occur rapidly in the acutely traumatized client. Quick assessment and action are needed for the best chance of survival. Trauma deaths can occur almost immediately at the time of the trauma, hours later, or days later primarily due to acute respiratory distress syndrome (ARDS), sepsis, or multiple organ failure. Following a traumatic injury, the injured sites are assessed, fluid replacements are prescribed, and medical and/or surgical interventions are performed.

Pathophysiology

Following a severe traumatic injury, there is cellular breakdown (catabolism) due to cell damage and hypoxia. In trauma, sodium shifts into cells and potassium shifts out of cells; fluid shifts from the intravascular (vessels) to the interstitial spaces and cells. These shifts can result in severe fluid and electrolyte imbalances. Kidney activity is altered during and after a severe traumatic injury. Decreased circulatory flow can decrease renal arterial flow and renal perfusion, thus diminishing renal function. With cellular breakdown and hypoxia, nonvolatile acids such as lactic acid increase in the vascular fluid, causing metabolic acidosis. Also, with decreased renal function, hydrogen ion retention occurs, thus contributing to the acidotic state that generally accompanies trauma and shock. Table 17-1 lists the physiologic changes that occur during trauma.

Table 17-1	Physiologic Changes Associated with Trauma
Physiologic Changes	**Causative Factors**
Potassium, sodium, chloride, bicarbonate	Potassium is lost from cells due to catabolism (cellular breakdown). As potassium leaves, sodium and chloride with water shift into the cells. The sodium pump does not function properly (see Chapter 6).
Fluid changes	Fluids along with sodium shift into cells and to the third space (interstitial space—at the injured site). The increased cellular and third-space fluids cause a vascular fluid deficit (dehydration) and hyponatremia.
	Serum osmolality may be normal or increased due to the fluid deficit and excess solutes other than sodium, such as potassium and urea. Remember, sodium influences the osmolality of plasma (see Chapter 1).
	The volume and composition of extracellular fluid (ECF) fluctuates depending on the number of cells injured and the body's ability to restore balance. Two to three days following injury, fluid shifts from the third space at the injured site back into the vascular space.
Protein changes	Trauma results in nitrogen loss due to increased protein catabolism, decreased protein anabolism, and/or a protein shift with water to the interstitial space. The colloid osmotic pressure is decreased in

(continues)

Table 17-1	Physiologic Changes Associated with Trauma—*continued*
Physiologic Changes	**Causative Factors**
Protein changes *continued*	the vascular fluid and increased in the interstitial fluid (tissues), which causes fluid volume deficit (vascular) and edema.
Capillary permeability	Increased capillary permeability causes water to flow into and out of the cells and into tissue spaces. This contributes to hypovolemia (fluid volume deficit).
Hormonal influence	ADH and aldosterone help to restore the ECF. A vascular fluid deficit and/or increased serum osmolality stimulates ADH secretion, which causes water reabsorption from the distal tubules of the kidneys. In certain traumatic situations (surgery, trauma, pain), SIADH (syndrome of inappropriate ADH) occurs and causes excess water reabsorption from the kidneys. Aldosterone is secreted from the adrenal cortex due to hyponatremia and stress. Aldosterone promotes sodium reabsorption from the renal tubules and is reabsorbed with water. Potassium is excreted.
Kidney influence	Kidney activity is altered during and after a severe traumatic injury. Sodium, chloride, and water shift to the injured site, which causes hypovolemia. Decreased circulatory flow can decrease renal arterial flow, which can cause temporary or permanent kidney damage. Decreased kidney function results in hyperkalemia.
Acid-base changes	With cellular breakdown and hypoxia from decreased perfusion, nonvolatile acids (acid metabolites), e.g., lactic acid, increase in the vascular fluid, causing metabolic acidosis. Kidneys conserve or excrete the hydrogen ion to maintain the acid-base balance. Decreased kidney function can cause hydrogen retention and acidosis. The lungs try to compensate for the acidotic state by blowing off excess CO_2—hyperventilation. Blowing off CO_2 decreases the formation of carbonic acid.

Etiology

Trauma can result from severe injury including massive blood loss from major arterial and venous vessels, injuries to the brain (epidural or subdural hematomas) or brain stem, ruptured spleen, liver lacerations, fractures to large bones, chest injury (hemopneumothorax), and crush injuries to bones, tissues, and organs of the body.

Clinical Manifestations

The clinical manifestations that frequently occur in traumatic injuries include changes in vital signs and/or behavioral, cardiac conduction, venous, neuromuscular, and integumentary changes. Laboratory test results are a guide to determine fluid, electrolyte, and acid-base changes that are occurring.

The pulse rate may be fast, irregular, or weak. The blood pressure decreases according to the blood volume and fluid deficit. With severe fluid loss, the pulse pressure is narrowed. Tachypnea, dyspnea, or deep and rapid breathing may be present.

To overcome the hypovolemic state caused by blood and fluid loss and fluid shift to the injured site and cells, antidiuretic hormone (ADH) is released. This is a compensatory mechanism to maintain the vascular fluid. The water reabsorption can be continuous for several days. Urine output is decreased due to excess production of ADH.

The client may be irritable, restless, and confused because of hypoxia and fluid and electrolyte losses. Integumentary changes may not be noted immediately following severe trauma with fluid losses. However, after several hours or a day, the skin turgor can be affected and mucous membranes may become dry. Table 17-2 lists the clinical manifestations related to trauma.

Clinical Management

Accurate clinical assessment is vitally important when planning and implementing care. Table 17-3 is a guide that may be used when assessing the client for fluid, electrolyte, and acid-base imbalances. To understand the significance of the assessment, the rationale helps to identify the type of imbalance present.

Table 17-2	Clinical Manifestations Related to Trauma
Clinical Manifestations	**Signs and Symptoms**
Vital Signs	Increased pulse rate (tachycardia)
Pulse	Irregular pulse rate, weak, thready pulse
Blood pressure	Blood pressure decreases when severe fluid loss occurs
	Pulse pressure narrows
Respiration	Increased breathing (tachypnea)
	Dyspnea
	Deep, vigorous breathing (Kussmaul breathing)
Temperature	Hypothermia commonly associated with shock. Septic shock causes hyperthermia.
Behavioral changes	Irritability, restlessness, and confusion
Cardiac conduction changes	ECG: T wave changes (inverted or peaked), ST segment changes, and cardiac dysrythmias (result of coronary ischemia or potassium imbalance)
Venous changes	Neck vein engorgement with cardiac tamporade or torsion pneumothorax
	No vein engorgement with fluid loss
Renal changes	Hourly urine output decreases
Neuromuscular changes	Muscular weakness
Integumentary changes	Poor skin turgor
	Dry mucous membrane
	Edema at injury site(s)
	Diaphoresis
	Draining wound, exudate
Laboratory Findings	
Electrolytes ↓ or ↑	Serum potassium, sodium, magnesium, chloride may be decreased or increased
Serum CO_2	Decreased CO_2 indicates metabolic acidosis; increased CO_2 indicates metabolic alkalosis or respiratory alkalosis
BUN ↑	Increased BUN indicates fluid loss or decreased renal function
Serum creatinine ↑	Increased serum creatinine indicates decreased renal function
Arterial blood gases: pH, $PaCO_2$, HCO_3	Decreased pH and HCO_3 indicate metabolic acidosis

Table 17-3	Assessment of Fluid, Electrolyte, and Acid-Base Imbalances in the Traumatically Injured Client

Observation	Assessment		Rationale
1. Vital signs: Pulse	Pulse rate Volume Pattern	____ ____ ____	Changes in vital signs (VS) are indicators of client's physiologic status. Several VS should be taken and the first reading acts as the baseline for comparison. Pulse rate and pattern should be monitored frequently. Pulse rate >120 may indicate hypovolemia and the possibility of shock. Full-bounding pulse can mean hypervolemia and an irregular pulse can mean hypokalemia.
Blood pressure	Admission BP Time Time	 ____ ____	Decrease in BP (systolic and diastolic) may not occur until severe fluid loss has occurred. Several BP readings should be taken, and the first BP reading acts as the baseline for comparison. A drop in systolic pressure can indicate hypovolemia. Pulse pressure (systolic minus diastolic) of <20 can indicate shock.
Respiration	Respiration Pattern	____ ____	Note changes in rate, depth, and pattern. A rate >32 can indicate hypovolemia. Deep, rapid, vigorous breathing can indicate acidosis as a result of cellular damage and shock. Hyperventilating (fast, shallow breathing) can be due to anxiety or hypoxia. Head injury can produce a wide variety of respiratory patterns.
Temperature	Temperature on admission	____	Hypothermia is a common finding in shock; an elevated temperature can indicate infection.

(continues)

Table 17-3	**Assessment of Fluid, Electrolyte, and Acid-Base Imbalances in the Traumatically Injured Client—*continued***	
Observation	**Assessment**	**Rationale**
2. Behavioral changes	Irritable ____ Apprehensive ____ Restless ____ Confused ____ Delirious ____ Lethargic ____	Irritability, apprehension, restlessness, and confusion are indicators of hypoxia and later of fluid and electrolyte imbalances (hypovolemia, water intoxication, and potassium imbalance).

3. Neurologic and neuromuscular signs	Sensorium
	  Confused ____
	  Semi-
	  conscious ____
	  Comatose ____
	Muscle
	  weakness ____
	Pupil dilation ____
	Tetany
	  Tremors ____
	  Twitching ____
	  Others ____
		Changes in sensorium can be indicative of fluid imbalance. Tetany can indicate a calcium and magnesium deficit. Hypocalcemia can occur with multiple transfusions of banked blood.

4. Fluid loss	Wound(s) ____
	Urine
	  Number of
	  voidings ____
	  Amount
	    ml/h ____
	    ml/8 h ____
	    ml/24 h ____
	  Color ____
	  Specific
	  gravity ____
	Vomitus
	  Number ____
	  Consistency ____
	  Amount ____
		Note the presence of an open draining wound. Kidneys regulate fluids and electrolytes. Monitoring the urine output hourly is most important. Oliguria can indicate a lack of fluid intake or renal insufficiency due to decreased circulation/circulatory collapse or hypovolemia.
		Frequent vomiting in large quantities leads to fluid, electrolyte (potassium, sodium, chloride), and hydrogen losses. Metabolic alkalosis can occur.

	Nasogastric
	tube
	  Amount—
	  ml/8h ____
	  Amount—
	  ml/24 h ____
		Gastrointestinal secretions should be measured. Large quantity losses of GI secretions can cause hypovolemia.

	Drain(s)
	  Number ____
	  Amount ____
		Excess drainage could contribute to fluid loss and should be measured if possible.

(continues)

Table 17-3	Assessment of Fluid, Electrolyte, and Acid-Base Imbalances in the Traumatically Injured Client—*continued*	
Observation	**Assessment**	**Rationale**
5. Skin and mucous membrane	Skin color Pale ____ Gray ____ Flushed ____	Pale and/or gray-colored skin can indicate hypovolemia or shock. Flushed skin can be due to hypernatremia, metabolic acidosis, or early septic shock.
	Skin turgor Normal ____ Poor ____	Poor skin turgor can result from hypovolemia/dehydration. This may not occur until 1–3 days after the injury.
	Edema—pitting peripheral Feet ____ Legs ____	Edema indicates sodium and water retention. Sodium, chloride, and water shift into the cells and to the injury site(s) (interstitial or third space).
	Dry mucous membranes ____ Sticky secretions ____	Dry, tenacious (sticky) secretions and dry membranes are indicative of dehydration or fluid loss. This may not occur until 1–3 days after the injury.
	Diaphoresis ____	Increased insensible fluid loss can result from diaphoresis (excess perspiration). Amount of fluid loss from skin can double.
6. Chest sounds and vein engorgement	Chest crackles ____	The chest should be checked for crackles due to overhydration (pulmonary edema) following fluid administration/resuscitation.
	Neck vein engorgement ____ Hand vein engorgement ____	Neck and hand vein engorgement are indicators of fluid excess. Crackles and vein engorgement can occur from excess IV fluids or rapid IV administration.
7. ECG (EKG)	T wave Flat ____ Inverted ____ Peaked ____	Flat or inverted T waves indicate cardiac ischemia and/or a potassium deficit. Peaked T waves indicate a potassium excess.

(continues)

Table 17-3	Assessment of Fluid, Electrolyte, and Acid-Base Imbalances in the Traumatically Injured Client—*continued*	
Observation	**Assessment**	**Rationale**
8. Fluid intake	Oral fluid intake Amount ml/8 h ____ ml/24 h ____	Oral fluids should not be given until the injury(s) can be assessed. If surgery is indicated, the client should be NPO.
	Types of IV fluids Crystalloids ____ Colloids ____ Blood ____	Crystalloids, i.e., normal saline, lactated Ringer's, are normally ordered first to restore fluid loss, correct shocklike symptoms, restore or increase urine output, and serve as a lifeline to administer IV drugs.
	Amount ml/8 h ____ ml/24 h ____ ml/h ____	Five percent dextrose in water can cause water intoxication (ICF volume excess) and is contraindicated as a resuscitation fluid in shock states.
9. Previous drug regimen	Diuretics ____ Digitalis ____ Steroids ____ Beta blockers ____ Calcium channel blockers ____	A drug history should be taken and reported to the physician. Potassium-wasting diuretics taken with a digitalis preparation can cause digitalis toxicity in the presence of hypokalemia. Steroids cause sodium retention and potassium excretion. Long-term steroid use can impair adrenal function in shock states and impair the client's ability to mount a stress response. A steroid bolus or "stress dose" is indicated for steroid-dependent clients. Beta blockers and calcium channel blockers block the effects of the sympathetic nervous system. They may block the compensatory mechanisms for shock.

(continues)

Table 17-3	Assessment of Fluid, Electrolyte, and Acid-Base Imbalances in the Traumatically Injured Client—*continued*	

Observation	Assessment		Rationale
10. Chemistry, hematology, and arterial blood gas changes	Electrolytes		Electrolytes should be drawn immediately after a severe injury and used as a baseline for future electrolyte results. (See Chapter 6 for normal values.)
	Serum	*Urine/24 h*	
	K ___	K ___	
	Na ___	Na ___	
	Cl ___	Cl ___	
	Ca ___		
	Mg ___		Urine electrolytes are compared to serum electrolytes. Normal range for urine electrolytes are: K 25–120 mEq/24 h Na 40–220 mEq/24 h Cl 150–250 mEq/24 h
	Serum CO_2	___	Serum CO_2 >32 mEq/L indicates metabolic alkalosis and <22 mEq/L indicates metabolic acidosis.
	Osmolality		Serum osmolality >295 mOsm/kg indicates hypovolemia/dehydration and <280 mOsm/kg indicates hypervolemia. Urine osmolality can be 100–1200 mOsm/kg with a normal range of 200–600 mOsm/kg.
	Serum	___	
	Urine	___	
	BUN	___	An elevated BUN can indicate fluid volume deficit or kidney insufficiency. Elevated creatinine indicates kidney damage. Normal range: BUN 10–25 mg/dl Creatinine 0.7–1.4 mg/dl
	Creatinine	___	
	Blood glucose	___	Blood sugar increases during stress (up to 180 mg/dl, or higher in diabetics).
	Hbg ___	Hct ___	Elevated hemoglobin and hematocrit can indicate hemoconcentration caused by fluid volume deficit (hypovolemia).

(continues)

Table 17-3	Assessment of Fluid, Electrolyte, and Acid-Base Imbalances in the Traumatically Injured Client—*continued*	
Observation	**Assessment**	**Rationale**
	Arterial blood gases (ABGs) pH _____ PaCO₂ _____ HCO₃ _____ BE _____	pH: <7.35 indicates acidosis and >7.45 indicates alkalosis. *PaCO₂ (respiratory component):* Norms 35–45 mm Hg Respiratory acidosis (↓ pH, ↑ PaCO₂) may occur due to inadequate gas exchange. A ↑ pH and ↓ PaCO₂ indicate respiratory alkalosis from hyperventilation. *HCO₃ (renal component):* Norms 24–28 mEq/L A ↓ HCO₃ and ↓ pH mean metabolic acidosis, which is the most common acid-base imbalance following injury from inadequate perfusion and lactic acid production. An ↑ HCO₃ and ↑ pH mean metabolic alkalosis. BE (base excess): Norms +2 to −2. Same as bicarbonate. A base excess of <-2 (also termed base deficit) is an indication of poor perfusion/inadequate resuscitation.

After an acute injury in which there is blood and fluid loss, intravenous therapy is initiated. Balanced electrolyte solutions (BES) such as normal saline solution (0.9% NaCl) and lactated Ringer's solution are usually started immediately. Oral fluids should not be given until the extent of the injury and the need for surgery is determined. Five percent dextrose in water (D_5W) is not the choice fluid replacement solution in trauma and shock states; it can cause water intoxication.

The client is typed and crossmatched for blood when significant blood loss occurs. Unless there is a significant loss of blood and fluid, the BES helps to restore fluid loss, increase circulation, and increase the blood pressure.

Excess and/or rapidly administered IV solutions can cause overhydration. Signs and symptoms of overhydration may include constant irritated cough, dyspnea, chest crackles, neck vein engorgement, and peripheral edema. A serum osmolality greater than 295 mOsm/kg indicates hypovolemia, and a serum osmolality less than 280 mOsm/kg indicates hypervolemia.

● SHOCK

Shock is the state of inadequate tissue perfusion that occurs when the hemostatic circulatory mechanism that regulates circulation fails. Shock can result from trauma because of a large loss of blood and fluid, which results in circulatory failure. Most shock-induced conditions are associated with trauma. A common feature of shock, regardless of the cause, is a low circulating blood volume in relation to vascular capacity. In a shock state, blood loss may not necessarily be from hemorrhaging but may result from "pooling" of blood in body cavities, limiting the amount of blood available to circulate. With shock, the cardiac output is insufficient to perfuse vital organs and tissues. There are four categories of shock: (1) hypovolemic, which includes hematogenic from hemorrhage; (2) cardiogenic; (3) septic; and (4) neurogenic.

Pathophysiology

The physiologic changes resulting from shock include a decrease in blood pressure; an initial increase in vasoconstriction of the blood vessels, particularly the skin, skeletal muscles, and kidneys but not the cerebral vessels; an increase in heart rate; a decrease in metabolism; and a decrease in renal function. Renal insufficiency can occur when hypotension is prolonged. Systolic blood pressure measurements must be 70 mm Hg and above to maintain kidney function and coronary perfusion.

When the blood pressure is low, the baroreceptors (pressure receptors) in the carotid sinus and aortic arch cause an increase in the systemic vasomotor activity that leads to vasoconstriction and cardiac acceleration to maintain homeostasis. The coronary arteries dilate with a decrease in blood volume. Inadequate oxygenation of cells leads to anaerobic metabolism and the formation of nonvolatile acids such as lactic acid. These changes result in an acid-base imbalance known as metabolic acidosis.

In early shock, fluid is shifted from the interstitial space to the intravascular space in order to compensate for the fluid deficit in the vascular system. As a result of this *early* shift, more fluid in the vascular system increases the venous return to the heart and increases the cardiac output. In *late* shock, fluid is forced from the intravascular space (blood vessels) back into the interstitial spaces (tissues). Table 17-4 describes the physiologic changes resulting from shock.

Etiology

Four types of shock—hypovolemic, cardiogenic, septic (also known as endotoxic or vasogenic), and neurogenic—are named for the clinical cause of the shock conditions. There are four classes of hypovolemic shock based on the amount of blood lost. With Class I there is approximately less than 1 1/2 units of blood loss. Class II may have up to 3 units or 1500 ml of blood loss. Severe shock occurs with Class III (3 to 4 units of blood loss) and Class IV (more than 4 units or 2000 ml of blood loss).

Table 17-5 describes the four types of shock, the clinical causes, and the rationale and physiologic changes that occur with each type. Hemorrhaging from injury or surgery, burns, or GI bleeding can cause hypovolemic shock. Cardiogenic shock may be caused by a myocardial infarction, cardiac failure, or cardiac tamponade. Severe bacterial infection and immunosuppressant therapy contribute to the development of septic shock. Neurogenic shock can result from high spinal anesthesia, severe emotional factors, or spinal cord injury.

Clinical Manifestations

Pale, cool skin; apprehension; restlessness; muscle weakness; a fall in blood pressure; tachycardia; tachypnea; and decreased urine output are characteristic signs and symptoms of the four types of shock. In shock, tachycardia is frequently seen before the blood pressure begins to fall. The increased heart rate is an early compensatory mechanism to increase circulation. A low pulse pressure (the difference between the systolic and diastolic pressures) of 20 mm Hg or less is indicative of impending shock. To maintain coronary

Table 17-4	**Physiologic Changes Resulting from Shock**
Physiologic Changes	**Rationale**
Arterial blood pressure: decreased	Reduced venous return to heart decreases cardiac output and arterial blood pressure (BP). Decrease in BP is sensed by pressoreceptorsin carotid sinus and aortic arch, which leads to immediate reflex increase in systemic vasomotor activity. (This center is found in the medulla.) Cardiac acceleration and vasoconstriction occur in order to maintain homeostasis with respect to blood pressure. This may be sufficient for early or impending shock.
Vasoconstriction of blood vessels: increased	Increased sympathetic nervous system activity causes vasoconstriction. Vasoconstriction tends to maintain blood pressure and reduce discrepancy between blood volume and vascular capacity (size). Vasoconstriction is greatest in skin, kidneys, and skeletal muscles and not as significant in cerebral vessels. Coronary arteries actually dilate with a decrease in blood volume. This is a compensatory mechanism to provide sufficient blood to the heart muscle (myocardium) for heart function.
Heart rate: increased	Heart rate is increased to overcome poor cardiac output and to increase circulation. Rapid, thready pulse is often one of the first identifiable signs of shock.
Metabolism: decreased	Fall in plasma hydrostatic pressure reduces urinary filtration. Unopposed plasma colloid osmotic pressure draws interstitial fluid into vascular bed. Blood loss results in loss of serum potassium, phosphate, and bicarbonate. Inadequate oxygenation of cells prevents their normal metabolism and leads to anaerobic metabolism and the formation of nonvolatile acids (acid metabolites), thus lowering serum pH values. With a fall in serum pH and a decrease in HCO_3, metabolic acidosis results. A rise in blood sugar is first seen due to release of epinephrine; later, blood sugar falls due to a decline in liver glycogen.
Kidney function: decreased	Low blood pressure causes inadequate circulation of blood to the kidneys. Renal ischemia is the result of a lack of perfusion to the kidneys. Renal insufficiency follows prolonged hypotension. Systolic blood pressure must be 70 mm Hg and above to maintain kidney function. One of the body's compensatory mechanisms in shock is to shunt blood around the kidneys to maintain intravascular fluid. Deficient blood supply makes tubule cells of kidneys more susceptible to injury. Urine output of less than 25 ml/h may be indicative of shock and/or decrease in renal function.

Table 17-5	Types and Clinical Causes of Shock	
Type of Shock	**Clinical Causes**	**Rationale and Physiologic Results**
Hypovolemic: Hematogenic (from hemorrhage)	Severe vomiting or diarrhea—acute dehydration Burns, intestinal obstruction, fluid shift to third space Hemorrhage that results from internal or external blood loss	Blood, plasma, and fluid loss from decreased circulating blood volume *Physiologic Results* 1. Decreased circulation 2. Decreased venous return 3. Reduced cardiac output 4. Increased afterload 5. Decreased preload 6. Decreased tissue perfusion
Cardiogenic	Myocardial infarction Severe arrhythmias Heart failure Cardiac tamponade Pulmonary embolism Blunt cardiac injury (formerly "cardiac contusion")	Because of these clinical problems, the pumping action of the heart is inadequate to maintain circulation (pump failure of myocardium). *Physiologic Results* 1. Decreased circulation 2. Decreased stroke volume 3. Decreased cardiac output 4. Increased preload 5. Increased afterload 6. Increased venous pressure 7. Decreased venous return 8. Decreased tissue perfusion

(continues)

Table 17-5	Types and Clinical Causes of Shock—*continued*	
Type of Shock	**Clinical Causes**	**Rationale and Physiologic Results**
Septic: Endotoxic Vasogenic	Severe systemic infections Septic abortion Peritonitis Debilitated conditions Immunosuppressant therapy	Septic shock is characterized by increased capillary permeability that permits plasma and fluid to pass into surrounding tissue. Often caused by a gram-negative organism. *Physiologic Results* 1. Vasodilatation and peripheral pooling of blood 2. Decreased circulation 3. Decreased preload 4. Decreased afterload, early shock and increased afterload, late shock 5. Decreased tissue perfusion
Neurogenic	Mild to moderate neurogenic shock: Emotional stress Acute pain Drugs: narcotics, barbiturates, phenothiazines High spinal anesthesia Acute gastric dilation Severe neurogenic shock: Spinal cord injury	Neurogenic shock is caused by loss of vascular tone. *Physiologic Results* 1. Decreased circulation 2. Vasodilatation and peripheral pooling of blood 3. Decreased cardiac output 4. Decreased venous return 5. Decreased tissue perfusion

circulation and renal function, the systolic pressure should be at least 70 mm Hg. Decreased central venous pressure (CVP), pulmonary artery pressure (PAP), and pulmonary capillary wedge pressure (PCWP) are present in all types of shock except cardiogenic shock. These pressures may be increased in cardiogenic shock.

Table 17-6 lists the clinical signs and symptoms and rationales related to the four types of shock.

Clinical Management

Immediate action needs to be taken when shock occurs so that it can be reversed. To maintain body fluid volume and particularly the intravascular fluid, fluid replacement must begin immediately for clients who are in shock or impending shock. Improvement of blood volume is needed to maintain tissue perfusion and oxygen delivery. The types of solutions for fluid replacement include crystalloids or balanced electrolyte (salt) solutions, and colloid solutions.

Crystalloids

Crystalloids expand the volume of the intravascular fluid. The two common types of crystalloids used for fluid replacement are normal saline solution (0.9% sodium chloride) and lactated Ringer's solution. Lactated Ringer's solution contains the electrolytes: sodium, potassium, calcium, and chloride with milliequivalents similar to plasma values. Normal saline solution (NSS) is a popular IV solution used for fluid replacement because it is iso-osmolar with approximately the same milliosmoles as plasma. Excess use of normal saline can increase the serum sodium and chloride levels. The lactate in the lactated Ringer's solution acts as a buffer to increase the pH, thus decreasing the acidotic state. Large quantities of lactated Ringer's solution may cause metabolic alkalosis. If the client has a liver disorder, the lactate is not metabolized into bicarbonate and lactic acid can result. Alternating the crystalloid solutions, such as normal saline solution and lactated Ringer's solution, usually maintains the body's electrolyte and acid-base balance. Table 17-7 lists the content of the two crystalloids that are used to replace fluid loss during shock.

The crystalloid 5% dextrose and water (D_5W) should NEVER be ordered for fluid replacement during shock. D_5W

Table 17-6 **Clinical Manifestations of Shock**

Signs and Symptoms	Types of Shock	Rationale
Skin: pale and/or cold and moist (except when caused by a spinal cord injury)	Hypovolemic Cardiogenic Neurogenic Septic (late)	Pale, cold, and/or moist skin results from increased sympathetic action. Peripheral vaso-constriction occurs and blood is shunted to vital organs. Skin is warm and flushed in early septic shock. Skin is warm and dry in neurogenic shock due to spinal cord injury.
Tachycardia (pulse fast and thready)	Hypovolemic Cardiogenic Septic	Increased pulse rate is frequently one of the early signs, except in neurogenic shock, in which the pulse is often slower than normal. Norepinephrine and epineph-rine, released by the adrenal medulla, increase the cardiac rate and myocardial contract-ibility. Tachycardia, pulse >100, generally occurs before arterial blood pressure falls.
Apprehension, restlessness	Hypovolemic Cardiogenic Septic Neurogenic	Apprehension and restlessness, early signs of shock, result from cerebral hypoxia. As the state of shock progresses, disorientation and confusion occur.
Muscle weakness, fatigue	Hypovolemic Cardiogenic Septic Neurogenic	Muscle weakness and fatigue, which occur early in shock, are the result of inadequate tissue perfusion.
Arterial blood pressure: early, a rise in or normal BP; late, a fall in BP	Hypovolemic Cardiogenic Septic Neurogenic	In early shock, blood pressure rises or is normal as a result of increased heart rate. As shock progresses, blood pres-sure falls because of a lack of cardiac and peripheral vaso-constriction compensation.
Pulse pressure: narrowed, <20 mm Hg		Narrowing of pulse pressure occurs because the systolic BP falls more rapidly than the diastolic BP.

(continues)

Table 17-6	Clinical Manifestations of Shock—*continued*	
Signs and Symptoms	**Types of Shock**	**Rationale**
Pressures: CVP, PAP, PCWP—decreased in hypovolemic, septic, neurogenic; increased in cardiogenic	Hypovolemic Cardiogenic Septic Neurogenic	Normal values: 1. Central venous pressure (CVP): 5–12 cm H_2O. With decreased blood volume, CVP <5 cm H_2O. 2. Pulmonary artery pressure (PAP): 20–30 mm Hg systolic, 10–15 mm Hg diastolic. With blood volume depletion or pooling of blood, PAP in hypovolemic <10 mm Hg, septic <10 mm Hg, neurogenic <10 mm Hg. In cardiogenic shock, PAP >30 mm Hg. 3. Pulmonary capillary wedge pressure (PCWP): 4–12 mm Hg. With blood volume depletion or peripheral pooling, the PCWP in hypovolemic, septic, and neurogenic <10 mm Hg and in cardiogenic >20 mm Hg.
Respiration: increased rate and depth (tachypnea)	Hypovolemic Cardiogenic Septic Neurogenic	Increased hydrogen ion concentration in the body stimulates the respiratory centers in the medulla, thus increasing the respiratory rate. Acid metabolites, e.g., lactic acid from anaerobic metabolism increases the rate and depth of respiration. Rapid respiration acts as a compensatory mechanism to decrease metabolic acidosis.
Temperature: subnormal	Hypovolemic Cardiogenic Neurogenic	Body temperature is subnormal in shock because of decreased circulation and decreased cellular function. In early septic shock, the temperature is elevated.
Urinary output: decreased	Hypovolemic Cardiogenic Septic Neurogenic	Oliguria (decreased urine output) occurs in shock because of decreased renal blood flow caused by renal vasoconstriction. Blood is shunted to the heart and brain. Urine output should be >25 ml/h.

Table 17-7	Crystalloids						
	mEq/L						
Crystalloids	**Na**	**K**	**Ca**	**Mg**	**Cl**	**Lactate**	**Gluconate**
0.9% NaCl (NSS)	154	—	—	—	154	—	—
Lactated Ringer's	130	4	3	—	109	28	—

is an iso-osmolar solution; if it is used continuously in large volumes, the solution in the body becomes hypo-osmolar. This can lead to intracellular fluid volume excess (water intoxication) or cellular swelling.

Intravenous solutions containing calcium, such as lactated Ringer's, should NOT be administered with blood transfusions. The calcium in the solution precipitates when it comes in contact with transfused blood. Normal saline solution (NSS) is the only solution used during blood transfusions.

Colloids

Colloids are substances that have a higher molecular weight than crystalloids and therefore cannot pass through the vascular membrane. Colloids increase intravascular fluid volume. When colloid therapy is used, less fluid is needed to reestablish the fluid volume in the vascular space. Table 17-8 lists the colloids that may be used for fluid replacement.

The colloids albumin 5%, plasma protein fraction (Plasmanate), and hetastarch increase the vascular volume to approximately the same amount that is infused. With low-molecular-weight dextran 40, the vascular fluid is expanded by one to two times the amount that is infused. With albumin 25%, the vascular volume is expanded four times the amount that is infused.

Crystalloids, Colloids, and Blood Products

Crystalloids are the first choice for treating hypovolemic shock. Crystalloids can restore fluid volume in the vascular and interstitial spaces and improve renal function; however, large quantities of crystalloids are needed. Excessive infusions of crystalloids might cause fluid overload in clients

Table 17-8 Colloids

Colloids*	Brand Names	Comments
Blood products	Packed RBCs Whole blood	Used to replace blood loss.
Albumin, 5% or 25%	Albuminar Plasbumin	Not used in acute shock; 1–4 ml/min.
Plasma protein fraction, 5%	Plasmanate	Rapid infusion rate can decrease blood pressure.
Hetastarch	Hespan	Synthetic starch similar to human glycogen. Very expensive.
Dextran 40	Dextran	Low-molecular-weight dextran 40 may prolong bleeding time.

*Colloid therapy is more expensive than crystalloid therapy.

who are elderly or who have heart disease. Frequently, a combination of crystalloids and colloids is used for fluid replacement. If severe blood loss occurs, blood transfusions may be necessary after infusion of 1 to 2 L of crystalloids. Each fluid replacement situation differs and each individual situation must be evaluated separately.

There are suggested formulas for restoring fluid loss, especially for clients in hypovolemic shock who have had some blood loss, moderate blood loss, or massive amounts of blood and body fluid loss. The simplest formula for fluid replacement is the 3:1 rule; for every 1 ml of blood lost, 3 ml of crystalloid solution are necessary to restore fluid volume. If hypotension persists despite 2 L of crystalloid solution replacement, a blood transfusion should be considered. When administering normal saline solution (NSS) or lactated Ringer's solution for hypovolemic shock, the IV solutions may be given rapidly at first to decrease the symptoms of shock. Later, the flow rate should be slowed. Table 17-9 lists the four classes of hypovolemic shock with their estimated amount of blood loss and percent of blood volume loss (% BV), changes in vital signs, pulse pressure, urine output, and types of fluid replacement.

Table 17-9	Classes of Hypovolemic Shock and Appropriate Fluid Replacement			
Characteristic Effects of Hypovolemic Shock	**Class I Mild Shock**	**Class II Moderate Shock**	**Class III Severe Shock**	**Class IV Severe Shock**
Blood loss	<750 ml or 1½ units	750–1500 ml or 1½–3 units	1500–2000 ml or 3–4 units	>2000 ml or >4 units
Blood loss (% BV)	<15%	15–30%	30–40%	>40%
Heart rate (bpm)	<100	>100	>120	>140
Blood pressure	Normal	Normal to slightly decreased	Decreased	Decreased
Pulse pressure	Normal or increased	Decreased from normal	Decreased 20–25 mm Hg	Decreased 20 mm Hg or less
Urine output	>30 ml/h	20–30 ml/h	5–15 ml/h	0–5 ml/h
Fluid replacement (3:1 rule) 3 ml replaced for 1 ml of blood loss	Crystalloid: NSS or lactated Ringer's	Crystalloid: NSS or lactated Ringer's	Crystalloid and blood	Crystalloid and blood

Vasopressors

Many years ago the first and foremost treatment of shock was to administer a vasopressor drug. The drug constricts the dilated blood vessels that occur with shock and raises the blood pressure. Vasopressors act as a temporary treatment for shock; if the cause of the shock is not alleviated, the progress of shock increases. Today, vasopressors are only used for severe shock or types of shock that do not respond to treatment. Note that vasopressors are *not* effective in the treatment of hypovolemic shock because constricting the blood vessels does not aid in the circulation of blood when the cause is most obvious, a lack of blood or fluid. Replacing blood or fluid volume loss should correct this type of shock. Table 17-10 outlines the clinical management for alleviating four types of clinical shock: hypovolemic, cardiogenic, septic, and neurogenic.

When vasopressors are used, cardiac dysrhythmias may occur. Levarterenol bitartrate (Levophed) is norepinephrine,

Table 17-10	Clinical Management of Shock States			
Hypovolemic Shock	**Cardiogenic Shock**	**Septic Shock**	**Neurogenic Shock**
1. O_2	1. O_2	1. O_2	1. O_2
2. IV fluids, such as	2. IV therapy is	2. IV therapy	2. IV therapy
a. Lactated Ringer's	limited when	crystalloids	3. Vasopressors,
b. Normal saline	pulmonary	3. Vasopressors	if necessary
c. Blood products	congestion is	for nonre-	4. Atropine for
3. No vasopressors	present and	sponsiveness	symptomatic
4. Electrolyte	venous	4. Blood	bradycardia
replacement	pressure is	cultures	
	elevated. Close	5. IV antibiotics	
	monitoring of		
	CVP and PCWP		
	3. Vasopressors, if		
	necessary		
	4. Antiarrythmics		
	Sodium		
	nitroprusside/		
	Nipride, nitro-		
	glycerin/NTG;		
	(decrease pre-		
	load and		
	decrease		
	afterload).		
	Intropic drugs		
	(e.g., dobuta-		
	mine amrinone/		
	Inocor)		
	Sedatives		
	Diuretics		

Note: Examples of vasopressors are (1) levarterenol bitartrate/Levophed, (2) dopamine hydrochloride/Intropin, (3) epinephrine infusion.

which is a strong vasopressor. It increases the blood pressure and cardiac output by constricting blood vessels. Epinephrine works in the same manner. Dopamine HCl (Intropin) is a catecholamine precursor of norepinephrine. It increases blood pressure and cardiac output. It also dilates renal vessels at a low dose, thus increasing renal blood flow and the glomerular filtration rate. Levophed causes vasoconstriction, which affects the renal arteries and can decrease renal function. Vasopressors are titrated according to the blood pressure and should be checked every 2 to 5 minutes.

Dobutamine is an adrenergic drug that moderately increases blood pressure by increasing the heart rate and cardiac output. Dobutamine is effective in increasing myocardial contractility.

● CLINICAL CONSIDERATIONS: TRAUMA AND SHOCK

1. In trauma and shock, check for signs and symptoms that may indicate hypovolemia and shock, such as restlessness, apprehension, confusion, tachycardia, narrowing of the pulse pressure (20 mm Hg or less), tachypnea, and cool and clammy skin.

2. Urinary output may be decreased. Report if urine output is less than 25 ml per hour or 200 ml per 8 hours. If the serum creatinine is elevated, renal dysfunction may be present due to a lack of renal perfusion related to shock.

3. Recognize that the hemoglobin, hematocrit, and BUN may be elevated during a hypovolemic state. With a large amount of blood loss, the hemoglobin drops, but not immediately.

4. Monitor intravenous therapy. The choice crystalloids are normal saline solution (NSS) and lactated Ringer's solution. Five percent dextrose and water should not be used to correct hypovolemia during shock.

5. Crystalloids are usually administered rapidly during early shock to increase blood pressure, hydrate the client, and increase urine output. Check for fluid overload in the young, older adult, and debilitated person. Signs and symptoms of overhydration are chest crackles, constant irritated cough, neck and/or hand vein engorgement, and dyspnea.

6. A simple formula for fluid replacement is the 3:1 rule; for every 1 ml of blood loss, 3 ml of crystalloid solution are needed to restore fluid volume. If hypotension persists despite 2 L of rapidly administered crystalloid solutions, blood transfusion is probably needed.

7. Colloids are used to treat shock when less fluid is needed.

8. Vasopressors are seldom used except to treat progressive shock and nonresponsive treatment to shock. Dopamine is the initial vasopressor of choice

because it does not affect renal arteries at a low dose. Other vasopressors cause vasoconstriction, thus decreasing blood flow to the kidneys and decreasing renal function.

9. Metabolic acidosis (lactic acidosis) frequently results from cellular damage and lack of fluid and nutrients to cells associated with severe hypovolemia and shock. In acidosis, the pH is below 7.35, HCO_3 is below 24 mEq/L, and base excess (BE) is less than -2.

● CLIENT MANAGEMENT

Assessment

● Check vital signs and report signs and symptoms that may indicate hypovolemia and shock, such as tachycardia, narrowing of the pulse pressure (20 mm Hg or less is an indicator of shock), tachypnea, and cool, clammy skin.

● Obtain a drug history. Report if the client is taking insulin, potassium-wasting diuretics, digoxin, steroid preparations, beta blockers, or calcium channel blockers.

● Assess the behavioral and neurologic status of the injured client and/or the client in shock. Irritability, apprehension, restlessness, and confusion are symptoms of a fluid volume deficit. Apprehension and restlessness are early symptoms of shock.

● Check urinary output. Less than 25 ml per hour or 200 ml per 8 hours may indicate fluid volume deficit or renal insufficiency. In severe shock, severe oliguria or anuria may occur.

● Check laboratory results, especially hemoglobin, hematocrit, arterial blood gases (ABG), serum electrolytes, BUN, and serum creatinine. Report abnormal findings.

Nursing Diagnoses

● *Deficient Fluid Volume,* related to traumatic injury and shock

● *Excess Fluid Volume,* related to massive infusions of crystalloids

● *Impaired Tissue Perfusion* (renal, cardiopulmonary, cerebral, and peripheral), related to decreased blood volume and circulation secondary to hypovolemia and shock

● *Impaired Urinary Elimination,* less than body requirement, related to fluid volume deficit and shock

Interventions

● Monitor vital signs. Compare the vital signs with those taken on admission and report differences immediately.

● Check skin color and turgor. Note changes; pallor; gray, cold, clammy skin; and poor skin turgor are symptoms of shock and fluid volume deficit.

● Monitor IV therapy. Crystalloids are usually administered rapidly initially to hydrate the client, increase blood pressure, and increase urine output. Normal saline solution (NSS) and lactated Ringer's solution are the crystalloids of choice.

● Auscultate the lungs for crackles. Overhydration from excessive fluids and rapid administration of IV fluids can cause pulmonary edema.

● Check for neck vein engorgement when overhydration is suspected.

● Check for pitting edema in the feet and legs. Weigh the client daily to determine if there is fluid retention.

● Monitor central venous pressure (CVP) and pulmonary capillary wedge pressure (PCWP), which are needed to adjust fluid balance. The norm for CVP is 5–12 cm/H_2O or 2–4 mm Hg (+ to −2), and for PCWP is 4–12 mm Hg. Keeping PCWP between 12 and 15 mm Hg in shock conditions provides the filling pressure required for adequate stroke volume and cardiac output. If PCWP drops below 10 mm Hg, administration of fluid is usually needed. If PCWP is greater than 18 mm HG, fluid restriction may be necessary.

● Monitor urine output. Hourly urine should be measured and if less than 25 ml/h, the IV fluid rate should be increased as ordered. Do not forget to check for overhydration when pushing fluids, IV or orally.

● Report systolic blood pressure of 80 mm Hg or less immediately. Kidney damage can occur due to poor renal perfusion during hypotensive states.

● Monitor laboratory results. Compare laboratory test results with those taken on admission.

● Monitor ECG readings and report arrhythmias (ST–T changes), which may be indicative of a potassium imbalance or cardiac ischemia.

● Monitor arterial blood gases (ABGs). Metabolic acidosis frequently results from cellular damage due to severe hypovolemia and shock. In acidosis, the pH is below 7.35, HCO_3 is below 24 mEq/L, and base excess (BE) is less than -2. Respiratory acidosis may also result due to the lungs' inability to excrete carbon dioxide.

Evaluation/Outcome

● Evaluate whether the cause of the shock has been controlled or eliminated.

● Verify that the client remains free of shocklike symptoms.

● Evaluate that the urine output is within normal range (600 to 1400 ml/per 24 hours).

● Evaluate the effects of IV therapy in controlling or alleviating shock.

● Determine that the laboratory results are within normal ranges.

CHAPTER 18

Burns and Burn Shock

Linda Bucher, RN, DNSc

INTRODUCTION

An estimated 2 million Americans seek medical care for burn injuries every year. Of these, 50,000 will be hospitalized and usually in an acute care setting that specializes in the care of burn victims. Care delivered in the first few hours after a burn injury is crucial to the patient's survival and functional recovery. Recovery from a major burn injury occurs over a lifetime.

PATHOPHYSIOLOGY

The pathophysiologic responses to a moderate or major burn are multisystem and occur in phases. The emergent/ resuscitative phase (shock phase) represents the first 48 hours after a burn injury and is characterized by burn shock and massive edema (fluid accumulation) at the site of the burn injury. The acute-wound coverage phase (stage of diuresis) of a burn injury begins with the reversal of the shock state and is characterized by diuresis (fluid remobilization). The acute-wound coverage phase ends with wound closure and represents the longest phase of a burn injury that is managed in the acute care setting. The rehabilitation phase (convalescent phase) of a burn injury begins on admission and continues throughout life. Table 18-1 summarizes the physiologic changes and the major lab findings associated with a major burn in the emergent/resuscitative phase of a burn injury.

Table 18-1	Multisystem Responses to Burn Injury in the Emergent/ Resuscitative Phase (0–48 hours)	
System	**Physiologic Change**	**Lab Findings**
Cardiovascular	Increased capillary permeability in area of burn injury due to inflammatory response; loss of plasma protein and electrolytes; increase in interstitial fluid → massive edema with decrease in intravascular volume → hypovolemia → decreased cardiac output, hypotension, tachycardia → burn shock.	Increased serum osmolality secondary to loss of vascular fluid and hemoconcentration. Elevated hematocrit secondary to dehydration and a greater loss of liquid blood components compared to hemolysis. Electrolytes: Decreased serum sodium and calcium secondary to movement of fluid from vascular space to interstitial space (edema). Increased serum potassium secondary to release of intracellular potassium from damaged tissues at burn site.
Respiratory	Edema and obstruction of the upper airway secondary to direct burn injury; direct damage to pulmonary tissue from inhalation of noxious gases → broncho-constriction, pulmonary edema, and respiratory distress; respiratory distress secondary to circumferential chest burns that limit chest excursion.	Decreased PaO_2 secondary to pulmonary damage and/or respiratory distress. Increased carboxyhemoglobin levels secondary to carbon monoxide (by-product of combustion) poisoning.

(continues)

Table 18-1	**Multisystem Responses to Burn Injury in the Emergent/ Resuscitative Phase (0–48 hours) —*continued***	
System	**Physiologic Change**	**Lab Findings**
Renal	Decreased urine output secondary to decreased renal blood flow, increased secretion of antidiuretic hormone (ADH) and aldosterone; acute renal failure secondary to burn shock; hemomyo-globinuria secondary to massive full-thickness burns or electrical burn injury → acute renal failure.	Elevated urine specific gravity secondary to hypovolemia. Elevated blood, urea, nitrogen (BUN), and creatinine secondary to acute renal failure. Hemoglobinuria secondary to release of free hemoglobin (from hemolysis at burn site) from massive burn injury. Myoglobinuria secondary to release of myoglobin from massive burn injury.
Gastrointestinal	Paralytic ileus secondary to burn shock; hypermetabolic state.	Metabolic acidosis secondary to the loss of bicarbonate ions that accompanies sodium loss. Elevated glucose secondary to release of catecholamines (stress response to burn injury). Decreased protein secondary to loss of protein at burn injury site.
Musculoskeletal	Development of compartment syndrome secondary to circumferential burns of the extremities.	Elevated creatine kinase enzymes due to massive tissue damage from burn injury.
Neurologic	Changes in level of consciousness, orientation; headache, seizures secondary to shock, hypoxia, elevated carboxyhemoglobin levels (smoke inhalation injury) and/or electrolyte imbalances.	

● ETIOLOGY

Most burns are preventable. The very young and the very old are at greater risk for experiencing and dying from a burn injury compared to young and middle-aged adults. Thermal burns are the most common type of burn injury and occur because of fires (e.g., motor vehicle crash), scalds (e.g., bath water), contact (e.g., iron), or steam (e.g., cooking). Chemical burns occur as a result of the ingestion of, contact with, or inhalation of acids (e.g., hydrochloric acid), bases (e.g., bleach), desiccants (drying agents) or vesicants (e.g., blistering gases). Electrical burns can result from exposure to high voltage (e.g., lightning) or low voltage (e.g., electrical outlet) energy sources. At times, neglect or abuse may account for a burn injury. Public education aimed at prevention (e.g., "Stop, Drop, Roll, Cool"; smoke detectors) has contributed to a decrease in the incidence and severity of burn injuries.

● CLINICAL MANIFESTATIONS

Classification of Burns

Burns are classified according to the depth of tissue involved. The skin consists of three layers: the epidermis, which is the outermost layer of skin; the dermis, known as the true skin and the location of the hair follicles, nerves, blood vessels, and sweat glands; and the subcutaneous tissue, which consists primarily of fatty tissue and blood vessels. Beneath the subcutaneous tissue lie the muscles and bones. Table 18-2 presents the characteristics of burns of varying depths.

Determination of Burn Size: Percentage of Body Surface Area (BSA) Burned

There are several methods used in non-burn care settings to estimate percentage of BSA burned. The palmar method uses the patient's palm (excluding fingers) to represent 1% of the total BSA. It is a quick method for estimating the percentage of total BSA burned in adults and children. The rule of nines is another easy method used to estimate total BSA burned. This method uses 9% or multiples of 9 in calculating the burned surface area. Figure 18-1 describes the rule of nines. The rule of nines is not appropriate for estimating burn size

Table 18-2	Classification and Defining Characteristics of Burns			
	Superficial (first degree)	**Superficial Partial-Thickness (first to second degree)**	**Deep Partial-Thickness (second degree)**	**Full-Thickness (third degree)**
Depth	Epidermal layer only	Epidermal layer and upper layers of dermis	Epidermis and most of dermis	Epidermis, dermis, subcutaneous tissue; may extend to muscle and bone
Physical Characteristics	Erythema, no blisters or edema; blanching with pressure	Blister formation; when blister erupts, wound is moist, bright cherry red or mottled in color; positive blanching with pressure	Slightly moist to dry; dark red to pale in color; may see blanching with pressure	Dry, leathery, firm; pearly white to waxy to charred; no blanching with pressure
Degree of Pain	Mild to moderate pain	Very painful	Very painful	Is sensitive to touch
Healing Time	3–5 days; injured epidermis peels away leaving healed tissue	10–21 days with minimal scarring	21–35 days with no infection; if infected, wound will convert to a full-thickness wound	Requires grafting, which may take months for wound to heal
Possible Causes	Sunburn, scald	Contact or flash burn	Chemical or flame burn	Flame or electrical burn

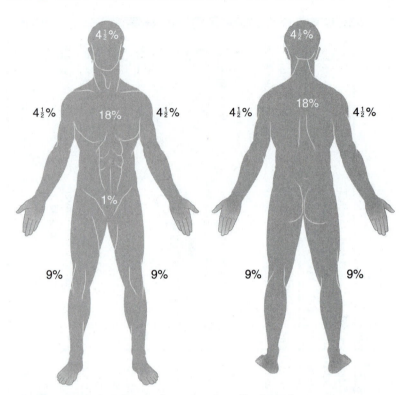

FIGURE 18-1 Rules of nines for estimation of body surface.

in children because a child's body has proportions that are different from an adult.

The Lund and Browder chart allows for the most accurate calculation of total BSA burned in children and adults. It accounts for changes in BSA across the life span as well as differences in burn severity (e.g., partial-thickness, full-thickness). This method is used to determine burn size in most burn care settings once the patient is stabilized.

Management of Burns

In 2001, the American Burn Association (ABA) revised the criteria for the care of burn victims. According to the ABA, burn victims meeting any of the following criteria should be referred to a burn center for optimal care:

● Second-degree burns covering > 10% BSA

● Any third-degree burns

● Any patient with any percentage of burn having any of the following:

  ● Potential or presence of airway or inhalation injury

  ● Any percentage of burn involving the face, hands, feet, joints, or perineum

  ● Any circumferential burn (e.g., burn surrounding an extremity)

  ● Any chemical or electrical burn

  ● Any patient with associated injuries (e.g., fractures) or preexisting medical problems (e.g., diabetes) that would complicate care, prolong recovery, or endanger life

  ● Any patient for whom neglect or abuse is suspected

CLINICAL MANAGEMENT

Patients with minor burns (e.g., superficial burns, partial-thickness burns < 10% of BSA) are generally managed by a primary care provider or in the emergency department. These patients rarely require hospitalization. Management of these burn wounds is focused on cleanliness, prevention of infection, and comfort. The burn should be cleansed gently with soap and water 2–3 times a day and then covered with a topical agent (e.g., silver sulfadiazine). Patients should also receive tetanus toxoid. Finally, oral analgesics (e.g., acetaminophen, ibuprofen) may be used to control the pain or discomfort.

Patients sustaining a major burn are generally treated in a burn care center. Management of these patients involves a multidisciplinary team that includes physicians, nurses, physical/occupational therapists, respiratory therapists, social workers, nutritionists, and counselors.

In the emergent-resuscitative phase (0–48 hours) care is focused on the management of airway-breathing-circulation (ABCs), fluid resuscitation, maintenance of electrolyte balance, aggressive pain management, and early wound care. Management of the patient's airway and breathing may range from the application of supplemental oxygen via a nasal cannula to endotracheal intubation and mechanical ventilation. Circulation is maintained by appropriate fluid resuscitation to prevent and/or treat burn shock and maintain electrolyte balance. Fluid resuscitation begins for any patient who has sustained a second-degree burn > 10% of BSA or any third-degree burn.

Several formulas have been developed for the initiation of fluid therapy in the emergent-resuscitative phase of burn care. The Parkland formula is the most common formula used in burn care centers. Table 18-3 describes how to calculate the intravenous fluid needs of a burn patient over the first 48 hours postburn. The end points of fluid resuscitation are urine output > 1.0 cc/kg/hour and stable vital signs.

Pain management is achieved through the use of intravenous narcotics. Initial wound care includes washing the wound surface with mild soap or aseptic solutions. Next, the wound is debrided of all nonviable tissue and an antibacterial agent (e.g., mafenide acetate) is applied. Finally, the wound is covered with an occlusive dressing.

The onset of the acute-wound coverage phase is marked by diuresis (fluid remobilization). The edema that occurs in the first 48 hours of the burn injury begins to resolve as the fluid that has accumulated in the interstitial space shifts back into the intravascular space. Hemodilution (decreased

Table 18-3	**Parkland Formula for Fluid Replacement during the Emergent-Resuscitative Phase of Burn Care**	
0–24 Hours	**24–48 Hours**	
4 cc lactated Ringer's solution × body weight in kilograms × percentage of BSA burned = 24-hour total fluid requirement ▪ Administer ½ of 24-hour total over first 8 hours postburn* ▪ Administer ¼ of 24-hour total over second 8 hours ▪ Administer ¼ of 24-hour total over third 8 hours	Dextrose and water Colloids (e.g., albumin) Titrate fluids down every 2 hours to maintain urine output at > 1 cc/kg/hour	

*First hour of this time period starts at the time of burn injury, not time of admission. For example, if the patient arrived at the burn center 45 minutes after the burn injury, the initial fluids (½ of the 24-hour total) would need to be infused over 7¼ hours.

hematocrit) may occur as a result of this fluid shift. Anemia (decreased red blood cell count) from hemolysis (destruction of red blood cells) at the burn site may become evident at this time. Intravenous therapy is usually limited during this time as the patient may actually be at risk for overhydration (fluid overload).

The risk for infection and sepsis is greatest during this phase and wound care becomes paramount. Additional management goals during this phase include ongoing pain control, nutritional support, and psychosocial support. Wound care techniques will vary based on the depth and location of the burn wound but will include wound debridement (excision of nonviable tissue) and the surgical grafting of donor skin or the placement of temporary wound coverings (e.g., Biobrane). Daily wound care involves wound assessment, and protection of the injured tissue, the granulation tissue, or new skin grafts. Antibiotics are ordered as needed and based on the results of wound cultures.

Wound care is often very painful and a source of great stress for patients. Patients are medicated before and during (as needed) wound care procedures with either intravenous or oral narcotics. Antianxiety, as well as complementary therapies (e.g., music therapy) may be helpful in managing the patient's stress and pain.

Patients with major burns require a greater number of calories to compensate for the hypermetabolic state that accompanies the burn injury. Early enteral (preferred) or parenteral nutrition is initiated to assist with wound healing. Nutritional support is discontinued once patients are able to consume 80–90% of the required calories.

A major burn injury will have a dramatic and permanent effect on the patient as well as the patient's family. Psychosocial support is critical and the patient and family will require assistance to deal with the complexities of the burn care and to adjust to the lifelong, psychological impact of the burn (e.g., change in appearance, inability to perform usual role functions).

The rehabilitation (convalescent) phase is the final phase of burn management and actually overlaps the first two phases. Starting at admission to the burn center, the goals for rehabilitation include the accomplishment of functional and cosmetic reconstruction, the achievement of the best functional status possible, and the return of the patient to a useful role in society. During this period, the patient will be taught home exercises and may be fitted with pressure appliances (e.g., Jobst garment) to reduce scarring and/or splints to prevent contractures.

●CLIENT MANAGEMENT

Assessment

- Obtain a thorough history of the burn injury, including time of injury, situation surrounding injury (e.g., child left alone in home), type of burn (e.g., thermal, electrical), and initial treatment measures.
- Obtain a complete health history from patient or patient's family.
- Complete a primary survey that includes an assessment of ABCs. Once ABCs are stabilized, obtain vital signs (blood pressure, pulse, respiratory rate, temperature) and a baseline weight.
- Perform a complete assessment of the burn injury including a determination of total BSA burned.
- Perform a complete head-to-toe assessment.

Nursing Diagnoses

- Deficient fluid volume, related to fluid shift to the burn area
- Risk for imbalanced fluid volume, related to fluid shift from burn area to vascular system and fluid resuscitation efforts
- Acute pain, related to burn injury
- Impaired skin integrity, related to burn injury
- Imbalanced nutrition, less than body requirements, related to hypermetabolic state postburn injury
- Risk for impaired gas exchange, related to inhalation injury, tracheal edema, bronchoconstriction
- Risk for infection, related to burn wounds
- Risk for disturbed body image, related to burn injury

● Risk for impaired urinary elimination, related to hypovolemia

Interventions

Deficient Fluid Volume

● Monitor vital signs and level of consciousness every 15 minutes to every hour during the first 48 hours.

● Report signs of impending burn shock: tachycardia, hypotension, decreased peripheral pulses, altered level of consciousness, oliguria.

● Administer intravenous fluids using Parkland formula or as ordered by physician.

● Monitor urine output every hour and urine specific gravity according to unit policy. Report urine output < 1cc/kg/hour.

● Monitor laboratory tests: electrolytes, BUN, creatinine, arterial blood gases, CBC and report abnormal findings or significant changes.

● Maintain strict intake and output, including daily weight.

● Replace electrolytes as ordered.

● Evaluate effectiveness of fluid resuscitation on tissue perfusion (e.g., urine output, mentation, peripheral pulses, blood pressure).

Risk for Imbalanced Fluid Volume

● Monitor vital signs every hour or more frequently if necessary.

● Monitor intake and output, including daily weight.

● Observe for signs of fluid overload: jugular vein distention, shortness of breath.

● Monitor breath sounds and report the presence of crackles and tachypnea.

● Monitor laboratory tests: electrolytes, BUN, creatinine, CBC, and report significant changes from baseline.

● Monitor urine output for increase or decrease in volume.

Evaluation/Outcome

● Fluid volume has been restored and maintained: vital signs are normal or at baseline for patient, positive skin turgor (in non-burn areas), urine output and urine specific gravity are within normal limits, mucous membranes are moist, laboratory values (e.g., electrolytes, BUN, creatinine, CBC) are within normal limits.

● Weight is stable.

● Breath sounds are clear or baseline for patient. Respiratory rate is within normal limits or baseline for patient.

● Patient is oriented to person, place, and time or at baseline orientation.

Gastrointestinal (GI) Surgical Interventions

Erlinda Wheeler, RN, PhD

INTRODUCTION

Fluid and electrolyte changes may occur in a client following a surgical procedure. Surgical interventions to correct gastrointestinal problems put the client at greater risk for fluid and electrolyte disturbances than other types of surgical procedures. Diagnostic testing and preparation for gastrointestinal (GI) surgery may further increase the client's risk for fluid, electrolyte, and acid-base imbalances. Postoperatively, the client may be NPO (nothing by mouth), have a gastrointestinal drainage tube, and have delayed peristalsis, which further contribute to the imbalances. Preexisting cardiopulmonary, endocrine, and renal conditions in conjunction with the use of diuretics, glucocorticoids, and insulin place the client undergoing GI surgery at a high risk for fluid, electrolyte, and acid-base imbalances. Assessment of these imbalances must begin preoperatively and continue postoperatively. Impairments in fluid volume status can occur rapidly; thus, astute assessment skills and timely interventions are essential to prevent or decrease potential complications.

ELECTROLYTE CONCENTRATION IN THE GASTROINTESTINAL TRACT

Electrolytes are most plentiful in the gastrointestinal tract. The concentration of sodium, potassium, and bicarbonate ions is higher in the intestines than in the stomach. Chloride

Table 19-1	Concentration of Electrolytes in the Stomach and Intestine (mEq/L)					
Area	Body Fluid	Na$^+$	K$^+$	Cl$^-$	HCO$_3^-$	
Stomach	Gastric juice	60.4	9.2	100*	0–14	H^{+*}
Small intestine	Intestinal juice	111.3*	20*	104.2*	31*	

*Electrolytes that are highly concentrated in these areas.

ion concentration is approximately the same in the intestines and stomach. However, the hydrogen ion is in higher concentration in the stomach and the bicarbonate ion concentration is higher in the intestines. A decrease in the number of hydrogen ions in the stomach can cause metabolic alkalosis, while a loss of the number of bicarbonate ions in the intestines can result in metabolic acidosis. Table 19-1 lists the concentrations of electrolytes in the stomach and intestine.

PATHOPHYSIOLOGY, ETIOLOGY, AND CLINICAL MANIFESTATIONS RELATED TO GI PROBLEMS

Clients undergoing a minor surgical procedure usually do not experience fluid, electrolyte, and/or acid-base disturbances. Following a major surgical procedure, sodium and water may be retained and potassium may be lost. Many clients undergoing gastrointestinal surgery experience fluid and electrolyte imbalances prior to surgery that often put them in a debilitated state. Vomiting and/or diarrhea are common conditions that may indicate a gastrointestinal problem that calls for surgical intervention. When fluids are lost, important electrolytes such as sodium, chloride, potassium, bicarbonate (intestine), and hydrogen (stomach) are also lost. Treatment of these fluid and electrolyte imbalances must be considered both prior to surgery and in conjunction with the concurrent fluid losses during the procedure. Replacement of fluid and electrolyte losses is necessary before, during, and following surgery.

Prolonged vomiting and/or diarrhea results in severe fluid volume deficit. This condition can lead to decreased urine output, tachycardia, and hypertension. The fluid loss results in a hemoconcentration, causing the hemoglobin, hematocrit, and BUN levels to rise. Fluid balance and adequate urine output need to be restored prior to surgery. If a gastric tube is inserted prior to surgery, fluid and electrolytes are lost through GI suctioning. Serum sodium and potassium levels may be decreased, normal, or elevated. The sodium, chloride, and potassium are lost because of vomiting, diarrhea, or GI suctioning; however, if the fluid volume deficit is severe, the hemoconcentration causes elevated serum electrolyte levels. With GI disturbances, hydrogen and chloride ions are lost from the gastric juices, resulting in metabolic alkalosis. Frequently, potassium is also lost, so the imbalance is hypokalemic alkalosis. Table 19-2 lists the causes, pathophysiologic changes, and clinical manifestations related to GI disturbances.

Table 19-2	Pathophysiologic Changes, Etiology, and Clinical Manifestations Related to Gastrointestinal Problems Prior to Surgery	
Etiology	**Pathophysiologic Changes**	**Clinical Manifestations**
Vomiting/diarrhea	ECF and ICF loss	Tachycardia
	Electrolyte loss (sodium, chloride, potassium, and hydrogen or bicarbonate)	Postural hypotension
		Dry mucous membrane
		Decreased skin turgor
	Acid-base imbalance (if severe)	Decreased urine output
	Hypokalemic alkalosis: loss of hydrogen and potassium from stomach	*Laboratory Changes*
		↑ Hemoglobin
		↑ Hematocrit
		↑ BUN
		↓, Normal, ↑ Sodium
	Metabolic acidosis: loss of bicarbonate from intestines	↓, ↑ Potassium
		↓ Bicarbonate (diarrhea)
Gastric suction	Prolonged GI suctioning: similar to vomiting	Laboratory changes similar to vomiting

⬤ CLINICAL MANAGEMENT

Clinical management of fluid, electrolyte, and acid-base imbalances for GI surgical clients can occur both preoperatively and postoperatively. Preoperative and postoperative management are addressed separately here.

Preoperative Management

Clients who are vomiting, have diarrhea, or are receiving gastric suctioning should be assessed for fluid and electrolyte imbalances. Fluid and electrolyte replacements are necessary prior to surgery to restore balance and maintain adequate urine output. Once signs, symptoms, and laboratory changes show fluid and electrolyte imbalances, identifying the sources of these imbalances is essential. Proper maintenance of body fluids and electrolytes decreases complications and promotes a speedy recovery period.

In healthy preoperative clients, long periods of being NPO prior to surgery are unnecessary. The usual practice is to keep the client NPO after midnight prior to surgery to prevent pulmonary aspiration. As a result of modern anesthesia, vomiting and aspiration rarely occur. The newer recommendations by the American Society of Anesthesiology (ASA) is to allow clear liquids up to 2 hours before elective surgery, depending on the type of surgery and the institution's policies.

Postoperative Management

During surgery fluid loss due to bleeding and/or shifting of intravascular fluid to the surgical site (third-space fluid) can cause a decrease in the volume of circulating vascular fluid. A balanced electrolyte (salt) solution such as lactated Ringer's is usually administered during the intraoperative period. Administration of blood or blood products is dependent on the amount of blood loss and condition of the client. Central venous pressure is monitored during the operative procedure in high-risk clients to determine fluid replacement.

Surgical procedures, anesthesia, trauma, and pain contribute to an increased release of the antidiuretic hormone (ADH). Excessive release of ADH is called the syndrome of inappropriate ADH or SIADH. Excess ADH release may persist for 12 to 24 hours after surgery. This causes fluid to be reabsorbed from the renal tubules and decreased urine output. Surgical procedures can also promote the increased secretion of aldosterone, resulting in sodium and fluid retention and potassium loss. Older adults and young children experiencing gastrointestinal surgical interventions are at the highest risk for the neuroendocrine response (ADH and aldosterone).

Gastric or intestinal intubation (tube passed into the stomach or intestines for suctioning purposes) is often performed before surgery. This alleviates vomiting due to an obstruction in the gastrointestinal tract or decompresses the stomach or bowel, or both, before and after the operative procedure.

Following abdominal surgery, a gastric or an intestinal tube is frequently inserted to remove secretions until peristalsis returns and to relieve abdominal distention. For gastric intubation, a Levine tube or Salem sump is inserted via the nose into the stomach. For an intestinal intubation, a Miller-Abbott tube or Cantor tube is inserted via the nose to the stomach and into the intestines. Intestinal tubes are longer than gastric tubes and they contain a small balloon filled with air or mercury that helps the tube move into the lower intestines. Urine output should be at least 25 ml/h and preferably 30 to 50 ml/h. Three liters or more of intravenous balanced salt solution are usually administered during the first 24 hours for fluid loss. Electrolytes are replaced according to the serum electrolyte levels.

Solid particles may accumulate and obstruct the gastrointestinal tubing. Irrigating the tube assures patency and proper drainage. Frequent irrigations using large amounts of water should be avoided to prevent electrolyte washout. Gastric tubes are irrigated at specific intervals with small amounts of normal saline solution to prevent electrolyte loss. Because suction removes fluids and electrolytes, oral fluid intake is restricted and parenteral therapy is initiated. Sips of water can alleviate the dryness in the mouth and lessen irritation in the throat, if allowed. However, one must be cautioned that water dilutes the electrolytes in the stomach and the suction then removes them.

A feeling of fullness, vomiting, and abdominal distention are signs and symptoms that peristalsis has not returned.

Checking periodically for bowel sounds is necessary to determine when peristalsis has returned.

An H_2 receptor antagonist (H_2 blocker) such as cimetidine (Tagamet), ranitidine (Zantac), or famotidine (Pepcid) is commonly administered to clients with a gastric tube. This group of drugs suppresses hydrochloric acid (HCl) production, thus minimizing the amount of HCl removed by gastric suction.

Coughing and deep breathing help to keep the lungs inflated and promote effective gas exchange. Inadequate ventilation due to pain, narcotics, and anesthesia causes alveolar collapse and eventually leads to CO_2 retention (respiratory acidosis). Table 19-3 lists the clinical management for clients following GI surgery.

CLINICAL CONSIDERATIONS: GASTROINTESTINAL (GI) SURGICAL INTERVENTIONS

1. Check for fluid and electrolyte imbalances prior to any type of surgery, especially gastrointestinal surgery. Indicators of fluid volume deficit are tachycardia, postural hypotension, dry mucous membranes, and poor skin turgor.

2. Monitor urinary output per hour, every 8 hours, and per day prior to and following surgery. Urine output may be decreased prior to surgery due to deficient fluid volume and may decrease following surgery because of SIADH.

3. Check laboratory test results for deficient fluid volume, i.e., increased hemoglobin, increased hematocrit, increased BUN (all caused by hemoconcentration), and increased/decreased serum potassium level, decreased/normal/elevated serum sodium level, decreased serum bicarbonate level (due to intestinal involvement).

4. Loss of hydrogen and chloride ions (hydrochloric acid) from gastric secretions causes metabolic alkalosis. Loss of bicarbonate from the intestinal secretions may cause metabolic acidosis.

5. The stomach and intestines are rich in electrolytes, especially sodium, chloride, potassium, hydrogen (stomach), and bicarbonate (intestine).

Table 19-3	Clinical Management for Pre- and Postoperative GI Surgery
Clinical Management	**Rationale**
Preoperative	
Fluid balance	Replace fluid loss. Three to five liters of balanced electrolyte solution (BES) may be necessary prior to surgery.
Electrolyte balance	Replace sodium and potassium as indicated by the serum electrolyte levels.
Urine output	Hourly urine output should be monitored. Urine output should not be less than 30 ml/hr.
Postoperative	
Fluid balance	Serum osmolality should be between 280 to 295 mOsm/kg. To determine serum osmolality, use the formula: $$2 \times \text{Serum sodium} + \frac{\text{BUN}}{3} + \frac{\text{Glucose}}{3} = \text{Serum osmolality}$$ A decreased serum osmolality may indicate hemodilution and an elevated serum osmolality indicates hemoconcentration. At least 3 liters of BES daily is indicated. Check for overhydration if the IV solution runs too fast.
Gastric or intestinal intubation	GI tubing should be patent. Plain water should not be used to maintain patency of tube; electrolytes are "washed out." Small amounts of saline solution or air may be indicated to maintain tube patency.
Electrolyte balance	Sodium and potassium gains or losses can be determined by periodically checking the serum electrolyte levels. Signs and symptoms of electrolyte imbalance should be reported.
Acid-base balance	Deep breathing and coughing improve gas exchange and prevent CO_2 retention and respiratory acidosis. Metabolic alkalosis may result from gastric suctioning because of the loss of the hydrogen and chloride ions (hydrochloric acid).
Peristalsis	Bowel sounds in the four quadrants should be checked to determine if peristalsis has returned. The gastrointestinal tube is usually removed when peristalsis has returned.
Medications H_2 blockers	Cimetidine, ranitidine, or famotidine suppresses the production of hydrochloric acid. The amount of HCl removed by gastric suction is diminished.

6. Intravenous fluid replacements for fluid volume deficits are balanced electrolyte solutions (BES) such as lactated Ringer's or normal saline solution (0.9% NaCl).

7. Avoid administration of 5% dextrose and water continuously. This isotonic IV solution becomes hypotonic when dextrose is rapidly metabolized leaving only the water, which dilutes the electrolyte levels.

8. Following abdominal surgery, peristalsis is decreased or absent. GI intubation is usually prescribed. Bowel sounds should be monitored to determine the presence of peristalsis.

● CLIENT MANAGEMENT

Assessment

● Prior to gastrointestinal surgery, assess for preexisting health problems and medications that can further increase the potential risk for fluid and electrolyte disturbances. Uncorrected preoperative hypovolemia and anemia may increase the risk for fluid and electrolyte disturbances postoperatively.

● Check the vital signs and use the results as a baseline for future comparisons. Deficient fluid volume may cause tachycardia, postural or orthostatic hypotension, and a decreased pulse pressure.

● Check intake, output, and weight. Urine output may decrease during a fluid volume deficit.

● Assess client's bowel sounds. Note if peristalsis is present prior to surgery.

● Assess for deficient fluid volume. Check serum osmolality; deficient fluid volume is present if the level is elevated.

● Check laboratory test results. Note if hemoglobin, hematocrit, and BUN are elevated; these are indicators of deficient fluid volume.

● If a gastric tube is inserted, check that the tube is draining.

Nursing Diagnoses

- Deficient fluid volume, related to gastrointestinal loss, decreased fluid intake, and/or fluid volume shift
- Pain, related to trauma from abdominal surgery
- Impaired tissue integrity, related to surgery, decreased or absence of bowel sounds, and decreased GI motility (peristalsis)
- Ineffective airway clearance, related to pain, ineffective coughing, deep breathing, and viscous mucous secretions
- Impaired urinary elimination, related to deficient fluid volume secondary to gastrointestinal disturbance

Interventions

- Monitor vital signs every 4 hours or more frequently if the client is unstable. Hypovolemia causes reflex tachycardia and postural hypotension.
- Check mucous membranes and skin turgor. Poor skin turgor with dry, scaly skin and dry mucous membranes indicate deficient fluid volume.
- Monitor urinary output. Report if the output is less than 600 ml per day. Urine output of 750 ml plus per day is preferable.
- Monitor laboratory results. Note if the hemoglobin, hematocrit, and BUN are elevated, which is indicative of hemocentration resulting from, deficient fluid volume.
- Monitor serum electrolyte results. Serum potassium is usually decreased because of deficient fluid volume; however, potassium may be increased because of hemoconcentration due to deficient fluid volume.
- Encourage coughing and deep breathing to improve alveolar expansion and mobilize secretions.
- Monitor intravenous flow rate. IV solutions that run too fast or a health status that does not warrant a large volume of fluids may cause the client to develop a fluid overload or overhydration.
- Monitor bowel sounds to determine the return of peristalsis.

● Check that the gastrointestinal tube is patent. Irrigate with normal saline solution or air according to the order.

Evaluation/Outcome

● Evaluate that the source of the ECFV problem has been eliminated or controlled.

● Evaluate the effectiveness of interventions (fluid and electrolyte replacement therapy, gastrointestinal intubation, medications, pain control measures, and so on) in balancing fluid needs and promoting comfort.

● Determine that the laboratory test results are within normal range.

● Monitor vital signs (particularly blood pressure and pulse rate) for stability.

● Evaluate renal function. Urine output is adequate and within normal volume.

CHAPTER 20

Increased Intracranial Pressure

Lisa Plowfield, RN, PhD

INTRODUCTION

Increased intracranial pressure is a life-threatening occurrence that requires close observation and rapid intervention to help prevent mortality and long-term adverse events. Intracranial pressure is that pressure within the intracranial cavity which is exerted by the volume of blood, cerebrospinal fluid, and brain tissue contained within the cavity. A small increase or decrease in any of these three components may have deleterious effects on brain structures and function. The health professional has a major responsibility in monitoring the neurologically impaired client for signs and symptoms of increasing intracranial pressure.

Because the brain is enclosed in the rigid cranial vault, a small increase in intracerebral fluid may result in a dramatic increase in intracranial pressure. Therefore, the health professional must closely monitor the neurologically impaired client for early signs of increasing intracranial pressure to help prevent adverse effects.

Chapter 20 discusses the physiology of intracranial pressure, the three types of intracerebral edema, factors that increase and decrease intracranial pressure, and associated complications that may occur with intracerebral hypertension. Signs and symptoms of increasing intracranial pressure along with management priorities and principles of fluid and electrolyte balance in the management of intracerebral hypertension are discussed.

● PATHOPHYSIOLOGY

An injury to the brain results in bleeding, swelling, and increased cerebral oxygen needs. Whenever any of the three components of the cranial vault increase in size or volume, the pressure within the closed cranial vault increases. Normal pressure is only maintained if an equal and opposite decrease in another of the components occurs. Three types of swelling occur within the brain.

Vasogenic edema is the most common type of fluid accumulation within the brain. It is essentially an extracellular edema. Vasogenic edema results from damage to the cerebral blood vessels causing increased capillary permeability. This allows a transudation of proteins and an influx of water from the extracellular space into the brain tissue. Causes of vasogenic edema include trauma, tumors, ischemia, and infection or abscess.

Cytogenic edema is intracellular. Increased capillary permeability results in an overall increase in water content within the brain and an inhibition of the sodium-potassium (Na-K) pump. This inhibition allows potassium to leave the cell and sodium chloride and water to enter the cell, causing the brain cells to swell.

Clinical causes of cytogenic edema include hypoxia from trauma or cerebral hemorrhage and hypo-osmolality.

Interstitial edema results from obstructive conditions such as hydrocephalus, brain tumors or infections that predispose the client to an excess of fluid in the brain, and a buildup of cerebrospinal fluid in the ventricles of the brain.

Intracranial pressure is also affected by cerebral blood flow. Regulators of blood flow within the central nervous system include CO_2, O_2, core body temperature, hydrogen ion concentration, and serum osmolality. Hypercapnia (an increase in $PaCO_2$) causes vasodilation, which results in an increase in intracranial pressure. Hypoxemia (a decrease in PaO_2) may also cause an increase in intracranial pressure.

An increase in core body temperature increases metabolism and results in an increase in intracranial pressure. A decrease in core body temperature causes a decrease in body metabolism and results in a decrease in intracranial pressure.

Prolonged hyperventilation causes excessive elimination of CO_2 and leads to respiratory alkalosis (increased pH and decreased $PaCO_2$). This may cause an increase in intracranial pressure.

Table 20-1	**Factors That Affect Cerebral Blood Flow**
Vasodilators	Excess CO_2
	Hypoxia
	Agitation
	Excessive movement
	Pain
	Fever
	Shivering
	Medications: peripheral vasodilators
Vasoconstrictors	Low levels of CO_2 (potent vasoconstrictor)
	High levels of O_2
	Medications: peripheral vasoconstrictors

Hypoventilation causes excessive retention of CO_2 and leads to respiratory acidosis (decreased pH and increased $PaCO_2$), which is far more dangerous than hyperventilation. Carbon dioxide is the most potent vasodilator known. As vasodilation increases, so does intracranial pressure. See Table 20-1 for factors that affect cerebral blood flow.

Serum osmolality is the number of formed particles in the serum and is an indication of serum concentration. Decreased serum osmolality indicates a fluid overload and may result in an increase in intracranial pressure.

Hypotonic fluids such as dextrose and water are generally avoided in the neurologically compromised client suspected of having an increase in intracranial pressure. Using intravenous fluids such as 5% dextrose in water (D_5W) results in the dextrose being metabolized, releasing free water which is absorbed by the brain cells, leading to cerebral edema.

● CLINICAL MANIFESTATIONS

Etiology

Causes of increased intracranial pressure include head trauma with both open and closed head injuries, intracranial tumors, intracranial hemorrhages, cerebrovascular accidents, and neurosurgery.

Table 20-2	Signs and Symptoms of Increasing Intracranial Pressure

Early Signs and Symptoms
  Headache
  Restlessness
  Confusion
  Visual disturbances
  Pupillary changes (size and response)
  Localizes painful stimuli
  Cranial nerve dysfunction
Progressive Signs and Symptoms
  Nausea, vomiting
  Muscle weakness (often unilateral)
  Increasing difficulty with arousal
  Decorticate and Decerebrate posturing to painful stimuli
Late Signs and Symptoms
  Vital sign alterations
    Bradycardia
    Decreased pulse pressure
    Respiratory pattern changes

Table 20-2 lists the early, progressive, and advanced clinical manifestations of increasing intracranial pressure. If early signs and symptoms of intracranial pressure are missed or unable to be controlled, progressive clinical manifestations occur.

If the progressive clinical manifestations of increasing intracranial pressure are not controlled, more deleterious effects are likely. The symptoms are those of decompensation. Once decompensation occurs, autoregulation (the compensatory alteration in the diameter of the intracranial blood vessels designed to maintain a constant blood flow during changes in cerebral perfusion pressure) is lost with progressively increased intracranial pressure.

In addition to the effects on brain metabolism and function, intracerebral hypertension has implications in the dysfunction of other major organ systems. Changes in the cardiopulmonary system include pulmonary crackles, S_3, atrial fibrillation, and hypotension. Hypotension drastically worsens cerebral edema because of a resultant decrease in cerebral perfusion pressure and compensatory fluid retention.

The development of stress ulcers and gastrointestinal bleeding may occur as a result of medical treatment.

● CLINICAL MANAGEMENT

Clinical management of intracerebral hypertension includes careful administration of fluids and electrolytes, maintaining an airway and adequate ventilation, medication administration, temperature control, and prevention of the Valsalva maneuver, which increases intracranial pressure.

Careful fluid management in the neurologically impaired client is essential. Hypotonic fluids such as dextrose and water are generally avoided. Physiological normal saline (0.09% NSS) or Ringer's solution are the preferred isotonic intravenous fluids.

Extracellular fluid volume is directly dependent upon total body sodium. The principal osmotic electrolyte of extracellular fluid is sodium (Na). Most clients with hyponatremia are hypoosmolar. The other major cation for fluid balance maintenance is potassium (K). It is essential to maintain normal Na and K levels in order to maintain normal serum osmolality. If the Na and K levels are not maintained within normal limits, the Na-K pump becomes defective. Potassium leaves the cell and Na, Cl, and water enter the cells.

Mannitol is an osmotic diuretic capable of relieving elevated intracranial pressure when given intravenously. Mannitol intravenous dosage is 0.25–1g/kg of body weight. Mannitol pulls intracellular fluid into the extracellular plasma and decreases intracranial pressure. Care must be taken to monitor for possible complications of pulmonary edema and water intoxication. An additional complication that can occur with the administration of osmotic diuretics to clients with intracranial hemorrhage is rebleeding. As the brain tissue shrinks from osmotic diuretics, rebleeding may occur.

Loop diuretics such as furosemide (Lasix) may be administered alone or in conjunction with osmotic diuretics to help eliminate excess fluid from the extracellular space.

Hyperventilation with a resultant decrease in $PaCO_2$ acts immediately to decrease cerebral blood flow and thus reduces intracranial pressure. When clients with increased intracranial pressure are mechanically ventilated, maintaining a $PaCO_2$ at 35 mm Hg with gentle hyperventilation is recommended. Due to the potent cerebral vasoconstriction that results from hyperventilation, excessive or prolonged hyperventilation may result in cerebral ischemia. Clients may need long-term mechanical ventilation to prevent respiratory acidosis, which is far more serious than respiratory alkalosis. Increased concentration of $PaCO_2$ in respiratory acidosis is a more potent vasodilator than is an increase in PaO_2 resulting from respiratory alkalosis.

Further measures to control or decrease intracranial pressure are aimed at preventing agitation, excessive movement, pain, and the Valsalva maneuver. Alert and cooperative clients should be encouraged not to cough, bend, stoop, lift, hold their breath, sneeze, or strain at bowel elimination. To prevent a transient increase in intracranial pressure, stool softeners are administered to help prevent straining with bowel movements. Sedatives and barbiturates may also be administered to alleviate agitation and pain. The head of the bed should be elevated 30°–45° to let gravity have its effect on reducing intracranial pressure. The head and neck should be midline with no flexion, extension, or rotation to promote jugular venous outflow.

Fever, shivering, pain, and agitation need to be managed effectively to avoid increasing intracranial pressure. Antipyretics, sedatives, and barbiturates may be used to avoid these events.

Clients with increased intracranial pressure are prone to seizures. Seizures may cause a transient increase in intracranial pressure, create safety issues for the client, or cause further hypoxia and hypercapnia. Preventive measures for seizure control include the administration and careful monitoring of anticonvulsant medications.

● CLIENT MANAGEMENT

Assessment

● Assess neurological status every 30–60 minutes. The most significant change that may indicate an increase in intracranial pressure is a change in the level of consciousness. Subtle changes initially include irritability, restlessness, and visual changes.

● Assess vital signs every 15–30 minutes for bradycardia, slowed and/or irregular respirations, hyperthermia, systolic hypertension, diastolic hypotension, and a widening pulse pressure. Careful monitoring of fluid balance is essential to help prevent cerebral hypertension. Hourly intake and output, careful monitoring of intravenous fluid rate, and daily weights are important assessment factors.

● Additional parameters to monitor include serum osmolality, arterial blood gases, and electrolytes. Decreased serum osmolality, increased $PaCO_2$, increased serum potassium, and decreased serum sodium may indicate an impending increase in intracranial pressure.

● Assess pulmonary sounds for crackles, heart sounds for an S_3, and an increase in skin turgor as indications for fluid retention.

● Clients with increased intracranial pressure may develop seizures. Assess for seizure activities and additional complications of cerebral hypertension such as rhinorrhea, otorrhea, and brain stem herniation.

● Administration and assessment of therapeutic effects of the following medications are essential: loop diuretics, osmotic diuretics, and anticonvulsants.

Nursing Diagnoses

● Ineffective tissue perfusion (cerebral), related to increased intracranial pressure
● Acute confusion, related to cerebral edema
● Ineffective breathing pattern, related to cerebral edema
● Risk for deficient fluid volume, related to diuretic therapy
● Risk for injury, related to potential for seizure activity

Interventions

● Monitor neurological status and vital signs. Compare with earlier findings to detect progression of increasing intracranial pressure. Check for subtle changes in behavior and cognitive response, irritability, restlessness, visual disturbances, and confusion may indicate the onset of increased intracranial pressure.

- Assess motor, sensory, and cranial nerve function to evaluate the progression or reduction of intracranial pressure.

- Monitor intake and output hourly. Monitor for dehydration and overhydration.

- Review serum osmolality, urine specific gravity, electrolytes, and arterial blood gases for hydration status and factors that exacerbate increased intracranial pressure.

- Maintain head of bed elevated 30–45 degrees and keep head and body aligned to prevent cerebral venous congestion.

- Administer pharmacologic agents that help alleviate increases in intracranial pressure.

- Monitor for seizure activity. Administer anticonvulsants as preventive measure.

Evaluation/Outcome

- Evaluate vital signs frequently for return to normal range and stability (observe for widening pulse pressure).

- Monitor pupillary reaction and ocular movements for return to normal functions of cranial nerves.

- Evaluate the effectiveness of interventions in reducing symptoms (disturbed LOC, arousability, irritability, agitation, memory loss, inability to follow simple commands) and other nonspecific early signs (headache, nausea, vomiting) of cerebral edema.

- Evaluate fluid balance (intake and output, daily weight, and intravenous fluid rate) and electrolyte levels (Na Cl, K, Ca) for return to normal range.

- Evaluate effectiveness of medications (loop diuretics, osmotic diuretics, steroids, anticonvulsants, etc.) in reducing edema and promoting a fluid balance.

- Monitor blood gases for normal/stable range to ensure adequate oxygenation.

Clinical Oncology

Julie Waterhouse, RN, PhD.

INTRODUCTION

Cancer is a disease caused by altered and uncontrolled cell growth. Cancer cells no longer look or function like normal cells and tissue. Cancer may occur in the form of a solid tumor (carcinoma or sarcoma) or may be present in the blood and bone marrow (leukemia) or in the lymph nodes (lymphoma). Solid tumor cells may spread from their original location to other tissue sites throughout the body. Fluid, electrolyte, and acid-base imbalances frequently occur due to the effects of the malignant cells and the side effects of cancer treatment. Chapter 21 discusses various fluid, electrolyte, and acid-base changes associated with cancer.

PATHOPHYSIOLOGY

Cancer is a group of diseases characterized by abnormal and uncontrolled cell growth. Cancer cells are malignant (capable of invading normal tissues and spreading to distant sites). Fluid and electrolyte disturbances occur frequently in individuals with cancer because of the nature of the malignant cell growth and the effects of therapies used to control or eliminate cancer.

Cancer may begin as an individual solid tumor (carcinoma or sarcoma) or may arise throughout the body in the blood-forming cells of the bone marrow (leukemia) or in the lymph nodes and channels (lymphoma). Wherever the cancer begins, the malignant cells are more primitive (anaplastic) than normal cells. They may be undifferentiated, or may differentiate in abnormal and bizarre ways.

This lack of normal differentiation causes some malignant cells to produce unusual proteins, antigens, hormones, enzymes, and other chemicals. In addition, because the malignant cells are abnormal, they do not respond to normal regulatory mechanisms such as hormonal and metabolic controls.

ETIOLOGY

The exact cause of cancer is not known. All cancers are believed to involve damage to one or more genes that control cell growth. This genetic damage may be caused by cigarette smoke, carcinogenic chemicals, radiation, viruses, diet, medications, and/or heredity. The cells with damaged growth control genes reproduce rapidly and independently, and further mutations occur as they reproduce. Sometimes the immune system recognizes and destroys the abnormal cells, but the cancer cells may evade or overwhelm the immune system and continue to grow and spread.

CLINICAL MANIFESTATIONS

One major consequence of the biochemical abnormalities seen in cancer cells is cachexia, a complex process manifested by anorexia, weight loss, wasting, weakness, anemia, fluid and electrolyte disturbances, and metabolism. Cachexia involves changes in the metabolism of proteins, lipids, and carbohydrates. For example, protein synthesis is diminished and insulin release is decreased. Glucose utilization is impaired also, and anaerobic metabolic pathways are used more often than the normal aerobic pathways. This produces higher than usual concentrations of lactic acid and may result in lactic acidosis.

Nitrogen transferred from body tissues to the tumor often leaves the client in negative nitrogen balance. Similarly, cancer clients often retain sodium, with a total of 120% that of healthy individuals. Sodium, however, is concentrated in the tumor and the serum sodium may be low (hyponatremia). The client with cancer may also experience a malabsorption syndrome, which involves inflammation, ulceration, decreased patency, and decreased secretions of the GI tract. These problems result in poor protein and fat absorption, which may compound fluid and electrolyte disturbances in cachexia.

A second major consequence of the primitive biochemical function of malignant cells is the abnormal secretion of hormones (ectopic hormone secretion). An example is bronchogenic cancer, which may secrete antidiuretic hormone (ADH), parathyroid hormone (PTH), insulin, or adrenocorticotropic hormone (ACTH). The resulting hormonal abnormalities may lead to fluid and electrolyte problems such as water intoxication (ICFVE), hyponatremia, hypokalemia, and hypophosphatemia. The most common of these hormonal abnormalities is the syndrome of inappropriate secretion of ADH (SIADH). This condition may develop gradually over weeks or months, or may be an acute development arising in days or even hours. Severe and/or acute instances of SIADH may be life threatening.

A third problem that commonly occurs in cancer clients in whom large numbers of malignant and normal cells are destroyed by radiation or chemotherapy is tumor lysis syndrome. In this oncologic emergency, cell breakdown allows the intracellular contents to spill into the vascular space. Release of purine nucleic acids from cells results in an increase in serum uric acid (hyperuricemia), while release of electrolytes such as potassium and phosphorus causes several electrolyte imbalances. Uric acid is poorly soluble in body fluids and is excreted primarily through the kidneys. Small increases above normal serum concentrations can cause uric acid precipitation in the renal tubules and collecting ducts and result in renal failure. This hyperuricemia, plus hyperkalemia, hyperphosphatemia, and hypocalcemia (because of the inverse relationship with phosphorus) may lead to life-threatening fluid and electrolyte complications.

A final major fluid and electrolyte problem that is frequently seen in patients with cancer is hypercalcemia. This metabolic disorder occurs when bone resorption (breakdown) exceeds bone formation, and the kidneys are unable to excrete the released calcium. Hypercalcemia is most common in patients with multiple myeloma, breast cancer, and lung cancer, usually occurring when tumors are advanced and difficult to treat. The majority of patients with cancer-related hypercalcemia have skeletal metastasis.

Less common fluid and electrolyte problems seen in cancer include lactic acidosis and hyperkalemia, which may occur during periods of uncontrolled malignant cell growth. Lactic acidosis is caused by rapidly growing malignant cells that metabolize excess glucose using anaerobic metabolism and produce lactic acid as a by-product. The resulting acidosis causes a compensatory shift of extracellular hydrogen ions and intracellular potassium. An even less common fluid balance problem can develop when cancer is treated with lymphokine-activated killer (LAK) cell therapy. This treatment causes increased vascular permeability leading to vascular leak syndrome. Severe edema and cardiovascular hypotension may result.

Table 21-1 lists the fluid and electrolyte disturbances commonly associated with cancer and cancer therapy. Also given are abnormal serum levels and the rationale for their occurrence.

●CLINICAL MANAGEMENT

The fluid and electrolyte disturbances listed in Table 21-1 can develop in almost any individual with cancer at any time during diagnosis, treatment, recovery, or terminal stages of the disease. Fluid and electrolyte problems are *most common,* however, with the following clinical conditions:

1. *Cachexia.* Severe anorexia, nausea, vomiting, and/or diarrhea combine with metabolic changes to cause numerous fluid and electrolyte imbalances.
2. *Ectopic hormone production.* Abnormal hormones (most commonly ADH) are secreted ectopically by the tumors, resulting in sodium and fluid abnormalities.
3. *Tumor lysis syndrome.* Large numbers of cells are destroyed by chemotherapy and/or radiation, causing changes in potassium, phosphorus, and uric acid levels.
4. *Hypercalcemia.* Rapid, widespread cell growth, usually with skeletal metastasis, disrupts calcium balance.

Cachexia

Cachexia may occur because of the effects of the malignancy itself and/or be caused by radiation, immunotherapy, and chemotherapy. Contributing problems include anorexia,

Table 21-1 Fluid and Electrolyte Disturbance in Cancer and Cancer Therapy

Fluid/Electrolyte Disturbance	Commonly Associated Cancer and Cancer Therapy	Defining Characteristics	Rationale/Comments
Hypercalcemia	Breast cancer, multiple myeloma, ovarian cancer, pancreatic cancer, leukemia, lymphoma, lung cancer, bladder cancer, kidney cancer, head and neck cancer, and prostate cancer	Serum calcium > 11 mg/dl	Hypercalcemia occurs in 10–20% of all cancer clients and in 40–50% of those with metastatic breast cancer or multiple myeloma. It is caused by bone destruction by metastatic tumors, elevated parathyroid hormone (PTH) levels related to some tumors, and elevated prostaglandin and osteoclast activating factor (OAF). Prolonged immobility is also a causative factor.

(continues)

Table 21-1	Fluid and Electrolyte Disturbance in Cancer and Cancer Therapy —*continued*		
Fluid/Electrolyte Disturbance	**Commonly Associated Cancer and Cancer Therapy**	**Defining Characteristics**	**Rationale/Comments**
Hyponatremia (usually associated with dehydration)	Lung cancer, pancreatic cancer, multiple myeloma, head and neck cancer, stomach cancer, brain cancer, colon cancer, ovarian cancer, and prostate cancer, aggressive diuretic therapy. High-dose cyclophosphamide/Cytoxan therapy; daunorubicin or cytosine chemotherapy (decreases blast cell count)	Serum sodium < 135 mEq/L	Hyponatremia is caused by liver, thyroid, and adrenal insufficiencies; renal failure, and congestive heart failure. A condition known as cerebral salt wasting is caused by some intracranial neoplasms. In this condition, the brain releases a postulated natriuretic factor or the neural innervation to the brain is altered. The result is the kidneys' inability to conserve sodium.
Syndrome of inappropriate antidiuretic hormone (SIADH)	Lung cancer, pancreatic cancer, brain cancer, ovarian cancer, colon, cancer, sarcoma, leukemia, prostate cancer, Hodgkin's disease, and other lymphomas, vincristine, cyclophosphamide chemotherapy	Serum sodium < 130 mEq/L, serum osmolality < 280 mOsm/kg	SIADH occurs because of increased release of ADH from posterior pituitary or ectopically from neoplastic tumors. The posterior pituitary then becomes impervious to the usual feedback control mechanism.

Hyperuricemia	Leukemias, lymphomas, multiple myeloma, any cancer treated aggressively with chemotherapy or radiation	Serum uric acid > 8.0 mg/dl, uric acid crystals in urine	Breakdown of large numbers of cells causes release of uric acid into the bloodstream (tumor lysis syndrome). Precipitation of uric acid in the kidneys results in gouty nephropathy, acute hyperuricemic nephropathy, and eventual renal failure. First signs of hyperuricemic renal failure may be nausea, vomiting, and lethargy. This type of renal failure may or may not be reversible. Symptoms of hyperuricemia include hematuria, flank pain, nausea, vomiting, and symptoms of renal failure.
Hypokalemia	Colon cancer, multiple myeloma, Hodgkin's disease, pancreatic cancer, stomach cancer, thyroid cancer, adrenal adenoma, adrenal hyperplasia tumors, and cancers that secrete adrenocorticotropic hormone (ACTH) ectopically	Serum potassium < 3.5 mEq/L	Dietary intake of potassium is deficient when the client is anorexic, vomiting, or NPO. Excessive diarrhea that leads to rapid potassium depletion occurs with many GI tumors, chemotherapy, radiation therapy to the lower abdomen, and antibiotic therapy.

(continues)

Table 21-1	Fluid and Electrolyte Disturbance in Cancer and Cancer Therapy —*continued*		
Fluid/Electrolyte Disturbance	**Commonly Associated Cancer and Cancer Therapy**	**Defining Characteristics**	**Rationale/Comments**
Hypokalemia, *continued*			Excessive urinary excretion may be caused by diuretics, hypercalcemia, hypomagnesemia, antibiotic therapy, ectopic ACTH secretion, nephrotoxicity due to chemotherapy or radiation, and renal tubular necrosis due to Hodgkin's disease, multiple myeloma, and acute blast crisis Ileostomy, colostomy, fistulas, and the diuretic phase of renal failure also contribute to hypokalemia.
Hypomagnesemia	Lung cancer, especially oat cell, ovarian cancer, and testicular cancer, total parenteral nutrition (TPN), *cis*-platinum chemotherapy	Serum magnesium < 1.5 mEq/L	Low magnesium level occurs most often in clients with severe diarrhea, vomiting, malabsorption syndrome, cachexia, ADH secretion, or renal disease. The *cis*-platinum and nephrotoxic antibiotics also contribute to hypomagnesemia.

Lactic acidosis	Hodgkin's disease, lymphoma, leukemia, lymphosarcoma, and lung cancer (especially oat cell with liver metastasis)	Arterial blood pH < 7.35, HCO_3 < 24 mEq/L, serum CO_2 < 22 mEq/L	Lactic acidosis (metabolic acidosis) occurs because rapidly growing malignant cells utilize large amounts of glucose. When the glucose is metabolized by the anaerobic pathway (glycolysis), pyruvic acid is the end product. When hypoxia exists, pyruvate is converted to lactic acid. Elevated serum lactic acid concentrations may exceed the liver's ability to metabolize and the kidneys' to excrete.
Hyperkalemia	Hodgkins' disease, lymphoma, leukemia, lung cancer (especially oat cell), and liver metastasis, aggressive chemotherapy	Serum potassium > 5.3 mEq/L	Intracellular-extracellular redistribution occurs during respiratory and metabolic acidosis (including lactic acidosis). Extracellular hydrogen ions shift into the cell in an attempt to raise serum pH. Intracellular potassium ions then shift out of the cell to compensate. Lysis of large numbers of malignant and normal cells during radiation and chemotherapy causes the release of massive amounts of potassium from destroyed cells (tumor lysis syndrome). Renal failure and hypoaldosteronism can cause renal retention of potassium.

(continues)

Table 21-1	Fluid and Electrolyte Disturbance in Cancer and Cancer Therapy —*continued*		
Fluid/Electrolyte Disturbance	**Commonly Associated Cancer and Cancer Therapy**	**Defining Characteristics**	**Rationale/Comments**
Hypophosphatemia	Leukemia, multiple myeloma, PTH-secreting tumors; total parenteral nutrition (TPN) (hyperalimentation)	Serum phosphorus < 2.5 mg/dl	Hypophosphatemia occurs with cancers that contain and secrete PTH (PTH normally regulates the rate of phosphorus reabsorption by the kidneys). Aggressive hyperalimentation/parenteral nutrition often induces hypophosphatemia because the phosphorus influx into cells is accelerated during carbohydrate metabolism. Malabsorption, sepsis, diuretics, corticosteroids, and thrombocytopenia are other contributing factors. Symptoms of hypophosphatemia are fatigue, weakness, anorexia, irritability, paresthesia, seizures, and coma.

| Decreased vascular volume (shift to the third space) | Liver cancer, including liver metastasis, stomach cancer, pancreatic cancer, colon cancer, and head and neck cancer | Serum albumin < 3.2 g/dl, decreased BP, increased H & H, increased BUN | Decreased vascular volume occurs when serum protein is decreased when tumor cells exude fluids, or when vascular permeability is increased by infection: Protein depletion occurs with anorexia/cachexia, nausea, and vomiting due to disease or therapy or to decreased protein synthesis in cancer clients. Some individuals with cancer have increased loss of protein via the GI tract, elevated basal metabolic rate due to disease or infection results in accelerated protein loss. Decreased serum protein leads to decreased blood volume and a drop in blood pressure. The client may have ample or excess extracellular fluid but is unable to retain it within the vascular space. Without treatment, cardiovascular failure and death result. |

(continues)

Table 21-1 **Fluid and Electrolyte Disturbance in Cancer and Cancer Therapy** *—continued*

Fluid/Electrolyte Disturbance	Commonly Associated Cancer and Cancer Therapy	Defining Characteristics	Rationale/Comments
Hypocalcemia/ hyperphosphatemia	Leukemia, lymphoma, and multiple myeloma; aggressive, chemotherapy and radiation	Serum calcium < 9 mg/dl, serum phosphorus > 4.5 mg/dl	Rapid cell lysis causes the release of large amounts of phosphate. Immature blast cells contain up to four times more phosphate than mature lymphocytes. The rise in serum phosphorus then causes a drop in serum calcium. Renal failure may result from precipitation of calcium phosphate in the kidneys. Symptoms include oliguria, anuria, azotemia, and tetany.

nausea, diarrhea, draining wounds, and fistulas. The most frequently encountered fluid and electrolyte disturbances are hypomagnesemia, hypokalemia, and decreased vascular volume.

Anorexia, nausea, and vomiting, decreased protein intake, diarrhea, malabsorption syndrome, and wound drainage increase protein loss in the cancer client. Low protein levels lead to decreased oncotic pressure (colloidal osmotic pressure) in the vascular system and result in decreased vascular volume. The basic goal of therapy in cancer clients with decreased vascular volume is to maintain blood pressure. Whole blood, packed red blood cells (RBCs), or albumin may be given to increase plasma oncotic pressure to restore fluid balance in the vascular space.

Hypomagnesemia may develop due to decreased intake caused by anorexia and vomiting or increased magnesium concentration in malignant cells. In addition, some pharmacologic agents (such as cisplatin, cyclosporin, and amphotericin) cause renal magnesium wasting. Hypokalemia is produced by decreased intake due to nausea or anorexia and increased loss by vomiting. Carefully prescribed and monitored hyperalimentation (TPN) can correct hypokalemia and hypomagnesemia and improve vascular volume.

Ectopic Hormone Production

Any malignant cells may secrete hormones ectopically (abnormally). The most commonly involved cancers and hormones are those listed in Table 21-2. Acute complications caused by ectopic hormone secretions in cancer clients include fluid and electrolyte imbalances, which are often severe and may result in death. The primary goal of therapy in cancer clients with ectopic hormone secretion is the eradication or reduction of the hormone-secreting tumor. If surgery, radiation, and/or chemotherapy do not eliminate the tumor and control the symptoms, long-term pharmacologic therapy may be ordered.

When malignant cells secrete antidiuretic hormone (ADH) ectopically, the cancer patient may develop the syndrome of inappropriate ADH (SIADH). SIADH involves decreased ability to secrete dilute urine, fluid retention, and dilutional hyponatremia. SIADH may be caused or exacerbated by chemotherapeutic agents such as cisplatin, cyclophosphamide, and

Table 21-2	Hormones Commonly Secreted Ectopically by Malignant Cells	
Hormones	**Type of Cancer**	**Common Associated Problems**
Antidiuretic hormone (ADH)	Lung (oat cell)	SIADH
	Pancreas	Hyponatremia
	Hodgkin's disease	Hypomagnesemia
	Prostate gland	
	Sarcoma	
Parathyroid hormone (PTH)	Lung	Hypercalcemia
	Leukemia	Hypophosphatemia
	Multiple myeloma	Hypomagnesemia
	Breast	
Adrenocorticotropic hormone (ACTH)	Lung (oat cell and non-oat cell)	Hypokalemia
Osteoclast activating factor (OAF)	Multiple myeloma	Hypercalcemia
	Lymphoma	
Prostaglandins (E series)	Breast	Hypercalcemia
	Kidney	
	Pancreas	

vincristine. Treatment of SIADH varies with the severity of the symptoms and the rapidity with which the condition develops.

● Mild SIADH

● Restriction of water and fluid intake to 500–1000 ml/day.

● Moderate to severe SIADH

● Saline infusion of 3–5% to restore serum sodium.

● Demeclocycline to interfere with the action of ADH on renal tubules.

● Lithium to induce diabetes insipidus (has serious side effects).

Extreme care should be taken when hyperosmolar saline (3–5% saline solution) is administered because it can raise the serum sodium level too rapidly and cause shrinkage of CNS neurons and neurologic dysfunction. Nonpeptide vasopressin V_2 receptor antagonists (which selectively block the action of ADH on the collecting ducts) are currently in clinical trials, and show promise as a major treatment for SIADH.

Tumor Lysis Syndrome

Following the destruction of large numbers of cells by chemotherapy, usually in leukemia or lymphoma, vast numbers of intracellular electrolytes enter the bloodstream. The cancer client can develop hyperuricemia, hyperkalemia, hypophosphatemia, and/or hypocalcemia. Renal failure or cardiac arrest may result. Drugs used for the management of these fluid and electrolyte imbalances include:

● Intravenous hydration to maintain urine output at 100 ml/hour or more.

● Allopurinol to decrease uric acid.

● Calcium gluconate IV infusion for hypocalcemia.

● Sodium bicarbonate to alkalinize the urine in hyperuricemia (uric acid is less soluble in acid urine).

● Diuretics such as furosemide (Lasix) or mannitol to promote excretion of uric acid and phosphates and minimize fluid retention.

Hypercalcemia

Individuals with cancer may experience severe electrolyte disturbances whenever rapid and widespread malignant cell growth occurs. The uncontrolled cell growth is marked by metastatic lesions (in carcinomas or sarcomas) or by multiple organ infiltration (in leukemias and lymphomas).

Metastatic lesions of the bone frequently cause hypercalcemia, which may develop rapidly and become severe very quickly. When an acute hypercalcemic crisis occurs, the mortality rate is extremely high (up to 50%). Management of mild and moderate hypercalcemia (<13 mg/dl) involves IV normal saline (NaCl 0.9%) to achieve adequate hydration and promote calcium excretion. For severe hypercalcemia the following drugs may be used:

● Furosemide (Lasix) to decrease tubular reabsorption of calcium.

● Steroids to increase calcium excretion.

● Calcitonin to inhibit bone resorption.

● Mithramycin to inhibit bone resorption.

● Biphosphonates to inhibit calcium release from bone.

● Gallium nitrate to make calcium dissolution more difficult.

● IV inorganic phosphates to inhibit calcium absorption and promote calcium deposition in bone and soft tissue. (This approach is used rarely except with chronic hypercalcemia due to severe potential side effects of calcium precipitation in lung, kidney, or heart tissues.)

CLIENT MANAGEMENT

Assessment

● Fluid and electrolyte balance must be monitored carefully in clients with any type of cancer and at all stages during diagnosis and treatment. Assessment is particularly important in clients during and immediately after treatment with chemotherapy, radiation, surgery, biologic response modifiers, or bone marrow transplantation. In addition, fluid and electrolyte problems are particularly common in clients dying from cancer.

● Assess for anorexia, nausea, vomiting, diarrhea, edema, weight loss or gain, neurological status, fatigue, and activity levels. Laboratory values of sodium, calcium, potassium, magnesium, and phosphorus should be checked and reported frequently. Arterial blood pH, serum albumin, and serum uric acid should also be assessed as indicated.

● Assessment of fluid and electrolyte disturbances is particularly difficult in individuals with cancer because symptoms of these disturbances (e.g., anorexia, vomiting, fatigue, diarrhea, and muscle weakness) mimic those of treatments, systemic effects of tumor growth, psychological responses to cancer, or general deterioration in advanced cancer.

Many fluid and electrolyte conditions in cancer clients can be prevented, reversed, or controlled. Table 21-3 provides an assessment guide for fluid and electrolyte imbalances in cancer clients. The blanks in the assessment column should be completed with the appropriate value, or checked to indicate presence of a sign or symptom. The comments column may be used for additional information or clarification.

Table 21-3	Assessment of Fluid and Electrolyte Imbalance	

Type of Primary Cancer: _____

Stage: _____ **Liver metastasis:** _____ **Bone metastasis:** _____

Observation	Assessment	Comments
Vital signs	Temperature	_____
	Pulse	_____
	Respiration	_____
	Blood pressure	_____
		_____
	Heart sounds	_____
	Peripheral pulses	_____
Intake	PO	_____
	IV infusions	_____
	Amounts	_____
Output	Amounts	_____
	Specific gravity	_____
	Urine osmolality	_____
	Polyuria	_____
	Oliguria	_____
	Anuria	_____
Weight and skin changes	Daily weight	_____
	Skin turgor	_____
	Skin temperature	_____
	Edema	_____
	Ascites	_____
GI changes	Anorexia	_____
	Nausea	_____
	Vomiting	_____
	Diarrhea	_____
	Constipation	_____
	Bowel sounds	_____
	Abdominal distention	_____
	Abdominal cramps	_____
	Fistula	_____
	GI suction	_____
	Draining tube	_____
Respiratory changes	Dyspnea	_____
	Hyperpnea	_____
	Chest crackles	_____
	Sputum	_____

(continues)

Table 21-3	Assessment of Fluid and Electrolyte Imbalance—*continued*

Type of Primary Cancer: _____
Stage: _____ **Liver metastasis:** _____ **Bone metastasis:** _____

Observation	Assessment		Comments
Neurologic changes	Headache	_____	
	LOC changes	_____	
	Irritability	_____	
	Disorientation	_____	
	Confusion	_____	
	Paresthesia	_____	
	Altered perception	_____	
	Seizures	_____	
	Coma	_____	
State of being	Alert	_____	
	Fatigue	_____	
	Lethargic	_____	
Muscular changes	Muscle weakness	_____	
	Hyporeflexia	_____	
	Hyperreflexia	_____	
	Muscle cramps	_____	
	Twitching	_____	
	Tetany signs	_____	
Body chemistry and hematology changes	Hemoglobin	_____	
	Hematocrit	_____	
	Platelets	_____	
	WBCs	_____	
	Differential	_____	
	Electrolytes:		
	Potassium	_____	
	Sodium	_____	
	Calcium	_____	
	Magnesium	_____	
	Chloride	_____	
	Phosphorus	_____	
	Serum osmolality	_____	
	Protein	_____	
	Albumin	_____	
	BUN	_____	
	Creatinine	_____	

(continues)

Table 21-3	Assessment of Fluid and Electrolyte Imbalance—*continued*	

Type of Primary Cancer: _____
Stage: _____ **Liver metastasis:** _____ **Bone metastasis:** _____

Observation	Assessment	Comments
	Uric acid	_____
	Lactate	_____
	ABGs:	
	pH	_____
	PaO$_2$	_____
	PaCO$_2$	_____
	HCO$_3$	_____
Chemotherapy	Drug	_____
	Dose, route	_____
	Side effects	_____
Radiation therapy	Dose	_____
	Times	_____
	Target area	_____

Nursing Diagnoses

● Deficient fluid volume, related to decreased serum protein, excessive sodium excretion, and/or decreased concentrating ability of renal tubules.

● Imbalanced nutrition, less than body requirements, related to anorexia, vomiting, diarrhea, wound drainage, and/or malabsorption.

● Excess fluid volume, related to dilutional hyponatremia and increased levels of ADH.

● Risk for injury, related to bone demineralization or alterations in potassium balance.

● Decreased cardiac output, related to increased serum potassium or calcium.

● Disturbed thought processes, related to altered electrolyte balance.

● Impaired urinary elimination, related to cell lysis and buildup of uric acid in the nephron.

Interventions

Deficient Fluid Volume

● Check frequently for signs and symptoms of dehydration. Signs such as rapid pulse and dry mucous membranes may be the first indication of deficient fluid volume.

● Check BP in supine and standing positions. Report a fall of more than 10 mm Hg diastolic. A drop of this extent may signal marked dehydration.

● Monitor intake and output, weight, pulse rate, serum electrolytes, and serum protein. These signs may be early indicators of deficient fluid volume.

● Maintain adequate hydration, with oral fluids if appropriate or with IV fluids as ordered. Fluids are necessary to replace or maintain the serum volume.

● Administer albumin, packed cells, whole blood, or other blood products as ordered. Albumin helps to maintain the colloid osmotic pressure of the blood and increase plasma volume. Administration of blood products helps to raise blood pressure and improve renal flow.

● Maintain or improve nutritional status, especially protein intake, if possible (see next nursing diagnosis). An adequate protein intake is essential to maintain normal colloidal pressure and retain fluid in the vascular space.

Imbalanced Nutrition:
Less Than Body Requirements

● Assess current and normal height and weight, diet history, caloric intake, anthropometric measurements, and physiologic factors such as difficulty swallowing or anorexia. This assessment facilitates identification of individuals with existing nutritional abnormalities or at high risk for nutritional problems. These data are also required to plan and monitor nutritional interventions.

● Monitor serum albumin, creatinine, lymphocyte count, and nitrogen balance. These values are the most likely to be affected in malnutrition related to cancer.

● Enhance oral nutrition by encouraging a high-protein, high-calorie diet fortified with commercial supplements. If adequate nutrition can be obtained orally, this route is safer and easier for the client.

● Encourage small, frequent feedings of calorie-dense and nonacidic foods. Cancer patients often experience an early sensation of fullness, so feedings should be small and spaced apart and should avoid empty calories.

● Administer medications to control or reduce nausea, vomiting, mouth pain, and diarrhea as needed. Medications that reduce these symptoms increase the client's potential intake and absorption of nutrients. Medications such as megestrol acetate or growth hormone may be ordered to stimulate appetite.

● Ease swallowing by implementing measures to relieve dryness of mucous membranes and/or reduce severity of stomatitis, such as oral hygiene, mouth rinses, and lubricants.

● Compensate for taste alterations by substituting fish, chicken, eggs, and cheese for meats; adding extra sweetness or flavorings. Reduce exposure to cooking smells as much as possible.

● If oral nutrition is inadequate, administer tube feedings through nasogastric, gastrostomy, or jejunostomy tube. The enteral route for provision of nutrition is preferable to the parenteral route.

● Assist in administration and monitoring of total parenteral nutrition if needed. The parenteral route for administering nutritional support is the least preferable due to the risk of complications, expense, and potential difficulties.

Excess Fluid Volume

● Monitor intake and output, urine specific gravity, breath sounds, heart sounds, peripheral pulses, edema, nausea, vomiting, anorexia, weakness, and fatigue. Heart failure, weakness, nausea, and vomiting can occur due to hyponatremia and water toxicity.

● Monitor serum electrolytes and notify physician of Na <120 mEq/L, K <3.5 mEq/L, Ca <8.5 mg/dl, or serum osmolality <280 mOsm/kg. Symptoms of hyponatremia and water toxicity begin near these levels.

- Monitor and report changes in LOC. Irritability, restlessness, confusion, convulsions, and unresponsiveness can occur. Place on seizure precautions if Na <110–120 mEq/L.

- Report weight gain of greater than 2 kg/day. Sudden weight gain may indicate fluid retention.

- Restrict fluid intake as ordered. Mild cases of SIADH may be controlled simply by restricting fluid intake.

- Administer hypertonic saline (3–5%) IV and drugs (demeclocycline or lithium carbonate) as ordered.

- Careful attention must be paid to fluid balance if drugs such as vincristine or cyclophosphamide are prescribed. Fluid restrictions worsen the risk of side effects for these drugs. Decrease dosage or discontinue the vincristine and cyclophosphamide chemotherapy, if ordered.

Risk for Injury

- Check for fatigue, apathy, depression, confusion, and weakness. These are neuromuscular symptoms of hypercalcemia and hypokalemia.

- Institute safety precautions to prevent accidental falls. Fractures are more likely because of bone demineralization and mental changes.

- Report new or worsening metastasis, especially bone metastasis. Hypercalcemia is more likely in the presence of bony metastasis, and can result in pathologic fractures. Hypokalemia can be caused by vomiting, diarrhea, nephrotoxicity, and hypercalcemia.

Decreased Cardiac Output

- Monitor potassium levels frequently, especially during and after aggressive radiation or chemotherapy, when hyperkalemia is most likely. Report potassium levels above 5.3 mEq/L. Cardiac dysrhythmias become more common as serum potassium increases above this level.

- Monitor serum calcium levels and notify the health care provider of calcium levels above 11 mg/dl. Elevated serum calcium is most common in the presence of skeletal metastasis and can lead to cardiac arrest.

● Carefully monitor cardiac rhythm and EKG pattern and report abnormalities. Peaked T waves are an early sign of hyperkalemia. Tachycardia, bradycardia, heart block, and cardiac arrest may follow. Calcium gluconate IVP may be ordered if EKG changes are present in hyperkalemia.

● Administer furosemide (Lasix) or other diuretics to promote excretion of potassium or to decrease tubular reabsorption of calcium. Insulin may be ordered to shift potassium into the cells.

● Administer Kayexalate in sorbitol PO or by enema to correct hyperkalemia. These agents cause a sodium-potassium ion exchange resulting in the excretion of excess potassium.

● Give calcitonin, mithramycin, biphosphates, steroids, or other medications as ordered to reduce serum calcium levels.

Disturbed Thought Processes

● Assess fluid and electrolyte balance frequently, particularly during periods of uncontrolled cell growth, tumor lysis, cachexia, ectopic hormone secretion, chemotherapy, and radiation. Fluid and electrolyte disturbances are most likely in cancer patients at these times, and many of these abnormalities (hypercalcemia, hypokalemia, hyponatremia, hypomagnesemia, etc.) can influence neuromuscular function.

● Administer agents to correct acidosis and/or electrolyte imbalance. Medicate for nausea, vomiting, diarrhea, or cardiac dysrhythmias as ordered. Control of these processes is necessary to prevent progression of neurological problems.

● Reorient to time, place, and person if confusion or disorientation is apparent. Impairment of thought processes can cause increased anxiety for the client and family.

● Check LOC, respiratory status, cardiac rhythm, renal function, and blood gases and report changes. Changes in these parameters may signal worsening of the fluid and electrolyte disturbance.

Impaired Urinary Elimination

● Administer intravenous hydration beginning 24 to 48 hours before treatment and at least 72 hours after treatment is completed. D_5 W/0.45 NS with $NaHCO_3$ mEq/L is usually recommended to alkalinize the urine. A pH of greater than 6 increases the solubility of uric acid.

● Monitor urinary output and urine color, clarity, hematuria, and specific gravity. It is particularly important to monitor these factors during and after chemotherapy, particularly in leukemia and lymphoma.

● Check for flank pain and medicate appropriately. Uric acid renal stones may cause acute, severe pain.

● Report signs of renal failure. Obstruction of urine flow by renal calculi can cause kidney damage and eventual renal failure.

● Report serum uric acid >8.0 mg/dl, urinary output <30 ml per hour, BUN >25 mg/dl, creatinine >1.2 mg/dl, or sudden weight gain with elevated BP, lung congestion, or edema.

● Administer allopurinol 100 mg/m^2 every 8 hours PO. Allopurinol reduces uric acid concentration by blocking conversion of uric acid precursors into uric acid.

● Teach the client and family dietary modifications to increase the alkalinity of the urine. Uric acid is more likely to precipitate in acidic urine.

Evaluation/Outcome

● Evaluate whether fluid balance has been restored/maintained through intake and output measures.

● Determine electrolyte balance by monitoring serum electrolyte tests.

● Monitor for signs and symptoms of fluid and electrolyte imbalances during anticancer therapy.

● Monitor weight frequently (losses can be common in client with cancer).

● Evaluate effectiveness of interventions through laboratory test findings and client's physical and mental status.

● Determine and document client's understanding of relevant signs, symptoms, and self-care.

Chronic Diseases with Fluid and Electrolyte Imbalances:
Heart Failure, Diabetic Ketoacidosis, and Chronic Obstructive Pulmonary Disease

Erlinda Wheeler, RN, PhD
Judith Herrman, RN, MS
Kathleen Schell, RN, DNSc

⬤ INTRODUCTION

A chronic disease, as defined by the U.S. National Center for Health Statistics, is a chronic condition that has a duration of three months or longer. Chronic conditions usually progress slowly over a long period of time. Chronic illnesses frequently do not occur as a single health problem, but are associated with multiple chronic health problems, e.g., a person with uncontrolled diabetes mellitus or chronic obstructive pulmonary disease (COPD) often develops heart failure (HF). This chapter addresses three common chronic diseases: (1) heart failure (HF), (2) diabetes mellitus (ketoacidosis), and (3) chronic obstructive pulmonary disease (COPD).

⬤ HEART FAILURE (HF)

Heart failure is a condition in which the heart is unable to adequately supply blood to meet the metabolic needs of the body. Left ventricular failure (heart failure) is the result of systolic or diastolic ventricular dysfunction. Right ventricular failure can be secondary to left ventricular failure or can result from pulmonary disease (cor pulmonale).

Pathophysiology

Heart failure is usually classified as left ventricular failure or right ventricular failure. Heart failure is most commonly caused by dysfunction of the left ventricle (systolic or diastolic dysfunction, or both). Systolic dysfunction can result from inadequate pumping of blood from the ventricle (pump failure) leading to decreased cardiac output. The left ventricle is unable to eject the normal stroke volume. Any condition that decreases myocardial contractility or increases afterload can cause systolic dysfunction (CAD, hypertension, dilated cardiomyopathy).

Diastolic dysfunction happens when there is inadequate filling of the ventricle during diastole, causing decreased blood volume in the ventricle and, therefore, decreased cardiac output. Inadequate filling of the ventricles is due to a decrease in ventricular compliance. Conditions causing diastolic dysfunction are ventricular hypertrophy, myocarditis, restrictive cardiomyopathy, and CAD.

Right ventricular failure can be secondary to left ventricular failure or pulmonary disease. Impairment of the right heart causes blood to back up in the systemic venous system, causing edema and eventually weight gain. Long-term heart failure usually involves both the right and the left ventricles. Table 22-1 lists the pathophysiologic factors associated with HF.

Etiology

Reasons that the heart fails include: (1) increased preload due to increased blood volume, (2) increased afterload because of increased pump resistance, and (3) decreased heart contractility. Causes of increased preload are mitral and/or aortic regurgitation and ventricular septal defects. Aortic stenosis and systemic hypertension cause pump resistance or increased afterload. Myocardial infarction and cardiomyopathy can cause decreased heart contractility. Table 22-2 lists the causes of left and right heart failure.

Table 22-1	Physiologic and Neurohormonal Changes Associated with Heart Failure
Physiologic Changes	**Rationale**
Cardiac output, CO (decreased)	Factors that influence CO are preload, afterload, myocardial contractility, and heart rate. Diseases (hypertension, CAD, ventricular hypertrophy, etc.) that adversely affect these factors decrease CO. Decrease in CO causes an increase in preload, afterload, contractility, and the heart rate to compensate for the failing heart.
Preload or left ventricular end-diastolic volume (LVEDV) (increased)	Increased volume in the ventricles after diastole will initially increase CO but can eventually lead to overstretching of the myocardium (ventricular dilatation) and cause contractility to decrease.
Afterload (increased)	Increased systemic vascular resistance is due to activation of the sympathetic nervous system stimulated by decreased CO and peripheral vascular resistance (PVR). Increased PVR leads to increased work for the heart to eject blood into the systemic circulation, leading to hypertrophy of the myocardium.
Myocardial contractility (decreased)	Contractility is affected by diseases (MI, myocarditis, cardiomyopathy) that affect myocyte activity, causing inefficient contraction of the ventricles. Increased preload and afterload will also affect contractility.
Heart rate (increased)	Tachycardia develops to compensate for decreased CO. Initially, cardiac output will increase, but eventually it causes less ventricular filling time.
Renal perfusion (decreased)	Decreased CO causes decreased renal blood flow.
Renin-angiotensin-aldosterone system activated	Decreased renal blood flow activates this system, causing vasoconstriction and sodium and fluid to be retained, leading to increased preload and afterload. Excess fluid dilutes sodium and can cause hyponatremia. Aldosterone can also cause loss of potassium in the urine, leading to hypokalemia.

(continues)

Table 22-1	Physiologic and Neurohormonal Changes Associated with Heart Failure—*continued*
Physiologic Changes	**Rationale**
Sympathetic nervous system (SNS) stimulated	Stimulation of SNS due to decreased CO causes tachycardia and increases systemic vascular resistance (BP) and the release of norepinephrine.
Left heart failure	Can be caused by either systolic or diastolic dysfunction or both. **Systolic dysfunction** is the inability of the left ventricle to pump enough blood to perfuse body tissues. **Diastolic dysfunction** is due to decreased compliance of the left ventricles leading to increased left ventricular end-diastolic pressure. Diseases affecting myocardial contractility, preload, and afterload lead to heart failure.
Right heart failure	Can result from left heart failure as a result of increased pressure on the left side. Pulmonary disease is also a cause of right heart failure.

Clinical Manifestations

The heart compensates for inadequate cardiac output by increasing the heart rate; thus, the blood pressure and respirations increase. The respiratory rate increases to improve the oxygen intake. Table 22-3 lists the clinical manifestations with rationales associated with HF. As the compensatory mechanisms fail to adequately control, left ventricular failure and/or pulmonary edema occurs, resulting in signs and symptoms similar to ECFVE or overhydration (constant, irritating cough, chest crackles, neck vein engorgement, and dyspnea). Right ventricular heart failure may also result. Symptoms include pitting edema in the extremities. Serum sodium and potassium levels may be normal or low due to hemodilution related to an excess of extracellular fluid. The serum osmolality may also reflect a low normal reading or decreased reading due to the ECFVE.

Table 22-2	Etiology of Heart Failure

Factors Affecting Heart Failure	Causes
Left Ventricular Failure (systolic and diastolic dysfunction)	
Increased preload	Mitral regurgitation
	Aortic regurgitation
	Ventricular septal defects
	Hypervolemia
Increased afterload	Systemic hypertension
	Aortic stenosis
	Hypertrophic cardiomyopathy
Myocardial dysfunction	Myocardial infarction
	Myocarditis
	Cardiomyopathy
	Coronary artery disease
	Dysrhythmias
Right Ventricular Failure	Pulmonary hypertension
	Left ventricular failure
	Myocardial infarction (right ventricular area)

Clinical Management

The main goals in the management of heart failure patients are to decrease oxygen demand of the body (promote rest) and to increase cardiac output. Increasing cardiac output involves decreasing preload, increasing myocardial contractility, and decreasing afterload. A low-sodium diet and fluid restriction are usually prescribed. The degree of sodium and fluid restriction is dependent on the severity of the heart failure.

The most common drug used to increase myocardial contractility and decrease tachycardia is digoxin. Digoxin is given for the first day or more in loading doses. Digoxin has a half-life of 36 hours, so digitalization (increased doses of digoxin) is needed to achieve a desired physiologic response. Digoxin is a cardiac glycoside (cardiotonic), which slows the ventricular contractions and increases the forcefulness of the contractions, thus increasing cardiac

Table 22-3	Clinical Manifestations Associated with HF
Clinical Manifestations	**Rationale**
Vital Signs (VS)	
Increased pulse rate (tachycardia)	Increased heart rate is a compensatory mechanism to improve circulation of the blood.
Increased respiration (tachypnea)	Respirations increase to increase oxygen intake for tissue oxygenation.
Increased blood pressure (hypertension)	When hypertension occurs, it is usually because of atherosclerosis. Noncirculating vascular fluid can also increase blood pressure.
Dyspnea	Difficulty breathing due to inadequate cardiac output and oxygen to the tissues, leading to increased breathing difficulty.
Fatigue with exertion or at rest	Inadequate blood flow and oxygen to the tissues.
Blood-tinged sputum; cough	Increased pulmonary capillary pressure causes blood from capillaries to enter the alveoli, leading to pulmonary edema.
Abnormal lung sounds (crackles)	Caused by fluid in the lungs; pulmonary edema.
Decreased urinary output	Decreased renal perfusion.
Edema	
Pulmonary	Caused by left ventricular heart failure. (Because of pump failure, fluid "backs up" in the pulmonary system, causing fluid congestion in the lung tissues.) Fluid inhibits adequate gas exchange (O_2 and CO_2). Signs and symptoms of pulmonary edema are similar to the signs and symptoms of overhydration.
Peripheral	May result from right ventricular heart failure. Fluids accumulate in the extremities due to the fluid back-up in the venous circulation.
Cyanosis	Cyanosis is a sign of hypoxia due to inadequate blood flow to body tissues.

(continues)

Table 22-3	Clinical Manifestations Associated with HF—*continued*
Clinical Manifestations	**Rationale**
Laboratory Results	
Plasma/serum sodium: increased (hypernatremia) or normal	Sodium retention in the extracellular fluid (ECF) usually occurs even when the serum sodium is within normal range or lower. Hemodilution can cause a normal or slightly lower serum sodium level.
Plasma/serum potassium: normal or decreased (hypokalemia)	The serum potassium level can be decreased with the use of potassium-wasting diuretics and due to hemodilution from fluid volume excess.
Plasma/serum magnesium: normal or decreased (hypomagnesemia)	Long-term use of potassium-wasting diuretics can cause both hypomagnesemia and hypokalemia.
Serum osmolality: < 280 mOsm/kg	Due to hemodilution. If the serum sodium level is increased, the serum osmolality increases.

output. The heart has to work harder to pump the blood against an increased vascular resistance (afterload). Diuretics decrease preload. Decreasing afterload and preload increases cardiac output. Diuretics are used to excrete sodium and water. Furosemide (Lasix) is a diuretic commonly administered intravenously and orally. This diuretic (a potassium-wasting diuretic) not only excretes sodium, but excretes potassium, calcium, and magnesium as well. When the serum potassium level decreases because of the use of potent potassium-wasting diuretics, ventricular dysrhythmias result from hypokalemia (K <3.2 mEq/L). Serum potassium and sodium levels need to be closely monitored. Serum digoxin levels have a narrow therapeutic range (0.5–2.0 mg/ml).

Other drug therapy used to control heart failure includes beta-adrenergic agonists, Ca^{++} channel blockers, phosphodiesterase inhibitors, angiotensin-converting enzyme (ACE) inhibitors, and vasodilators. Both beta-adrenergic agonists and ACE inhibitors increase cardiac output. Cardiac glycosides, sympathomimetics (beta-adrenergic agonists), and phosphodiesterase (PDE) inhibitors are three positive inotropic group agents that exert an effect on the heart by increasing myocardial contractility. Table 22-4 lists the drug categories and doses used to manage heart failure.

Clinical Considerations: Heart Failure (HF)

1. Know the signs and symptoms of heart failure. The more common clinical manifestations are dyspnea, crackles, edema, tachycardia, and neck vein engorgement.

2. For quick assessment of overhydration because of heart failure, check for hand vein engorgement. Lower the hand below the heart level until the hand veins are engorged; then raise the hand above the heart level. If the hand veins remain engorged above the heart level for 10 to 15 seconds, fluid volume excess is likely to be present.

3. Serum sodium and potassium should be monitored. If the client is taking digoxin and a potassium-wasting diuretic such as furosemide (Lasix), daily potassium supplements should be administered. If the client is taking digoxin and furosemide or hydrochlorothiazide, hypokalemia (serum potassium loss) is likely to occur. Hypokalemia enhances the action of digoxin and can cause digitalis toxicity (slow, irregular pulse, anorexia, nausea, vomiting, and visual disturbances).

4. Check for signs and symptoms of hypokalemia; e.g., dizziness, muscular weakness, abdominal distention, diminished peristalsis, and dysrhythmia.

5. Monitor vital signs and ECG for changes during clinical management. Note if the client is having difficulty breathing.

6. For clients having difficulty breathing, elevate the head of the bed. This position lowers the diaphragm and increases the air space.

7. The client with HF should not use table salt unless otherwise indicated.

Table 22-4	Medications for the Control of HF

Drug	Rationale
Digitalis Preparation Digoxin	Digoxin exerts a positive inotropic action on the heart, increasing the contractility of the myocardium. To increase the blood level of digoxin when first used, a digitalization program over 24 hours is prescribed; e.g., 1.0–1.5 mg dose divided over 24 hours, then maintenance doses of 0.125–0.25 mg are prescribed daily. A serum digoxin level of >2.0 mg/ml causes digitalis toxicity; therefore, the serum level needs to be closely monitored. Signs and symptoms of digitalis toxicity include anorexia, nausea, vomiting, diarrhea, bradycardia (pulse rate <60), and visual disturbances.
Diuretics **Loop or High-Ceiling** Furosemide (Lasix)	Diuretics increase urine output, which decreases fluid volume. A loop diuretic is usually prescribed for severe HF. Furosemide moves large volumes of fluid for excretion. It is effective even when the glomerular filtration rate (GFR) is low.
Thiazide Hydrochlorothiazide (HydroDiuril)	Thiazide diuretics are prescribed for mild to moderate HF. Thiazides are not effective when the GFR is low. Loop and thiazide diuretics cause potassium (K) loss; thus, potassium supplements should be given and the serum potassium levels should be closely monitored. Hypokalemia causes ventricular dysrhythmias.
Sympathomimetics (Beta-Adrenergic Agonists) Dopamine Dobutamine	Beta adrenergics stimulate the beta cells in the heart, increasing myocardial contractility and cardiac output. Dopamine and dobutamine have a strong positive inotropic effect (increase contractility) and can decrease afterload. These agents dilate renal blood vessels; thus, urine output is increased. However, high doses of

(continues)

Table 22-4	Medications for the Control of HF

Drug	Rationale
Sympathomimetics (Beta-Adrenergic Agonists), continued	dopamine can stimulate the alpha$_1$-adrenergic receptors, which can cause an increase in vascular resistance and an increase in afterload, which decreases cardiac output. Dobutamine does not activate the alpha$_1$ receptors. Both agents are used for short-term treatment of acute HF.
Phosphodiesterase Inhibitors Amrinone lactate (Inocor) Milrinone (Primacor)	These agents exert a positive inotropic effect on the heart. They increase myocardial contractility and promote vasodilation, thus decreasing afterload. They are used primarily for short-term (<24 hours) drug therapy for severe HF.
Angiotensin-Converting Enzyme (ACE) Inhibitors Captopril (Capoten) Enalapril (Vasotec)	ACE inhibitors promote vasodilation by inhibiting angiotensin II, a potent vasoconstrictor that stimulates the release of aldosterone, causing sodium and water retention. By blocking angiotensin II, cardiac output, stroke volume, and renal blood flow are increased. Adverse effects include hypotension, hyperkalemia due to a decrease in aldosterone, and a cough of unknown origin. ACE inhibitors should not be used with potassium supplements.
Vasodilators Nitroglycerin Sodium nitroprusside Prazosin HCL (Minipress)	Vasodilators are helpful for short-term treatment of HF. Nitrates such as nitroglycerin affect the veins, thus decreasing pooling of blood and pulmonary congestion. With nitrates, hypotension and reflex tachycardia may result. Sodium nitroprusside and prazosin can cause venous and arterial dilation. These agents decrease both preload and afterload. With use of vasodilators, the blood pressure needs to be monitored closely.

● CLIENT MANAGEMENT FOR HF

Assessment

- Obtain baseline vital signs and ECG to determine abnormal changes and for comparison with future vital signs and ECG readings.

- Assess for signs and symptoms of left ventricular heart failure (overhydration or pulmonary edema), i.e., constant, irritating cough, dyspnea, neck and/or hand vein engorgement, chest crackles.

- Check serum electrolyte levels, especially potassium and sodium. Use baseline electrolyte results for comparison with future serum electrolytes.

Nursing Diagnoses

- Excess fluid volume, related to decreased cardiac output related to impaired excretion of Na and H_2O.

- Impaired breathing patterns, related to transudation of fluid into the lung tissues.

- Impaired tissue integrity, related to fluid accumulation in the extremities and buttocks.

- Decreased cardiac output, related to cardiopulmonary insufficiency.

Interventions

- Auscultate lung areas to detect abnormal breath sounds, such as crackles due to lung congestion (pulmonary edema).

- Monitor vein engorgement by checking hand veins for fluid overload. Lower the hand below the heart level until the hand veins are engorged, then raise the hand above the heart level. If the hand veins remain engorged above the heart level after 15 seconds, fluid volume excess is most likely present.

- Check the feet and ankles daily in the early morning before the client rises. If edema is present, the reason is probably due to cardiac and/or renal dysfunction.

- Instruct the client not to use table salt to season foods. Salt contains sodium, which can cause water retention. Suggest other ways to enhance flavor of foods.

- Instruct the client to eat foods rich in potassium (fruits, vegetables) if the client is taking a potassium-wasting diuretic and digoxin. Hypokalemia enhances the action of digoxin and can cause digitalis toxicity (slow, irregular pulse, anorexia, nausea, vomiting).

- Assess for signs and symptoms of hypokalemia.

- Monitor breathing patterns. Note the presence of dyspnea, shortness of breath, rapid breathing, and wheezing.

- Elevate the head of the bed 30° to 75° to lower the diaphragm and increase alveoli spaces for gas exchange.

- Encourage the client to change positions frequently. Edematous tissue can break down due to hypoxia and constant pressure on skin surface.

- Provide skin care, especially to edematous areas, at least twice daily.

Evaluation/Outcome

- Evaluate the therapeutic effect of interventions to correct the underlying cause of HF.

- Remain free of signs and symptoms of heart failure.

- Evaluate the effectiveness of medications in reducing pulmonary and/or peripheral edema, and cardiac symptoms.

- Evaluate the dietary intake, and fluid intake and output.

- Evaluate that a support system is available for the client.

DIABETES MELLITUS (DM) AND DIABETIC KETOACIDOSIS (DKA)

The pathophysiological changes and the signs and symptoms of diabetes mellitus (DM) result from an absolute or relative deficiency of insulin. Insulin is used by the body to transport glucose into the cells to be used in metabolism. Destruction of the beta cells of the pancreas, the cells responsible for the production of insulin, from either autoimmune or other processes, results in the insulin insufficiency. Over 15 million people in the United States are affected by some form of diabetes mellitus. Two of the most common types of diabetes mellitus are Type 1 diabetes mellitus, resulting from an absolute insulin deficiency; and Type 2 diabetes mellitus, resulting from a relative lack of insulin. Type 1, previously known as insulin-dependent or juvenile onset diabetes mellitus, and Type 2, previously referred to as non-insulin-dependent or adult onset diabetes mellitus require very different methods of treatment. The cornerstones of treatment of Type 1 DM are insulin, diet, exercise, and stress management; for Type 2 DM management includes diet/weight control, oral hypoglycemic agents, exercise, and, in rare cases, insulin supplementation.

Diabetic ketoacidosis (DKA) is often associated with Type 1 diabetes mellitus, and results from a severe or complete deficit of insulin secretion. DKA is characterized by a blood sugar exceeding 300 mg/dl, ketosis, a blood pH <7.30, and a bicarbonate level <14 mEq/L. Hyperosmolar hyperglycemic state (HHS) is characterized by a blood sugar >500 mg/dl, dehydration, and a serum osmolality <300 mOsm/kg.

Pathophysiology

A cessation or deficit of insulin secretions limits the body's utilization of glucose. With an insulin deficit, the cells are starved of important nutrients. Fat and protein catabolism (breakdown) occurs to provide the body with needed energy. Fatty acids are released from the breakdown of adipose (fat) tissue. Acids are further broken down into ketonic acids (ketones) and acetoacetate (acetone). Because the liver cannot oxidize the excess ketones, the ketone bodies accumulate in the blood. The acetone is excreted by the lungs.

Table 22-5 describes the pathophysiologic factors associated with diabetic ketoacidosis.

Etiology

Many clients with diabetes mellitus are undiagnosed. Their first presentation with the disease is in acute diabetic ketoacidosis. Untreated diabetes mellitus can lead to diabetic ketoacidosis as a result of the high blood sugar levels and lack

Table 22-5	Pathophysiologic Changes Associated with Diabetic Ketoacidosis
Pathophysiologic Changes	**Rationale**
Ketosis	Failure to metabolize glucose leads to an increase in fat catabolism and ketone bodies. Ketosis occurs when there is an excess of ketone bodies (ketonic acids) in the blood. Ketosis leads to diabetic ketoacidosis. Ketones (strong acids) combine with the sodium, causing sodium depletion. Ketone bodies are excreted as ketonuria.
Increased lactic acid	Cellular breakdown due to a lack of nutrients to the cells causes the release of lactic acid from the cells.
Increased hydrogen ions	Hydrogen ions are reabsorbed from the kidney tubules back into circulation as the bicarbonate ions are excreted. An increase in hydrogen ion concentration increases the acidotic state.
Hyperosmolality	An elevated blood sugar increases the hyperosmolality of the extracellular fluid. Because of hyperosmolality, osmotic diuresis occurs, causing the kidneys to excrete bicarbonate, potassium, and phosphorus. Also, hyperosmolality leads to the withdrawal of cellular fluid and cellular dehydration occurs.
Glycosuria	An elevation of the blood sugar, >180 mg/dl, increases the glucose concentration in the glomeruli of the kidneys. When the concentration of glucose in the glomeruli exceeds the renal threshold for tubular reabsorption, glycosuria results. Increased glucose concentration acts as an osmotic diuretic, causing diuresis.
Dehydration (cellular and extracellular)	Cellular dehydration occurs due to increased glucose concentration in the blood. Extracellular fluid increases because of the cellular fluid shift and then decreases due to osmotic diuresis. With a cellular fluid shift, potassium is lost from the cells; the extracellular potassium level may be within normal range or elevated.

of nutrients to the cells. Ketosis due to cellular breakdown causes the blood pH and bicarbonate levels to decrease, resulting in ketoacidosis. Selected acute stressors such as trauma, infection, major surgical interventions, myocardial infarction, some medications, and select medical conditions can trigger the occurrence of diabetic ketoacidosis.

Hyperosmolar hyperglycemic state (HHS) develops in middle-age or older individuals. It is usually associated with Type 2 diabetics. HHS develops more slowly than DKA. The blood sugar levels and BUN are usually greater than those with DKA. Clients with HHS usually do not develop ketosis; the reason for this is unknown. Stress or injury can precipitate a hyperosmolar hyperglycemic state. Table 22-6 indicates the causes of DKA and HHS.

Table 22-6	Causes of Diabetic Ketoacidosis and Hyperosmolar Hyperglycemic State
Categories	**Causes**
Diabetic Ketoacidosis	
Insulin deficiency	Undiagnosed DM, Type I
	Omission of prescribed insulin
Acute incidence	Infection
	Trauma
	Major surgical interventions
	Pancreatitis
	Gastroenteritis
Miscellaneous	Hyperthyroidism
	Steroids (glucocorticoids)
	Adrenergic agonists
Hyperosmolar hyperglycemic state (HHS)	
Insulin deficiency	Undiagnosed DM, Type 2
Incidences	Stress
	Infection
	Renal or cardiovascular disease
Miscellaneous	Continuous use of total parenteral nutrition (TPN)
	Steroids

Clinical Manifestations

The most common symptoms of DKA are extreme thirst, polyuria, weakness, and fatigue. Hyperglycemia induces osmotic diuresis. Dehydration results from diuresis; the skin is dry with poor skin turgor, and the lips are parched.

Potassium, sodium, magnesium, phosphorus, and bicarbonate imbalances usually result from DKA. As cells break down because of a lack of nutrients, excess potassium moves from the cells into the extracellular compartments. When the acidotic state is corrected, potassium reenters the cells and hypokalemia may result. During early fluid loss, the sodium level may be elevated because of an increase in the aldosterone secretion (sodium-retaining hormone) response. However, with continuous diuresis, the serum sodium level is decreased. The hemoglobin and hematocrit elevate in response to the fluid volume deficit (hemoconcentration). Table 22-7 describes the signs and symptoms and laboratory results related to DKA.

Classic signs and symptoms of a hypoglycemic reaction (insulin shock) include nervousness; dizziness; cold, clammy skin; headache; irritability; visual changes; fatigue; hunger; tachycardia; and slurred speech. These symptoms occur when the blood sugar is 50 mg/dl or lower.

Clinical Management

Treatment modalities for DKA include: (1) vigorous fluid replacement, (2) insulin replacement, and (3) electrolyte correction. Osmotic diuresis can cause a fluid volume deficit of 4 to 8 liters of body fluid. In such a case, immediate restoration of fluid loss is essential.

Fluid Replacement

In the first 24 hours, 80% of the total water and salt deficit should be replaced. There is less urgency for the other electrolytes because the rate of assimilation of the intracellular electrolytes is limited during the acidotic state. Administration of potassium must be included, but *not in early treatment* (unless indicated), because an elevated serum potassium can be toxic.

For the first hour, 1 to 2 liters of crystalloid (normal saline solution [0.9% NaCl] or lactated Ringer's solution) may

Table 22-7 Clinical Manifestations of DKA

Signs and Symptoms	Rationale
Extreme Thirst *Polyuria*	Elevated blood sugar and ketones increase the serum osmolality, causing thirst and osmotic diuresis.
Weakness, Fatigue	Reduced cellular metabolism results in low energy levels.
Nausea, Vomiting	Continuous vomiting causes a loss of body fluids and electrolytes. The body attempts to compensate for acidosis with the vomiting of acidic gastric contents. Dehydration results.
Vital Signs Temperature elevated or N	Infection causes an elevated temperature; dehydration can cause a slightly elevated temperature.
Pulse rapid	With a loss of body fluid, the heart beats faster to compensate in order to maintain circulation. Tachycardia of greater than 140 bpm denotes a severe fluid loss.
Blood pressure slightly to severely decreased	With early fluid loss from diuresis, the blood pressure decreases by 10–15 mm Hg.
Respiration rapid, vigorous breathing	Kussmaul breathing is a compensatory mechanism to decrease H_2CO_2 (acid) by blowing off CO_2.
Poor Skin Turgor; Dry, Parched Lips; Disorientation, Confusion	Dehydration frequently results in these symptoms: poor skin turgor; dry, parched lips; and confusion.
Abdominal Pain with Tenderness	Abdominal pain usually indicates severe ketoacidosis.
Laboratory Test Results Blood sugar 300–800 mg/dl	Blood sugar level is high; at times, it is not as high as hyperosmolar hyperglycemic state (HHS). Sugar is not metabolized and utilized by the cells.

(continues)

Table 22-7	Clinical Manifestations of DKA —*continued*
Signs and Symptoms	**Rationale**

Electrolytes Potassium N, ↓, ↑	Potassium in the cells is low, but the serum potassium level may be high due to a hemoconcentration. Normal or low levels can also occur.
Sodium N, ↓, ↑	Sodium is lost because of diuresis. Serum levels can be elevated due to dehydration.
Magnesium N, ↓, ↑ Chloride N, ↓ Phosphorus low N or ↓	Magnesium and phosphorus react the same as potassium. Chloride is excreted with sodium and water.
CO_2 ↓	The serum CO_2 is a bicarbonate determinant. With the loss of bicarbonate, the serum CO_2 is greatly decreased (<14 mEq/L).
Serum osmolality 300–350 mOsm/kg	Fluid loss (dehydration) increases the serum osmolality.
Hematology Hemoglobin, hematocrit ↑ WBC ↑	Because of fluid loss, hemoconcentration results, increasing hematocrit levels. Hemoglobin levels may be increased or decreased dependent upon concurrent anemia and hemoconcentration. Elevated white blood cells can indicate an infection.
Arterial Blood Gases (ABGs) pH ↓ $PaCO_2$ ↓ HCO_3 ↓	The pH is low in the acidotic state. The $PaCO_2$ may be decreased as the lungs are expelling CO_2 (compensatory mechanism). The bicarbonate is lost through diuresis with an increase in hydrogen and ketone (acid) levels.
Urine Glycosuria Ketonuria	Glucose and ketones spill into the urine.

Note: N = normal; ↑ = elevated; ↓ = decreased; bpm = beats per minute

be rapidly infused to reestablish the fluid volume balance. This may be followed by 1 liter every hour for the next two hours or as indicated. Rapid fluid replacement decreases the hyperglycemic state by causing hemodilution. ECF is restored directly through intravenous therapy; however, a fluid overload in the ECF space should be avoided. Rapid replacement of fluids must be vigilantly monitored to avoid overhydration. Cerebral edema in children and pulmonary edema in older adults must be carefully watched for and treated soon after detection. ICF replacement occurs over approximately two days.

Insulin Replacement

Ten to fifteen years ago, massive doses of insulin were administered for the treatment of DKA. Today, less insulin is used when correcting DKA. Preferably, regular insulin is given through an intravenous line with a bolus dose followed with a continuous infusion. A standard guideline for IV insulin replacement is an insulin bolus of 0.15 U/kg, followed by 0.1 U/kg per hour continuous IV infusion until blood sugar reaches 250 mg/dl. If the blood sugar does not fall, the infusion can be increased to 0.2 U/kg per hour. It is important to monitor the client's hydration status throughout insulin infusion. Refer to the accompanying box for an example of this guideline.

A client weighs 154 pounds or 70 kg. The order reads regular insulin bolus of 0.15 U/kg and 0.1 U/kg/hour in continuous normal saline solution. Using the standard guideline for an insulin bolus (0.15 × weight in kgs):

0.15 U × 70 kg = 10.5 units

Followed by the standard guideline for IV continuous infusion (0.1 U × 70 kg = 7 U/hr). The patient would receive 10.5 units of insulin in a bolus followed by 7 units of insulin per hour in an IV of normal saline solution. When the blood sugar level reaches 250 mg/dl, the IV solution is generally changed to 5% dextrose in water. This prevents the possible occurrence of a hypoglycemic reaction. As the acidosis state is corrected, insulin is utilized more rapidly by the body for metabolizing sugar (glucose).

The longer the acidosis persists, the more resistant the person is likely to be to insulin, and more insulin administration may be required.

Electrolyte Correction

Potassium (K) replacement should start approximately six to eight hours after the first dose of insulin has been administered (intravenously or intramuscularly) and as the acidotic state is being corrected. Potassium replacement is dependent upon adequate renal function, and, therefore, the client must have voided in order to begin replacement. Serum potassium levels should be taken frequently. Potassium moves back into cells as the fluid imbalance and the acidotic state are corrected.

Magnesium, phosphate, and bicarbonate serum levels should be closely monitored. If the serum magnesium level is low, hypokalemia is not fully corrected until the magnesium level is corrected.

There is some controversy related to phosphate replacement when treating DKA. Phosphates are needed for neuromuscular function; thus, serum phosphorus should be monitored along with the other electrolytes.

Another controversial issue is the use of bicarbonate therapy in the treatment of DKA. Generally, replacement of fluids and insulin corrects the acidotic state. If the pH falls below 7.0, bicarbonate replacement is usually prescribed.

A summary of the clinical management of diabetic ketoacidosis is presented in Table 22-8.

Clinical Considerations: Diabetes Mellitus (DM) and Diabetic Ketoacidosis (DKA)

1. Check for signs and symptoms of hyperglycemia and hypoglycemia. With hyperglycemia and DKA, extreme thirst, polyuria, weakness, and fatigue usually occur. The common signs and symptoms of hypoglycemia are cold, clammy skin; nervousness; weakness; dizziness; tachycardia; slurred speech; headache; irritability; visual changes; fatigue; hunger; and decreased blood pressure.

2. Assess urine output. Polyuria occurs in uncontrolled diabetes mellitus and diabetic ketoacidosis. Check urine for glycosuria and ketonuria. When blood sugar is >180 mg/dl, glycosuria usually occurs.

3. Check the serum osmolality using the formula:

$$2 \times \text{Serum Na} + \frac{\text{BUN}}{3} + \frac{\text{Glucose}}{18} = \text{serum osmolality}$$

Table 22-8	Treatment Modalities for Diabetic Ketoacidosis
Categories	**Treatment Modalities**
Fluid replacement	First 24 hours: 80% water and salt deficit replacement.
	First hour: 1 to 2 liters of crystalloid (normal saline solution [0.9% NaCl] or lactated Ringer's).
	Second and third hour: 1 liter per hour as indicated. Avoid fluid overload.
	Blood sugar reaches 250 mg/dl; IV fluids are switched to D_5W to avoid a possible hypoglycemic reaction.
	ICF replacement occurs in about two days.
Insulin replacement	Suggested replacement:
	initial bolus of regular insulin: 0.15 U/kg.
	Hourly in IV fluids: 0.1 U/kg until the blood sugar level reaches 250 mg/dl.
	If acidosis persists, insulin resistance is occurring: More insulin administration may be needed.
Electrolyte replacement	Potassium: Replacement is initiated about six to eight hours after the first dose of insulin, and when adequate renal function has been confirmed. Monitor serum K levels frequently.
	Magnesium, phosphate, and bicarbonate: Monitor serum levels closely. Replace as indicated.
	Bicarbonate replacement is usually not indicated unless the pH is <7.1. Replacement of fluids and insulin normally corrects the acidotic state.

If the serum osmolality is >296 mOsm/kg, hemoconcentration or fluid loss is occurring due to polyuria.

4. Check for signs and symptoms of fluid loss, i.e., poor skin turgor; dry, parched lips; dry, warm skin; dry mucous membranes; increased pulse rate; and decreased blood pressure.

5. Monitor blood sugar levels. A client with diabetes mellitus should check blood sugar level daily using a glucometer or other approved testing device. Daily

insulin dose(s) may need to be increased or decreased according to blood sugar levels.

6. Monitor arterial blood gases (ABGs), particularly pH and HCO_3, when diabetic ketoacidosis is suspected. Diabetic acidosis or metabolic acidosis can occur in severely uncontrolled diabetes mellitus, Type 1. A decrease in arterial pH and HCO_3 determines the severity of the acidotic state.

7. When correcting DKA, large volumes of intravenous fluids are administered. Check that a fluid overload or hypervolemia is not occurring. Signs and symptoms of hypervolemia include constant, irritating cough, dyspnea, chest crackles, and vein engorgement.

● CLIENT MANAGEMENT FOR DKA

Assessment

● Obtain the client's history of diabetes mellitus.

● Check for abnormal vital signs such as tachycardia, slightly decreased blood pressure, deep rapid breathing (Kussmaul respirations), and slightly elevated or high temperature. These can indicate dehydration and a possible acidotic state.

● Check urine for glycosuria and ketonuria. These are additional indicators of DKA.

● Assess urine output. Polyuria is an indicator of hyperglycemia and osmotic diuresis.

Nursing Diagnoses

● Deficient fluid volume, related to hyperglycemia and osmotic diuresis (polyuria).

● Imbalanced nutrition, less than body requirements, related to insufficient utilization of glucose and nutrients.

● Ineffective tissue perfusion (renal, cardiopulmonary, peripheral), related to deficient fluid volume and lack of glucose utilization.

● Excess fluid volume, related to excessive administration of IV fluids.

● Risk for injury, cells and tissues, related to glucose intolerance and infections secondary to DKA.

Interventions

● Monitor vital signs. Changes that can be indicative of fluid loss or dehydration and acidosis include rapid, thready pulse rate; slightly decreased systolic blood pressure; rapid and deep breathing (Kussmaul respiration); and a slightly elevated temperature.

● Check for other signs and symptoms of fluid loss such as poor skin turgor; dry, parched lips; dry, warm skin; and dry mucous membranes.

● Check the serum osmolality. Serum osmolality >296 mOsm/kg can indicate hemoconcentration due to fluid loss.

● Monitor blood sugar level. Levels greater than 200 mg/dl indicate hyperglycemia. Increased blood sugar levels can cause osmotic diuresis.

● Observe for signs and symptoms of hypokalemia and hyperkalemia (see Chapter 5).

● Instruct clients to monitor their blood sugar level and/or urine to detect glycosuria. For testing blood sugars, the use of a glucometer or some other approved testing device is suggested.

● Administer normal saline solution and/or a Ringer's solution as prescribed to reestablish ECF.

● Administer regular insulin intravenously as prescribed in a bolus and in IV fluids to correct insulin deficiency (see suggested guidelines in Table 22-8).

● Observe for signs and symptoms of a hypoglycemic reaction (insulin reaction or shock) from possible overcorrection of hyperglycemia. The symptoms include cold, clammy skin; nervousness; weakness; dizziness; tachycardia; low blood pressure; headache; irritability; visual changes; fatigue; hunger; and slurred speech.

● Monitor urine output, heart rate, blood pressure, and chest sounds for abnormalities. Fluid deficit limits tissue perfusion and decreases circulatory volume and nutrients available to the vital organs.

● Monitor arterial blood gases (ABGs), particularly the pH, $PaCO_2$, and HCO_3. A decrease in arterial pH and HCO_3 determines the severity of the acidotic state.

Evaluation/Outcome

● Evaluate the therapeutic effect of interventions in correcting diabetic ketoacidosis. Serum osmolality, serum electrolytes, and the arterial blood gases are within normal ranges.

● The client remains free of signs and symptoms related to diabetic ketoacidosis.

● Evaluate the effectiveness of fluid, insulin, and electrolyte replacements.

● Determine that the urine output has returned to normal daily range.

CHRONIC OBSTRUCTIVE PULMONARY DISEASE (COPD)

Chronic obstructive pulmonary disease (COPD) is a chronic lung disease associated with airflow obstruction or limitation that is not fully reversible. The fourth leading cause of chronic morbidity and mortality in the United States, COPD includes emphysema and chronic bronchitis. Although chronic bronchitis is considered more a disease of the bronchial airways and emphysema is defined as lung parenchymal destruction with airspace enlargement, these two types of COPD commonly coexist. Asthma was removed from this group of diseases by the American Thoracic Society in 1995 because it is better characterized by inflammation with activation of complex cellular and chemical mediators than obstruction. However, asthmatics may develop COPD.

Pathophysiology

The physiologic changes associated with most types of COPD include: (1) thickening of bronchial walls caused by submucosal edema and excess mucous secretion, (2) loss of elastic recoil of lung tissue, and (3) destruction of the alveolar septa that promote overdistention and dead air space. Airway obstruction is greatest on expiration.

With advanced COPD, respiratory acidosis occurs. Because of hypoventilation, carbon dioxide is retained. Water combines with CO_2 to produce carbonic acid and a decrease in pH, resulting in respiratory acidosis. With inadequate gas exchange, CO_2 retention or hypercapnia is increased. Reduced oxygen in the blood is frequently caused by airway obstruction and alveolar hypoventilation. The thickened alveolar capillary membrane reduces oxygen diffusion. Table 22-9 lists the pathophysiologic changes and rationale associated with COPD conditions.

Etiology

Established causes of COPD include cigarette smoking, occupational exposure to dusts, gases, and fumes, and alpha$_1$-antitrypsin deficiency. A deficiency in the protein alpha$_1$-antitrypsin, which inhibits specific proteolytic enzymes in the lung, is a common genetic cause of emphysema. Other factors that have been implicated as probable causes include frequent childhood respiratory infections, living in a densely air-polluted environment, living in a low-socioeconomic environment, and exposure to secondhand smoke. Table 22-10 lists the established and probable causes of COPD.

Clinical Manifestations

Symptoms of COPD commonly develop in the 5th decade of life, when individuals present with a chronic productive cough or an acute chest illness. Clients typically have a history of two packs per day for 20 years or longer of smoking. Dyspnea is more likely during the 6th or 7th decade, and it often becomes the dominant symptom. Dyspnea on exertion leads to deconditioning and a vicious cycle of shortness of breath, activity intolerance, and increased sputum production. Clients experience orthopnea and require a forward-bending posture to sit and/or a semisitting position to sleep. Other classic manifestations of COPD include use of accessory respiratory muscles, a barrel-shaped chest, and digital clubbing. Table 22-11 lists the signs and symptoms of early to advanced COPD.

Table 22-9	Pathophysiologic Changes in Chronic Obstructive Pulmonary Disease (COPD)
Pathophysiologic Changes	**Rationale**
Decreased elasticity of bronchiolar walls (loss of elastic recoil)	Loss of elastic recoil causes a premature collapse of airways with expiration. Alveoli become overdistended when air is trapped in the affected lung tissue and dead air space is increased. Overdistention leads to rupture and coalescence of several alveoli.
Alveolar damage	Chronic air trapping and airway inflammation lead to weakened bronchiolar walls and alveolar disruption. Coalescence of adjacent alveoli results in bullae (parenchymal air-filled spaces >1 cm in diameter). The total area of gas exchange is greatly reduced and pulmonary hypertension may develop.
Mucous gland hyperplasia and increased mucous production	Oversecretion of mucus is commonly found in bronchitis and advanced emphysema. Increased mucous production can cause mucous plugs, which lead to airway obstruction.
Inflammation of bronchial mucosa	Inflammatory infiltration and edema of the bronchial mucosa commonly occur in bronchitis, but are also found in advanced emphysema. Edema and infiltration cause thickening of bronchiolar walls.
Airway obstruction	This condition is caused primarily by narrowed bronchioles, edema, and mucous plugs. Obstruction is greatest on expiration. During inspiration bronchial lumina widen to admit air; the lumina collapse during expiration.
CO_2 retention Increased $PaCO_2$ >45 mm Hg (hypercapnia) Norms: 35–45 mm Hg	Accumulation of carbon dioxide (CO_2) concentration in the arterial blood from inadequate gas exchange is the result of hypoventilation.

(continues)

Table 22-9	Pathophysiologic Changes in Chronic Obstructive Pulmonary Disease (COPD)—*continued*
Pathophysiologic Changes	**Rationale**
Respiratory acidosis	CO_2 retention results from hypoventilation. Water combines with CO_2 to produce carbonic acid, and with increased CO_2 retention respiratory acidosis occurs [$(H_2O) + CO_2 = H_2CO_3$]. The arterial blood gases reflect pH <7.35; $PaCO_2 > 45$ mm Hg.
Hypoxemia	Hypoxemia, or reduced oxygen (O_2) in the blood, is frequently caused by airway obstruction and alveolar hypoventilation. The thickened alveolar capillary membrane reduces O_2 diffusion.
Cor pulmonale (right heart failure due to pulmonary hypertension)	Destruction of alveolar tissue leads to hypoxic vasoconstriction and a reduction of the size of the pulmonary capillary bed. Pulmonary hypertension occurs when 2/3 to 3/4 of the vascular bed is destroyed. The workload of the right ventricle is then increased, thus causing right ventricular hypertrophy and eventually right heart failure.
Increased red blood cell (RBC) count	Secondary polycythemia occurs as a compensatory mechanism with prolonged hypoxemia. Hemoglobin and hematocrit are increased to enhance O_2 transport.
Alpha$_1$-antitrypsin deficiency	A genetic predisposition to alpha$_1$-antitrypsin deficiency is present. An antitrypsin or trypsin inhibitor is produced in the liver. A deficit of antitrypsin allows proteolytic enzymes (released in the lungs from bacteria or phagocytic cells) to damage lung tissue. The result is emphysema.

Table 22-10	Causes of COPD

Established Causes	Probable Causes
Smoking	Exposure to secondhand smoke
Occupational exposure to dusts, gases, and fumes	Frequent childhood respiratory infections
Alpha₁-antitrypsin deficiency	Living in a densely air-polluted environment
	Living in a low-socioeconomic environment

Table 22-11	Clinical Manifestations of COPD

Signs and Symptoms	Rationale
Cough (productive)	A cough is usually associated with bronchitis because of the excessive secretion of the mucous glands. In emphysema a cough is associated with respiratory infection or cardiac failure. Bacterial growth in retained mucous secretions leads to repeated infections and a chronic cough.
Dyspnea	Difficulty in breathing and shortness of breath following exertion are early signs of COPD. In advanced COPD, dyspnea occurs with little or no exertion.
Vital Signs	
Increased heart rate and blood pressure	Hypoxia stimulates the peripheral chemoreceptors, primarily the carotid bodies. Signals are sent to the respiratory muscles, which in turn trigger this "pulmonary reflex" in attempt to increase cardiac output and decrease hypoxemia.
Prolonged expiration	Loss of elasticity of lung tissue causes bronchioles to collapse during normal expiration.
Accessory muscle use	Activated when the diaphragm becomes significantly depressed. These muscles contract, increasing negative intrapleural pressure and offsetting increased airway resistance.

(continues)

Table 22-11	Clinical Manifestations of COPD —*continued*
Signs and Symptoms	**Rationale**
Barrel-Shaped Chest (AP diameter > lateral diameter)	This is the result of loss of lung elasticity, chronic air trapping, and chest wall expansion with chest rigidity. It may also be compounded by dorsal kyphosis which results from a bent-forward position used to facilitate breathing. Shoulders are elevated and the neck appears to shorten. Accessory muscles of respiration are used for breathing.
Chronic Fatigue	Fatigue, an early sign of COPD, is caused by hypoxia and the increased effort required to move air into and out of the lungs.
Cyanosis	In advanced COPD, marked cyanosis is due to poor tissue perfusion, which results from hypoxemia.
Clubbing of Nails	Clubbing of nails is commonly seen in association with hypoxemia and polycythemia. It may be due to capillary dilation in an attempt to draw more oxygen to the fingertips.
Palpation	
Hyperresonant percussion notes	Reflect increased lung inflation from air trapping.
Decreased fremitus	Transmission of vibrations is obstructed.
Breath Sounds	
Decreased	Reduced airflow and increased lung inflation.
Crackles	Air passing through fluid in airways.
Wheezes	Air passing through narrowed airways.
Spirometry Results	
Forced expiratory volume exhaled in one second (FEV_1) < 80% predicted FEV_1 to forced vital capacity (FVC) ratio < 70% predicted	Narrow airways and increased airway resistance decrease ability to exhale completely. Considered the "gold standard."

(continues)

Table 22-11	Clinical Manifestations of COPD —*continued*
Signs and Symptoms	**Rationale**
Decreased Pulmonary Diffusion Capacity (carbon monoxide single-breath technique)	Destruction of alveolar walls causes a decrease in the diffusion of test gas from alveoli into blood.
Laboratory Results Arterial blood gases (ABGs) pH < 7.35 $PaCO_2 > 45$ mm Hg $HCO_3 > 28$ mEq/L $PaO_2 < 70$ mm Hg BE $> +2$ (respiratory acidosis with metabolic compensation)	Increased CO_2 retention and water cause an excessive amount of carbonic acid. As a result of too much carbonic acid in the blood, acidosis develops and the pH is decreased. The $PaCO_2$ is the respiratory component of the ABGs. A decreased pH and an increased $PaCO_2$ indicate respiratory acidosis. The PaO_2 may be normal or greatly reduced, depending on the degree of distortion of ventilation/ perfusion ratio. An increased bicarbonate (HCO_3) level indicates metabolic compensation to neutralize or decrease the acidotic state. A normal HCO_3 (24–28 mEq/L) indicates no compensation.
Hemoglobin (Hgb) and Hematocrit (Hct) Increased (hemoglobin may increase to 20 g)	Increased Hgb and Hct are due to hypoxemia. More hemoglobin can carry more oxygen. An elevated hemoglobin is a sign that cyanosis is more likely.
Electrolytes: Potassium, low to low normal Sodium, normal to slightly elevated	The serum potassium level may be 3.0–3.7 mEq/L and can be the result of poor dietary intake related to breathlessness, potassium-wasting diuretics, or chronic use of steroids (e.g., cortisone). Usually the sodium level is normal, but it can be elevated due to cardiac failure, excess IV saline infusions, or chronic use of steroids.

Diagnosis of COPD is primarily confirmed through a history and physical, arterial blood gas analysis, pulmonary function tests (including measurements of lung volumes, flow volume curves, and diffusion capacity), and serum alpha$_1$-antitrypsin levels. Chest x-rays can rule out other chest diseases and show marked hyperinflation and a flattened diaphragm in advanced emphysema.

Major complications of COPD include hypercapnea, respiratory acidosis, and hypoxemia. Respiratory infection results from bacterial growth in retained mucous secretions. Cor pulmonale, a later complication caused by hypoxemia, pulmonary hypertension, and right ventricular failure, is evidenced by increasing dyspnea, fatigue, weakness, jugular venous distention, an enlarged and tender liver, gastrointestinal disturbances, and dependent edema.

Clinical Management

Low-flow oxygen is frequently prescribed for hypoxemic clients with a PaO$_2$ less than or equal to 55 mm Hg and an oxygen saturation level $<89\%$. Oxygen therapy also decreases pulmonary hypertension and, thus, cardiac workload. When a nasal O$_2$ cannula or transtracheal catheter is used, the flow rate should be 1 to 2 liters per minute. If a high concentration of oxygen is delivered, the hypoxic respiratory drive is decreased.

Hydration is important in the management of COPD. Increased fluids aid in liquifying secretions and ease in the expectoration of mucous secretions. Increased fluid intake is contraindicated if right heart failure or cor pulmonale are present. Bronchodilators are useful to dilate the bronchial tubes, enhance mucociliary clearance of mucus, and improve ventilation.

Three types of chest physiotherapies are frequently prescribed. These include: (1) chest clapping for loosening thick, tenacious mucous secretions, (2) diaphragmatic breathing for increasing alveolar ventilation, and (3) pursed-lip breathing to prevent airway collapse. Table 22-12 lists the treatment modalities for COPD.

A pharmacologic stepped approach is recommended for COPD clients. Beta$_2$ agonists are used for mild symptoms. If symptoms become moderate, a cholinergic antagonist is added. If symptoms persist, methylxanthines are also given.

Table 22-12 Clinical Management of COPD

Management Methods	Rationale
Smoking Cessation	Smoking cessation will slow the rate of decline in FEV_1 and decrease the production of coughing and sputum.
Oxygen (O_2) if PaO_2 55 mm Hg or less or evidence of tissue hypoxia, cor pulmonale, or altered mental status	Low-flow O_2: 1–2 L/min with a nasal cannula, transtracheal catheter, or other devices that focus on O_2 with delivery on inspiration. Noninvasive and invasive mechanical ventilation may be indicated during exacerbations of COPD.
Hydration	Fluid intake should be increased to 2–3 L/day to thin secretions and ease expectoration unless cor pulmonale and/or right heart failure is present.
Bronchodilators Beta$_2$ agonists (e.g., albuterol, terbutaline) Anticholinergics (e.g., ipratropium) Methlxanthines (e.g., theophylline)	These agents dilate bronchioles, enhance mucociliary clearance, and improve ventilation. Depending on the agent, bronchodilators can be administered orally, intravenously, and through inhalers (with or without spacers) and nebulizers. Side effects may include tachycardia, cardiac dysrhythmias, changes in BP, tremor, agitation, insomnia, and nausea/vomiting.
Antibiotics	When a respiratory infection is present, antibiotics are usually given, orally or intravenously. *Streptococcus pneumoniae* and *Haemophilus influenzae* are common bacteria in this client population.
Vaccinations	A one-time pneumococcal and an annual or biannual influenza vaccine decrease the incidence of serious illnesses and death.
Chest Physiotherapy	Postural drainage, chest clapping, and vibration loosen the thick, tenacious mucous secretions that must be expectorated. Deep breathing and coughing should follow. Diaphragmatic breathing improves tidal volume and increases alveolar ventilation. Pursed-lip breathing prevents airway collapse so that trapped air in the alveoli can be expelled.

(continues)

Table 22-12	Clinical Management of COPD —*continued*
Management Methods	**Rationale**
Exercise	Exercises that are muscle group specific are used to strengthen respiratory muscle, arm, and leg strength. Improves respiratory status, endurance, and state of well-being.
Complementary and Alternative Therapies	Practicing relaxation techniques, biofeedback, and/or undergoing hypnosis helps to decrease anxiety, fear, and panic. Decreased dyspnea can result.
Nutritional Support with Attention to Electrolytes	Malnutrition is associated with wasting of respiratory muscles. Diaphragmatic functioning decreases with hypophosphatemia, hyperkalemia, hypocalcemia, and hypomagnesemia.
Pulmonary Rehabilitation Program	A multidisciplinary approach to exercise training, nutrition counseling, patient education, and psychosocial support. These programs improve survival and quality of life, reduce respiratory symptoms, increase exercise tolerance, decrease need for hospitalizations, and increase psychological functioning.

For worsening symptoms unresponsive to current therapy and for severe exacerbations, corticosteroids (oral, inhaler, or intravenous) are added to the regimen. Antibiotics are indicated for infection.

Clinical Considerations: Chronic Obstructive Pulmonary Disease (COPD)

1. Recognize signs and symptoms of COPD, such as dyspnea, prolonged expiration, wheezing, diminished breath sounds, use of accessory muscles, barrel-shaped chest, cough, and chronic fatigue.

2. Monitor arterial blood gases (ABGs). A decreased pH (<7.35) and an increased $PaCO_2$ (>45 mm Hg) are indicative of the acid-base imbalance respiratory

acidosis. The compensatory (metabolic) mechanism that brings the pH close to normal value is the HCO_3.

Hypoxemia with a PaO_2 less than or equal to 55 mm Hg is an indication for low-flow oxygen therapy.

3. Chest physiotherapy is helpful to mobilize secretions and improve ventilation. Types of chest physiotherapy include: chest clapping (loosens thick, tenacious mucous secretions), diaphragmatic breathing (increases alveolar ventilation), and pursed-lip breathing (prevents airway collapse).

4. Overuse of pressurized bronchodilator aerosols can cause a rebound effect.

5. COPD clients should avoid people with respiratory infections, air pollution, excess dust, pollen, and extreme hot or cold weather, all of which could cause breathlessness.

6. Hydration is important to liquify tenacious mucous secretions. Small feedings for COPD clients help prevent breathlessness that could occur when consuming large feedings.

7. Low-flow oxygen (1 to 2 liters per minute with a nasal O_2 cannula, transtracheal catheter, or ventimask with 24 or 28%) is suggested. Oxygen administration that is too high can decrease the hypoxic respiratory drive. Noninvasive and invasive mechanical ventilators may be needed to decrease CO_2 retention and aid in ventilation.

●CLIENT MANAGEMENT OF COPD

Assessment

● Obtain a client history of respiratory-related problems such as dyspnea at rest and on exertion, increasing shortness of breath, wheezing, fatigue, and activity intolerance.

● Assess for history of risk factors such as exposure to tobacco smoke, occupational dusts, gases and fumes, and air pollution. Determine if client has a history of numerous respiratory infections, or a family history of alpha$_1$-antitrypsin deficiency.

● Inspect for use of accessory muscles, barrel-shaped chest, clubbing, and cyanosis.

- Percuss and auscultate the lung areas noting decreased fremitus, hyperresonance, decreased lung expansion, diminished breath sounds, crackles, and wheezing.
- Check vital signs for baseline reading to compare with future vital sign readings.
- Check the arterial blood gas (ABG) report. Compare results with the norms: pH 7.35 to 7.45, $PaCO_2$ 35 to 45 mm Hg, HCO_3 24 to 28 mEq/L, BE −2 to +2, PaO_2 80–100 mm Hg. Consider the COPD client's normal PaO_2 level.

Nursing Diagnoses

- Impaired gas exchange, related to alveolar damage, the collapse of the bronchial tubes, particularly the bronchioles, and excessive mucous production.
- Ineffective airway clearance, related to excess mucous secretions and the constriction of the bronchial tubes, fatigue, and ineffective cough secondary to COPD.
- Ineffective breathing patterns, related to airway obstruction, diaphragm flattening, and fatigue.
- Ineffective tissue perfusion, related to hypoxemia.
- Activity intolerance, related to breathlessness and fatigue.
- Imbalanced nutrition, less than body requirements, related to breathlessness.
- Anxiety related to breathlessness, dependence on others and the treatment regime.
- Self-care deficit, related to the inability to take part in ADL because of dyspnea or breathlessness.
- Ineffective coping, related to breathlessness and lifestyle changes.
- Risk for injury, lungs, related to smoking and respiratory infections.
- Knowledge deficit regarding disease process, treatment, and lifestyle changes, related to unfamiliarity with information sources.
- Sleep pattern disturbance, related to dyspnea.
- Fatigue, related to change in metabolic energy or hypoxemia.

● Altered thought processes related to hypoxemia, hypercarbia, or sleep deprivation.

● Altered sexuality, related to extreme fatigue.

● Risk for hopelessness.

Interventions

● Monitor ABG and pulse oximetry. A marked decrease in pH and a marked increase in $PaCO_2$ indicates respiratory acidosis. A decrease in PaO_2 (< 55 mm Hg) and O_2 saturation (< 89%) indicates severe hypoxemia. Supplemental oxygen therapy may be necessary.

● Monitor vital signs. Report increase in pulse rate and changes in the rate of respiration. Labored breathing is a common sign of a respiratory problem.

● Check the electrolytes and hematology findings. Phosphorous, potassium, magnesium, and calcium play a role in respiratory muscle functioning. Elevated hemoglobin and hematocrit indicate hypoxemia.

● Monitor breath sounds and lung expansion by auscultating and percussing lung fields.

● Assist with the use of aerosol bronchodilators. Check breath sounds before and after use of aerosol treatments. Overuse of pressurized bronchodilator aerosol can cause a rebound effect.

● Check breath sounds for fine and coarse crackles and wheezes. Provide chest physiotherapy (chest clapping) for coarse crackles and have client deep breathe and cough to clear bronchial secretions.

● Instruct the client on how to do breathing exercises, e.g., pursed-lip breathing to prevent airway collapse, and diaphragmatic breathing to increase alveolar ventilation.

● Monitor fluid and food intake. Hydration is important to liquify tenacious mucous secretions. Frequent small feedings may be necessary.

● Instruct the client to recognize early signs of respiratory infections, e.g., color change in sputum, elevated temperature, and coughing. Recommend annual influenza vaccinations.

● Encourage the client to limit activities that increase the body's need for oxygen.

● Teach client exercises that increase respiratory muscle, arm, and leg strength.

● Encourage the client to try mild exercises in the afternoon or when breathlessness is not severe. Avoid exercise in early mornings when mucous secretions are increased and after meals when energy is needed for digestion.

● Teach client energy conservation principles. Encourage client to pace activities, alternating low- and high-energy tasks. Intersperse activities with adequate rest periods. Instruct client to minimize talking and avoid breath-holding during activities. Organize living space so that items used most often are within easy reach.

● Encourage smoking cessation.

● Refer to support groups, a pulmonary rehabilitation program, community agencies, and/or assistance programs.

Evaluation/Outcome

● Evaluate the therapeutic effects of interventions (breathing exercises, chest clapping, rest, bronchodilators, oxygen therapy, etc.) to correct or control COPD.

● Evaluate that the laboratory findings and other diagnostics indicative of COPD have improved or stabilized.

● Client demonstrates a stabilization of COPD signs and symptoms; client experiences few or no exacerbations of the disease.

● Client maintains adequate nutrition.

● Client uses breathing exercises and energy conservation techniques in daily life.

● Client verbalizes knowledge of medication actions and side effects; client demonstrates correct technique for medication via nebulizers or inhalers.

● Client accesses appropriate resources to maintain health and well-being.

Appendix A

Common Laboratory Tests and Values for Adults and Children

Hematology	Color-Top Tube	Reference Values	
		Adult	Child
Bleeding time		Ivy's method: 3–7 minutes	Same as adult
		Duke's method: 1–3 minutes	
Carboxyhemoglobin (CO)—See Chemistry.			
Clot retraction	Red	1–24 h	Same as adult
Coagulation time (CT)		5–15 min	Same as adult
		Average: 8 min	
Erythrocyte sedimentation rate (ESR)	Lavender	<50 years old (Westergren)	Newborn:
		Male: 0–15 mm/h	0–2 mm/h
		Female: 0–20 mm/h	4–14 years old:
		>50 years old (Westergren)	0–10 mm/h
		Male: 0–20 mm/h	
		Female: 0–30 mm/h	
		Wintrobe method:	
		Male: 0–9 mm/h	
		Female: 0–15 mm/h	
Factor assay	Blue		
I Fibrinogen		200–400 mg/dl	Same as adult
		Minimum for clotting: 75–100 mg/dl	
II Prothrombin		Minimum hemostatic level:	
		10%–15% concentration	
III Thromboplastin		Variety of substances	

IV Calcium		4.5–5.5 mEq/L or 9–11 mg/dl	
V Proaccelerin labile factor		Minimum hemostatic level: 50%–150% activity; 5%–10% concentration	Same as adult
VI		Not used	
VII Proconvertin stable factor		Minimum hemostatic level: 65%–135% activity; 5%–15% concentration	
VIII Antihemophilic factor (AHF)		Minimum hemostatic level: 55%–145% activity; 30%–35% concentration	
IX Plasma thromboplastin component (PTC Christmas factor)		Minimum hemostatic level: 60%–140% activity; 30% concentration	
X Stuart factor, Prower factor		Minimum hemostatic level: 45%–150% activity; 7%–10% concentration	
XI Plasma thromboplastin antecedent (PTA)		Minimum hemostatic level: 65%–135% activity; 20%–30% concentration	
XII Hageman factor		0% concentration	
XIII Fibrinase, fibrin stabilizing factor (FSF)		Minimum hemostatic level: 1% concentration	
Fibrin degradation products (FDP)	Red	2–10 µg/ml	Not usually done
Fibrinogen	Blue	200–400 mg/dl	Newborn: 150–300 mg/dl Child: same as adult
Hematocrit (Hct)	Lavender	Male: 40%–54%; 0.40–0.54 SI units Female: 36%–46%; 0.36–0.46 SI units	Newborn: 44%–65% 1–3 years old: 29%–40% 4–10 years old: 31%–43%

(continues)

Reference Values

Hematology	Color-Top Tube	Adult	Child
Hemoglobin (Hb or Hgb)	Lavender	Male: 13.5–17 g/dl Female: 12–15 g/dl	Newborn: 14–24 g/dl Infant: 10–17 g/dl Child: 11–16 g/dl
Hemoglobin electrophoresis	Lavender		
A_1		95%–98% total Hb	
A_2		1.5%–4.0%	
F		<2%	Newborn: 50%–80% total Hb Infant: 2%–8% total Hb Child: 1%–2% total Hb
C		0%	
D		0%	
S		0%	
Lymphocytes (T & B) assay	Lavender (2 tubes)	T cells: 60%–80%, 600–2400 cells/µl B cells: 4%–16%, 50–250 cells/µl	
Partial thromboplastin time (PTT)	Blue	PPT: 60–70 seconds APTT: 25–40 seconds	
Plasminogen	Blue	2.5–5.2 U/ml 3.8–8.4 CTA	
Platelet aggregation and adhesion	Blue	Aggregation in 3–5 minutes	

Test	Tube	Adult Value	Pediatric Value
Platelet count (thrombocytes)	Lavender	150,000–400,000 µL (mean, 250,000 µL) SI units: 0.15–0.4 × 10^{12}/L	Premature: 100,000–300,000 µL Newborn: 150,000–300,000 µL Infant: 200,000–475,000 µL Same as adult
Prothrombin time (PT)	Blue or black	11–15 seconds or 70%–100% Anticoagulant therapy: 2–2.5 times the control in seconds or 20%–30%	
RBC indices (mil/µL)	Lavender	Male: 4.6–6.0 Female: 4.0–5.0	Newborn: 4.8–7.2 Child: 3.8–5.5
MCV (cuµ)		80–98	Newborn: 96–108 Child: 82–92
MCH (pg)		27–31	Newborn: 32–34 Child: 27–31
MCHC (%)		32–36	Newborn: 32–33 Child: 32–36
RDW (Coulter S)		11.5–14.5	
Reticulocyte count	Lavender	0.5%–1.5% of all RBCs 25,000–75,000 µL (absolute count)	Newborn: 2.5%–6.5% of all RBCs Infant: 0.5%–3.5% of all RBCs Child: 0.5%–2.0% of all RBCs

(continues)

Reference Values

Hematology	Color-Top Tube	Adult	Child
Sickle cell screening	Lavender	0	0
White blood cells (WBC)	Lavender	4,500–10,000 μL	Newborn: 9,000–30,000 μL 2 years old: 6,000–17,000 μL 10 years: 4,500–13,500 μL
White blood cell differential	Lavender		
Neutrophils		50%–70% of total WBCs	29%–47%
Segments		50%–65%	
Bands		0%–5%	
Eosinophils		0%–3%	0%–3%
Basophils		1%–3%	1%–3%
Lymphocytes		25%–35%	38%–63%
Monocytes		2%–6%	4%–9%
Immunohematology (Blood Bank)			
Coombs direct	Lavender	Negative	Negative
Coombs indirect	Red	Negative	Negative
Cross matching	Red	Absence of agglutination (clumping)	Same as adult
Rh typing	Red	Rh+ and Rh−	Same as adult

Chemistry	Color-Top Tube	Reference Values	
		Adult	Child
Acetaminophen	Red	Therapeutic: 5–20 µg/ml; 31–124 µmol/L (SI units) Toxic: >50 µg/ml; >305 µmol/L (SI units) >200 µg/ml, possible hepatoxicity	Therapeutic: same as adult
Acetone (ketone bodies)	Red	Acetone: 0.3–2.0 mg/dl; 51.6–344 µmol/L (SI units) Ketones: 2–4 mg/dl	Newborn: slightly higher than adult Infant and child: same as adult
Acid phosphatase (ACP)	Red	0.0–0.8 U/L at 37°C (SI units)	6.4–15.2 U/L
Adrenocorticotropic Hormone (ACTH)	Lavender	7–10 AM: 15–80 pg/ml; 4 PM: 5–30 pg/ml, 10 PM to Midnight: <10 pg/ml	
Alanine aminotransferase (ALT, SGPT)	Red	10–35 U/L	Same as adult
Albumin	Red	3.5–5 g/dl	Infant: could be twice as high
Alcohol	Red	0%	
Aldolase (ALD)	Red	3–8 U/dl (Sibley-Lehninger) 22–59 mU/L at 37°C (SI units)	Infant: 12–24 U/dl Child: 6–16 U/dl

(continues)

Reference Values

Chemistry	Color-Top Tube	Adult	Child
Aldosterone	Red or green	Fast: <16 mg/dl; 4–30 mg/dl (sitting position)	3–11 years: 5–70 mg/dl
Alkaline phosphatase (ALP)	Red	41–136 U/L	Infant: 40–300 U/L
ALP[1]		20–130 U/L	Child: 60–270 U/L
ALP[2]		20–120 U/L	Older child: 50–230 U/L
Alpha$_1$-antitrypsin	Red	78–200 mg/dl 0.78–2.0 g/L	Newborn: 145–270 mg/dl Infant and child: same as adult
Alpha-fetoprotein (AFP)	Red	(see table below)	
Ammonia	Green	Toxic level: >500 ng/ml 15–45 µg/dl 11–35 µmol/L (SI units)	Newborn: 64–107 µg/dl Child: 21–50 µg/dl
Amylase		30–170 µ/L Isoenzymes: S: 45–70% P: 30–55%	

Weeks of Gestation	Serum (ng/ml)	Amniotic Fluid (µg/ml)
14	7–50	11.0–32.0
15	7–60	5.5–31.0
16	10–72	5.7–31.5
17	11–90	3.8–32.5
18	14–94	3.6–28.0
19	24–112	3.7–24.5
20	31–122	2.2–15.0

Test	Tube Color	Normal Value (Adult)	Normal Value (Child)
Angiotensin-converting enzyme (ACE)	Red or green	11–67 U/L	Not usually performed
Anion gap	Lavender	10–17 mEq/L	
Antidiuretic hormone (ADH)		1–5 pg/ml	
Arterial blood gases (See *Others*)		1–5 ng/L	
Ascorbic acid (vitamin C)	Gray or red	0.6–2.0 mg/dl (plasma)	0.6–1.6 mg/dl (plasma)
		34–114 μmol/L (SI units, plasma)	
		0.2–2.0 mg/dl (blood)	
		12–114 μmol (SI units, serum)	
Aspartate aminotransferase	Red	0–35 U/L	Newborn: four times normal level
			Child: same as adult
(AST, SGOT)		Average 8–38 U/L	
Bilirubin (indirect)	Red	0.1–1.0 mg/dl	
		1.7–17.1 μmol/L (SI units)	
Bilirubin (total and direct)	Red	Total: 0.1–1.2 mg/dl; 1.7–20.5 μmol/L (SI units)	Newborn, total: 1–12 mg/dl; 17.1–205 μmol/L (SI units)
		Direct (conjugated): 0.1–0.3 mg/dl; 1.7–5.1 μmol/L (SI units)	Child, total: 0.2–0.8 mg/dl
Blood urea nitrogen (BUN)	Red	5–25 mg/dl	Infant: 5–15 mg/dl
			Child: 5–20 mg/dl
BUN/creatinine ratio	Red	10:1 to 20:1	

(continues)

Chemistry	Color-Top Tube	Reference Values	
		Adult	Child
Calcitonin	Green or lavender	Male: <40 pg/ml Female: <25 pg/ml	Newborn: usually higher
Calcium (Ca)	Red	4.5–5.5 mEq/L 9–11 mg/dl 2.3–2.8 mmol/L (SI units)	Child: <70 pg/ml Newborn: 3.7–7.0 mEq/L; 7.4–14 mg/dl Infant: 5.0–6.0 mEq/L; 10–12 mg/dl Child: 4.5–5.8 mEq/L; 9–11.5 mg/dl
Ionized calcium (iCa)		4.4–5.9 mg/dl 2.2–2.5 mEq/L 1.1–1.24 mmol/L	
Carbamazepine	Red	Therapeutic: 4–12 μg/ml; 16.9–50.8 μmol/L (SI units) Toxic: > 12–15 μg/ml; > 50.8–69 μmol/L (SI units)	
Carbon dioxide combining power (CO_2)	Green	22–30 mEq/L 22–30 mmol/L (SI units)	20–28 mEq/L
Carbon monoxide (CO)	Lavender	< 2.5% saturation of Hb	
Carboxyhemoglobin (may be done in hematology)		2%–9% saturation of Hb (smokers)	Same as adult

Test	Tube color	Values
Carotene	Red	40–130 µg/dl
Catecholamines	Green or lavender	60–200 mg/dl; 0.74–3.72 µmol/L (SI units); Positive for pheochromocytoma: > 1000 pg/ml
Epinephrine		Supine: < 50 pg/ml; Sitting: < 60 pg/ml; Standing: < 90 pg/ml
Norepinephrine		Supine: 110–410 pg/ml; Sitting: 120–680 pg/ml; Standing: 125–700 pg/ml
Dopamine		Supine and standing: < 87 pg/ml
Ceruloplasmin (Cp)	Red	18–45 mg/dl; 180–450 mg/L (SI units); Infant: <23 mg/dl or normal; Child: 30–65 mg/dl
Chloride (Cl)	Red	95–105 mEq/L; 95–105 mmol/L (SI units); Newborn: 94–112 mEq/L; Infant: 95–110 mEq/L; Child: 98–105 mEq/L
Cholesterol	Red	Desirable level: < 200 mg/dl; Moderate risk: 200–240 mg/dl; High risk: > 240 mg/dl; Infant: 90–130 mg/dl; 2–19 years: Desirable level: 130–170 mg/dl; Moderate risk: 171–84 mg/dl; High risk: > 185 mg/dl

(continues)

Reference Values

Chemistry	Color-Top Tube	Adult	Child
Cholinesterase	Green	0.5–1.0 U (RBC) 3–8 U/ml (plasma) 6–8 IU/L (RBC) 8–18 IU/L at 37°C (plasma)	Same as adult
Copper (Cu)	Red or green	Male: 70–140 µg/dl: 11–22 µmol/L (SI units) Female: 80–155 µg/dl; 12.6–24.3 µmol/L (SI units) Pregnancy: 140–300 µg/dl	Newborn: 20–70 µg/dl Child: 30–190 µg/dl Adolescent: 90–240 µg/dl
Cortisol	Green	8 AM–10 AM: 5–23 µg/dl; 138–635 nmol/L (SI units) 4 PM–6 PM: 3–13 µg/dl; 83–359 nmol/L (SI units)	8 AM–10 AM: 15–25 µg/dl 4 PM–6 PM: 5–10 µg/dl
Creatinine phosphokinase (CPK)	Red	Male: 5–35 µg/ml; 30–180 IU/L, 55–170 U/L at 37°C (SI units) Female: 5–25 µg/ml; 25–150 IU/L; 30–135 U/L at 37°C (SI units)	Newborn: 65–580 IU/L at 30°C Child: Male: 0–70 IU/L at 30°C Female: 0–50 IU/L at 30°C
Creatinine	Red	0.5–1.5 mg/dl 45–132.3 µmol/L (SI units)	Newborn: 0.8–1.4 mg/dl Infant: 0.7–1.7 mg/dl 2–6 years: 0.3–0.6 mg/dl, 24–54 µmol/L (SI units) 7–18 years: 0.4–1.2 mg/dl, 36–106 µmol/L (SI units)

Cryoglobulins	Red	Negative
Disseminated intravascular coagulation (DIC) screening test		See *Part III, Hematologic Conditions.*
Dexamethasone suppression test	Green	Cortisol: 8 AM <10 μg/dl
Digoxin	Red	Therapeutic: 0.5–2 ng/ml; 0.5–2 nmol/L (SI units)	Therapeutic: Infant: 1–3 ng/ml; 1–3 nmol/L (SI units)
D-xylose absorption	Red	Toxic: > 2 ng/ml; > 2.6 nmol/L (SI units) 25–40 mg/dl/2h Older adult same as adult	Toxic: >3.5 ng/ml 30 mg/dl/1h

Estetrol (E₄) Red

Pregnancy:

Weeks of Gestation	pg/ml
20–26	140–210
30	350
36	900
40	>1050

Estradiol (E₂)	Red	Female: Follicular phase: 20–150 pg/ml Midcycle: 100–500 pg/ml Luteal: 60–260 pg/ml Postmenopausal: <30 pg/ml Male: 15–50 pg/ml	3–10 pg/ml

(continues)

Reference Values

Chemistry	Color-Top Tube	Adult	Child
Estriol/E$_3$	Red	Pregnancy: **Serum** Weeks of Gestation — ng/dL 25–28 — 25–165 29–32 — 30–230 33–36 — 45–370 37–38 — 75–420 39–40 — 95–450	1–10 years: <10 pg/ml
Estrone (E$_1$)	Red	Female: 2 Follicular phase: 30–100 pg/ml Ovulatory phase: >150 pg/ml Luteal phase: 90–160 pg/ml Postmenopausal: 20–40 pg/ml	
Estrogen	Red	Male: 10–50 pg/ml Female: Early menstrual cycle: 60–200 pg/ml Midcycle: 120–440 pg/ml	1–6 years: 3–10 pg/ml 8–12 years: <30 pg/ml
Fasting blood sugar (FBS)	Gray or red	Male: 40–155 pg/ml 70–110 mg/dl (serum) 60–100 mg/dl (blood)	Newborn: 30–80 mg/dl Child: 60–100 mg/dl
Feasting blood sugar (*See Postprandial blood sugar.*)			

Test	Tube	Adult	Child
Ferritin	Red	Female: 10–125 ng/ml 10–125 µg/L (SI units) Male: 35–300 ng/ml 35–300 µg/L (SI units)	Newborn: 20–200 ng/ml Infant: 30–200 ng/ml 1–16 years: 8–140 ng/ml
Folate (folic acid) (may be done by nuclear medicine)	Red	3–16 ng/ml (bioassay) >2.5 ng/ml (RIA; serum) 200–700 ng/ml (RBC)	Same as adult
Follicle-stimulating hormone (FSH)	Red	Pre/postovulation: 4–30 mU/ml Midcycle: 10–90 mU/ml Postmenopausal: 40–170 mU/ml Male: 4–25 mU/ml	5–12 mU/ml
Gamma-glutamyl transferase (GGT)	Red	Male: 4–23 IU/l Female: 3–13 IU/L; 4–33 U/L at 37°C (SI units)	
Gastrin	Red or lavender	Fasting: < 100 pg/ml	Not usually performed
Glucose-6-phosphate dehydrogenase (G-6-PD) (may be done in hematology)	Lavender or green	8–18 IU/gHb 125–281 U/dl (packed RBC) 251–511 U/dl (cells) 1211–2111 mIU/ml (packed RBC)	Same as adult
Glucose—fasting blood sugar (*See Fasting blood sugar.*)			
Glucagon	Lavender	50–200 pg/ml	

(continues)

Chemistry	Color-Top Tube	Reference Values	
		Adult	**Child**

Glucose tolerance test (GTT) — Gray or red

Time	Serum (mg/dl)	Blood (mg/dl)	Child (6 years or older)
Fasting	70–110	60–100	Same as adult
0.5 hour	<160	<150	
1 hour	<170	<160	
2 hour	<125	<115	
3 hour	Fasting level	Fasting level	

Growth hormone — Red
Male: <5 ng/ml
Female: <10 ng/ml
Child: <10 ng/ml

Hexosaminidase — Red
Total: 5–20 U/L
A: 55%–80%

Human chorionic gonadotropin (HCG) — Red
Nonpregnant female: <0.01 IU/ml

Pregnant (Weeks)	Values
1	0.01–0.04 IU/ml
2	0.03–0.10 IU/ml
4	0.10–1.0 IU/ml
5–12	10–100 IU/ml
13–25	10–30 IU/ml
26–40	5–15 IU/ml

			ng/mL	
Human immunosuppressive virus (HIV)	Red	Negative		
Human leukocyte antigen (HLA)	Green	Histocompatibility match		
Human placental lactogen (HPL)	Red or green	**Weeks of Gestation**		
		8–27	4.6 µg/ml	
		28–31	2.4–6.0 µg/ml	
		32–35	3.7–7.7 µg/ml	
		36–40	5.0–10.0 µg/ml	
Immunoglobulins (*See Serology.*)	Red			
Insulin	Red	5–25 µU/ml		
Iron	Red	50–150 µg/dl; 10–27 µmol/L (SI units)		Infant (6 months–2 years): 40–100 µg/dl Newborn: 100–270 µg/dl
Iron-binding capacity (IBC, TIBC)	Red	250–450 µg/dl		Infant (6 months–2 years): 100–350 µg/dl Child: same as adult
Lactic acid	Green	Arterial blood: 0.5–2.0 mEq/L; <11.3 mg/dl Venous blood: 0.5–1.5 mEq/L; 8.1–15.3 mg/dl Critical: >5 mEq/L; >45 mg/dl		
Lactic dehydrogenase (LDH/LD)	Red	100–190 IU/L; 70–250 U/L		Newborn: 300–1500 IU/L Child: 50–150 IU/L

(continues)

Chemistry	Color-Top Tube	Reference Values	
		Adult	**Child**
LDH isoenzymes	Red		
LDH₁		14%–26%	
LDH₂		27%–37%	
LDH₃		13%–26%	
LDH₄		8%–16%	
LDH₅		6%–16%	
Lactose tolerance test	Gray	20–50 mg/dl rise from fasting blood glucose	
Lead	Lavender or green	10–20 µg/dl	10–20 µg/dl
		20–40 µg/dl (acceptable)	20–30 µg/dl (acceptable)
LE cells (Lupus) also in hematology	Red or green	Negative	
Lecithin/sphingomyelin ratio (L/S; amniotic fluid)		1:1 before 35 weeks of gestation	
		L: 6–9 mg/dl	
		S: 4–6 mg/dl	
		4:1 after 35 weeks of gestation	
		L: 15–21 mg/dl	
		S: 4–6 mg/dl	
Leucine aminopeptidase (LAP)	Red	8–22 mU/ml, 12–33 IU/L; 75–200 U/ml	
Lipase	Red	20–180 IU/L	Infant: 9–105 IU/L at 37°C
		14–280 mU/ml	Child: 20–136 IU/L at 37°C
		14–280 U/L (SI units)	

Lipoproteins (*See Cholesterol, Phospholipids, and Triglycerides.*)			
Lithium	Red	0	0
		Therapeutic: 0.8–1.2 mEq/L	
		Toxic: >2 mEq/L	
Luteinizing hormone (LH)	Red or lavender	Pre/postovulation: 5–30 mIU/ml	6–12 years: <10 mIU/ml
		Midcycle: 50–150 mIU/ml	13–18 years: <20 mIU/ml
		Postmenopause: >35 mIU/ml	
		Male: 5–25 mIU/ml	
Magnesium (Mg)	Red	1.5–2.5 mEq/L; 1.8–3.0 mg/dl	Newborn: 1.4–2.9 mEq/L
			Child: 1.6–2.6 mEq/L
Myoglobin	Red	12–90 µg/L; 12–90 ng/ml	
Nifedipine	Red	Therapeutic: 50–100 ng/ml	
		Toxic: >100 ng/ml	
		Toxic level: >200 ng/ml	
5'Nucleotidase (5'N)	Red	<17 U/L	
Osmolality	Red	280–300 mOsm/kg	270–290 mOsm/kg
Parathyroid hormone (PTH)	Red	PTH: 11–54 pg/ml	
		C-Terminal PTH: 50–330 pg/ml;	
		N-Terminal PTH: 8–24 pg/ml	
Pepsinogen I	Red	124–142 ng/ml	Premature: 20–24 ng/ml
			<1 year: 72–82 ng/ml
			1–2 years: 90–106 ng/ml
			3–6 years: 80–104 ng/ml
			7–10 years: 77–103 ng/ml
			11–14 years: 96–118 ng/ml
			(continues)

Reference Values

Chemistry	Color-Top Tube	Adult	Child
Phospholipids	Red	150–380 mg/dl	
Phosphorus (P) (inorganic)	Red	1.7–2.6 mEq/l 2.5–4.5 mg/dl	Newborn: 3.5–8.6 mg/dl Infant: 4.5–6.7 mg/dl Child: 4.5–5.5 mg/dl
Postprandial blood sugar (feasting: PPBS)	Gray or red	<140 mg/dl 2 hours (plasma) <120 mg/dl 2 hours (blood) Older adult: <160 mg/dl 2 hours (plasma); <140 mg/dl 2 hours (blood)	Same as adult
Potassium (K)	Red	3.5–5.3 mEq/L 3.5–5.3 mmol/L (SI units)	Infant: 3.6–5.8 mEq/L Child: 3.5–5.5 mEq/L
Progesterone	Red	Female: Follicular phase: 0.1–1.5 ng/ml Luteal: 2–28 ng/ml Pregnancy: First trimester: 9–50 ng/ml Second trimester: 18–150 ng/ml Third trimester: 60–260 ng/ml Male: <1.0 ng/mL	

Prolactin (PRL)	Red or lavender	Nonpregnant: Follicular phase: 0–23 ng/ml Luteal: 0–40 ng/ml Postmenopausal: <12 ng/ml Pregnancy: First trimester: <80 ng/ml Second trimester: <160 ng/ml Third trimester: <400 ng/ml Male: 0.1–20 ng/ml Pituitary adenoma: >100–300 ng/ml
Prostate-specific antigen (PSA)	Red	Normal: 0–4 ng/ml BPH: 4–19 ng/ml Prostate cancer: 10–120 ng/ml
Protein	Red	6.0–8.0 g/dl
Protein electrophoresis	Red	Albumin: 3.5–5.0 g/dl; 52%–68% of total protein Premature: 4.2–7.6 g/dl Newborn: 4.6–7.4 g/dl Infant: 6.0–6.7 g/dl Child: 6.2–8.0 g/dl Globulin: 1.5–3.5 g/dl; 32%–48% of total protein Premature: 3.0–4.2 g/dl Newborn: 3.5–5.4 g/dl Infant: 4.4–5.4 g/dl Child: 4.0–5.8 g/dl

(continues)

Reference Values

Chemistry	Color-Top Tube	Adult	Child
Renin	Lavender	Normal sodium diet: supine: 0.2–2.3 ng/ml; upright: 1.6–4.3 ng/ml. Restricted salt diet: upright: 4.1–10.8 ng/ml	3–5 years: 1.0–6.5 ng/ml 5–10 years: 0.5–6.0 ng/ml
Salicylate	Red	0 Therapeutic: 15–30 mg/dl Toxic: Mild: >30 mg/dl Severe: >50 mg/dl	0 Toxic: >25 mg/dl
Serotonin	Lavender	50–175 ng/mL; 10–30 μg/dl; 0.29–1.15 μmol/L (SI units)	
Sodium (Na)	Red	135–145 mEq/L 135–142 nmol/L (SI units)	Infant: 134–150 mEq/L Child: 135–145 mEq/L
T₃	Red	80–200 ng/dl	Newborn: 90–170 ng/dl Child, 6–12 years: 115–190 ng/dL
Testosterone	Red or green	Male: 0.3–1.0 μg/dl; 300–1000 ng/dl Female: 0.03–0.1 μg/dl; 30–100 ng/dl	Male adolescent: >0.1 mg/dl Male, 12–14 years old: >100 ng/dl

Test	Tube	Values	
Theophyline	Red	Therapeutic: Adult: 5–20 µg/ml; 28–112 µmol/L (SI units) Elderly: 5–18 µg/ml Toxic: Adult: >20 µg/ml; >112 µmol/L (SI units) Older adult same as adult	Therapeutic: Premature: 7–14 µg/ml Neonate: 3–12 µg/ml Child: same as adult Toxic: Premature: >14 µg/ml Neonate: >13 µg/ml Child: same as adult
Thyroid-binding globulin (TBG)	Red or green	10–26 µg/dl	
Thyroxine (T_2)	Red	4.5–11.5 µg/dl (T_4 by column) 5–12 µg/dl (T_4 RIA) 1.0–2.3 ng/dl (Thyroxine iodine)	Newborn: 11–23 µg/dl 1–4 months: 7.5–16.5 µg/dl 4–12 months: 5.5–14.5 µg/dl 1–6 years: 5.5–13.5 µg/dl 6–10 years: 5–12.5 µg/dl
Transferrin	Red	200–430 mg/dl; 2–4.3 g/L (SI units) Pregnancy (full term): 300 mg/dl	Newborn: 125–275 mg/dl
Transferrin percent saturation	Red	Male: 30%–50% Female: 20%–35%	
T_3 resin uptake (may be done by nuclear medicine)	Red	25–35 relative % uptake	Not usually done

(continues)

Reference Values

Chemistry	Color-Top Tube	Adult	Child
Tricyclic antidepressants			
Triglycerides	Red	10–150 mg/dl 0.11–2.09 mmol/L (SI units)	Infant: 5–40 mg/dl Child: 10–135 mg/dl
Uric acid	Red	Male: 3.5–8.0 mg/dl Female: 2.8–6.8 mg/dl	2.5–5.5 mg/dl
Vancomycin	Red	Therapeutic range: Peak: 20–40 μg/ml Trough: 5–10 μg/ml Toxic level: >40 μg/ml	
Vitamin A	Red	30–95 μg/dL; 1.05–3.0 μmol/L (SI units); 125–150 IU/dl	1–6 years: 20–43 μg/dl; 0.7–1.5 μmol/L (SI units) 7–12 years: 26–50 μg/dl 13–19 years: 26–72 μg/dl
Vitamin B₁	Red	10–60 ng/ml; 5.3–8.0 μg/dl	
Vitamin B₆	Lavender	5–30 ng/ml; 20–120 nmol/L (SI units)	
Vitamin B₁₂	Red	200–900 pg/ml	Newborn: 160–1200 pg/ml
Vitamin C (See *Ascorbic acid*.)			
Vitamin D₃	Red or green	1,23 dihydroxy: 20–76 pg/ml 25-hydroxy: 10–55 ng/ml	
Vitamin E	Red	5–20 μg/ml; 0.5–1.8 mg/dl; 12–42 μmol/L (SI units)	3–15 μg/ml; 0.3–1.0 mg/dl; 7–23 μmol/L (SI units)

	Color-Top Tube	Adult	Child
Zinc	Navy-blue	60–150 µg/dl; 11–23 µmol/L (SI units)	
Zinc	Urine	150–1250 µg/24 h	
Zinc protoporphyrin (ZPP)	Green or lavender	15–77 µg/dl	Same as adult
		Average: <35 µg/dl; <0.56 µmol/L (SI units)	

		Reference Values	
Serology	**Color-Top Tube**	**Adult**	**Child**
Adenovirus antibody	Red	Negative	Negative
Anti-DNA	Red	<1:85	<1:60 <1:70
Antiglomerular basement membrane antibody (AGBM)	Red	Negative	
Antimitochondrial antibody (AMA)	Red	Negative at 1:5 Positive: >1:160	
Antimyocardial antibody	Red	None detected	
Antinuclear antibodies (ANA)	Red	Negative at 1:20 dilution	Negative
Antistreptolysin O (ASO)	Red	100 IU/ml; <160 Todd U/ml	Newborn: similar to mother's 2–5 years: <100 IU/ml 12–19 years: <200 IU/ml; <200 Todd U/ml

(continues)

Serology	Color-Top Tube	Reference Values	
		Adult	Child
Carcinoembryonic antigen (CEA) (may be done by nuclear medicine)	Red or lavender	<2.5 ng/ml (nonsmokers) <3.5 ng/ml (smokers)	Not usually done
Chlamydia test	Red	<1:16	
Cold agglutinins (CA)	Red	1:8 antibody titer	Same as adult
Complement (total)	Red	75–160 U/ml; 75–160 kU/L (SI units)	
Complement C_3	Red	Male: 80–180 mg/dl; 0.8–1.8 g/L (SI units) Female: 76–120 mg/dl; 0.76–1.2 g/L (SI units)	Not usually done
Complement C_4	Red	15–45 mg/dl; 150–450 mg/l (SI units)	Not usually done
C-reactive protein (CRP)	Red	0	0
Cryoglobulins	Red	Up to 6 mg/dl	Negative
Cytomegalovirus (CMV) antibody	Red	Negative to <0.30	
Encephalitis virus antibody	Red	Titer: <1:10	
Enterovirus group	Red	Negative	
Febrile agglutinins	Red	Febrile group: titers *Brucella:* <1:20 *Tularemia:* <1:40 *Salmonella:* <1:40 *Proteus:* <1:40	Same as adult
FTA-ABS (fluorescent treponemal antibody absorption)	Red	Negative	Negative

Test		Adult value	Child value
Haptoglobin	Red	60–270 mg/dl 0.6–2.7 g/L (SI units)	Newborn: 0–10 mg/dl Infant: 1–6 months: 0–30 mg/dl, then gradual increase
HB$_s$ Ab	Red	Negative	Negative
HB$_c$ Ab	Red	Negative	Negative
Hepatitis A virus (HAV)	Red	None detected	
Hepatitis B surface antigen (HB$_s$Ag)	Red	Negative	Negative
Herpes simplex virus (HSV)	Red	<1:10	
Heterophile antibody	Red	<1:28 titer	
Immunoglobulins (Ig)	Red		Same as adult

				1–3 years old	**7–11 years old**
Total Ig		900–2200 mg/dl			
IgG		800–1800 mg/dl		400–1500 mg/dl	700–1700 mg/dl
IgA		100–400 mg/dl		300–1400 mg/dl	600–1450 mg/dl
IgM		50–150 mg/dl		20–150 mg/dl	50–200 mg/dl
IgD		0.5–3 mg/dl		20–100 mg/dl	30–120 mg/dl

Test		Adult value	Child value
Legionnaire antibody test	Red	Negative	
Lyme antibody test	Red	Titer <1:256	
Mumps antibody	Red	Negative or <1:8 titer	Same as adult
Rabies antibody test	Red	IFA: <1:16	
Rapid plasma reagin (RPR)	Red	Negative	Negative
Rhematoid factory (RF)	Red	<1:20 titer	Not usually done

(continues)

Serology	Color-Top Tube	Reference Values	
		Adult	**Child**
Rubella antibody detection (HAI or HI)	Red	<1:8 titer susceptible 1:10–1:32 titer, past rubella exposure 1:32–1:64 titer, immunity >1:64 titer, definite immunity	Same as adult
Thyroid antibodies (TA)	Red	Negative or <1:20 titer	Not usually done
TORCH test	Red	Negative	Negative
Toxoplasmosis antibody test	Red	No infection: <1:4 Infected: >1:256	
Venereal disease research laboratory (VDRL)	Red	Negative	Negative

Urine Chemistry	Reference Values	
	Adult	**Child**
Aldosterone	6–25 µg/24 h	Not usually done
Amylase	4–37 U/L/2h	Not usually done
Ascorbic acid tolerance (4-, 5-, or 6-hour sample)	Oral: 10% of administered amount IV: 30%–40% of administered amount	Not usually done
Bilirubin and bile	Negative to 0.02 mg/dl	Same as adult
Calcium (Ca)	100–250 mg/24 h (average calcium diet) 2.50–6.25 mmol/24 h	Same as adult

Catecholamines		Lower level than adult—weight difference
Epinephrine	<100 µg/24 h	
Norepinephrine	<0.59 µmol/24h (SI units)	
Cortisol	0–14 µg/dl (random) <20 ng/24 h <100 ng/24 h	
Creatinine clearance	24–105 µg/24 h 85–135 ml/min	Similar to adult
Creatinine	Male: 20–26 mg/kg/24 h; 0.18–0.23 mmol/kg/24 h (SI units) Female: 14–22 mg/kg/24 h; 0.12–0.19 mmol/kg/24 h (SI units)	

Estriol (E$_3$)

Pregnant:

Weeks of Gestation	mg/24 h
25–28	6–28
29–32	6–32
33–36	10–45
37–40	15–60

Estrogens (total)	Female: Preovulation: 5–25 µg/24 h Follicular phase: 24–100 µg/24 h Luteal phase (menstruation): 22–80 µg/24 h Postmenopause: 0–10 µg/24 h Male: 4–25 µg/24 h	<12 years: 1 µg/24 h >12 years: same as adult
Estrone (E$_1$)	Female: Follicular phase: 4–7 µg/24 h Ovulatory phase: 11–30 µg/24 h Luteal phase: 10–22 µg/24 h Postmenopausal: 1–7 µg/24 h	

(continues)

Reference Values

Urine Chemistry	Adult	Child
Follicle-stimulating hormone (FSH)	Follicular: 2–15 IU/24 h Luteal phase: 4–20 IU/24 h Menopause: >50 IU/24 h	<10 mUU/24 h (prepubertal)
Human chorionic gonadotropin (HCG)	Positive for pregnancy: no agglutination Negative for pregnancy: agglutination	Not usually performed
17-Hydroxycorticosteroids (17-OHCS)	Male: 3–12 mg/24 h Female: 2–10 mg/24 h	Infant: <1 mg/24 h 2–4 years: 1–2 mg/24 h 5–12 years: 2–6 mg/24 h
5-Hydroxyindoleacetic acid (5-HIAA)	Random: negative 24 hours: 2–10 mg/24 h	Not usually performed
Ketone bodies (acetone)	Negative	Negative

17-Ketosteroids (17-KS)	Male: 5–25 mg/24 h
	Female: 5–15 mg/24 h
	>65 years: 4–8 mg/24 h
		Infant: 1 mg/24 h
		1–3 years: <2 mg/24 h
		3–6 years: <3 mg/24 h
		7–10 years: <4 mg/24 h
		10–12 years:
		  Male: <6 mg/24 h
		  Female: <5 mg/24 h
		Adolescent:
		  Male: <3–15 mg/24 h
		  Female: <3–12 mg/24 h

Myoglobin	None detected	

Osmolality	50–1200 mOsm/kg	Newborn: 100–600 mOsm/kg
	Average: 200–800 mOsm/kg	Child: same as adult
Phenylketonuria (PKU)	Not usually done	PKU: negative (positive when serum phenylalanine is 12–15 mg/dl)
		Guthrie: negative (positive when serum phenylalanine is 4 mg/dl)
Porphobilinogen	Random: negative	Same as adult
	24 hour: 0–2 mg/24 h	
Porphyrins		
Coproporphyrins	Random: 3–20 μg/dl	0–80 μg/24 h
	24 hours: 50–160 μg	
Uroporphyrins	Random: negative, 24 hours: <30 μg	10–30 μg/24 h
Potassium (K)	25–120 mEq/24 h	17–57 mEq/24 h
	25–120 mmol/24 h (SI units)	
Pregnanediol	Male: 0.1–1.5 mg/24 h	0.4–1.0 mg/24 h
	Female: 0.5–1.5 mg/24 h (proliferative phase); 2–7 mg/24 h (luteal phase); 0.1–1.0 mg/24 h (postmenopausal)	

Pregnancy:

Weeks of Gestation	mg/24 h
10–19	5–25
20–28	15–42
29–32	25–49

(continues)

Reference Values

Urine Chemistry	Adult	Child
Pregnanetriol	Male: 0.4–2.4 mg/24 h Female: 0.5–2.0 mg/24 h	Infant: 0–0.2 mg/24 h Child: 0–1.0 mg/24 h
Protein	0–5 µg/24 h	
Sodium (Na)	40–220 mEq/24 h	Same as adult
Uric acid	250–500 mg/24 h (low-purine diet)	Same as adult
Urinalysis		
pH	4.5–8.0	Newborn: 5–7 Child: 4.5–8
Specific gravity (SG)	1.005–1.030	Newborn: 1.001–1.020 Child: Same as adult
Protein	Negative	Negative
Glucose	Negative	Negative
Ketones	Negative	Negative
RBC	1–2/low-power field	Rare
WBC	3–4	0–4
Casts	Occasional hyaline	Rare
Vitamin B$_1$	100–200 µg/24 h	

Reference Values

Others	Adult	Child
Urobilinogen	Random: 0.3–3.5 mg/dl	Same as adult
	0.05–2.5 mg/24 h	
	0.5–4.0 Ehrlich units/24 h	
	0.09–4.23 μmol/24 h (SI units)	
Bleeding time	Ivy's method: 3–7 minutes	Same as adult
Arterial blood gases (ABGs)		
pH	7.35–7.45	7.36–7.44
$PaCO_2$	35–45 mm Hg	Same as adult
PaO_2	75–100 mm Hg	Same as adult
HCO_3	24–28 mEq/L	Same as adult
BE	+2 to −2 (∓ 2 mEq/L)	Same as adult
Cerebrospinal fluid (CSF)		
Pressure	75–175 mm H_2O	50–100 mm H_2O
Cell count	0–8 mm^3	0–8 mm^3
Protein	15–45 mg/dl	15–45 mg/dl
Chloride	118–132 mEq/L	120–128 mEq/L
Glucose	40–80 mg/dl	35–75 mg/dl
Culture	No organism	No organism
Chloride (sweat)	<60 mEq/L	<50 mEq/L
Semen examination	60–150 millim/ml	Not usually done
	Volume: 1.5–5.0 ml	
	Morphology: >75% mature spermatozoa	
	Motility: >60% actively mobile spermatozoa	

From *Laboratory and Diagnostic Tests with Nursing Implications* (6th ed.), by J. L. Kee, 2002, East Rutherford, NJ., Prentice Hall Health. Reprinted with permission.

Appendix B

Foods Rich in Potassium, Sodium, Calcium, Magnesium, Chloride, and Phosphorus

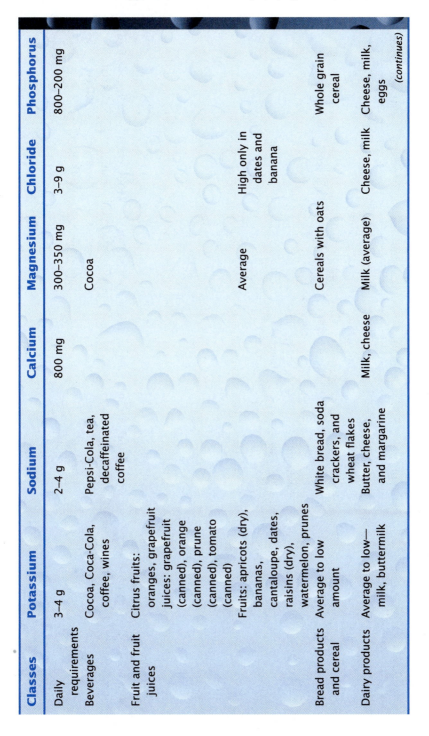

Classes	Potassium	Sodium	Calcium	Magnesium	Chloride	Phosphorus
Daily requirements	3–4 g	2–4 g	800 mg	300–350 mg	3–9 g	800–200 mg
Beverages	Cocoa, Coca-Cola, coffee, wines	Pepsi-Cola, tea, decaffeinated coffee		Cocoa		
Fruit and fruit juices	Citrus fruits: oranges, grapefruit juices: grapefruit (canned), orange (canned), prune (canned), tomato (canned)					
	Fruits: apricots (dry), bananas, cantaloupe, dates, raisins (dry), watermelon, prunes			Average	High only in dates and banana	
Bread products and cereal	Average to low amount	White bread, soda crackers, and wheat flakes		Cereals with oats		Whole grain cereal
Dairy products	Average to low—milk, buttermilk	Butter, cheese, and margarine	Milk, cheese	Milk (average)	Cheese, milk	Cheese, milk, eggs

(continues)

Classes	Potassium	Sodium	Calcium	Magnesium	Chloride	Phosphorus
Nuts	Almonds, Brazil nuts, cashews, and peanuts	Low, except if salted	Brazil nuts (moderate)	Almonds, Brazil nuts, peanuts, and walnuts		Peanuts
Vegetables	Baked beans, carrots (raw), celery (raw), dandelion greens, lima beans (canned), mustard greens, tomatoes, spinach *Note:* Nearly all vegetables are rich in potassium when raw; but K will be lost if water used in cooking is discarded.	Average to low Celery (high average)	Baked beans, kale, mustard and turnip greens, broccoli	Green, leafy	Spinach, celery	Dry beans
Meat, fish, and poultry	Average—meats High average—sardines, codfish, scallops	Corned beef, bacon, ham, crab, tuna fish, sausage (pork) Low in poultry	Salmon, meats	Fish, shrimp Low in poultry Low in meats Egg, average	Eggs, crabs, fish (average), turkey	Beef, pork, fish, chicken, turkey

Classes	Potassium	Sodium	Calcium	Magnesium	Chloride	Phosphorus
Miscellaneous	Catsup (average), spices, potato chips, and peanut butter	Catsup, mayonnaise, potato chips, pretzels, pickles, dill, olives, mustard, Worcestershire sauce, celery salt, salad dressing—French and Italian	Molasses	Chocolate and chocolate bars, chocolate syrup Molasses Table salt		

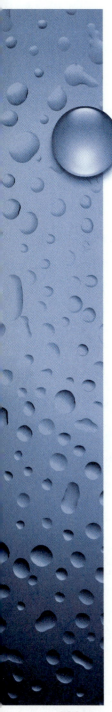

Appendix C

Clinical Pathways:
Newborn Hyperbilirubinemia
Heart Failure

Christiana Care
Visiting Nurse Association

Page 1 of 5
Newborn Hyperbilirubinemia
Home Care Pathway

Client Name:_____
Admission #:_____
ID #:_____

Outcomes: 1. Newborn's weight stabilizes and begins to rise.
2. Bilirubin level decreases.
3. Newborn has normal skin reactions to phototherapy.

KEY
✓ = Done   Ø = None   NA = Not Applicable   I = Instructed   R = Reinstructed   V = Variance   A= Achieved

Admission	Discharge
1. OASIS	Outcomes Met: 1. Y___ N___ V___ 2. Y___ N___ V___ 3. Y___ N___ V___
2. Client / Family Data	
3. HCFA Certification	Discharged to : Family _____ Other ____ ED_____
4. Consent to Treat	Rehospitalized ___ Reason:_____
5. Client payment responsibilities	Plans for discharge (include MD follow - up):_____
6. Medication List	
7. DME used & company name:_____	
8. Bilirubin level on hospital discharge (or most recent level):_____	
9. DAT=	
10. Additional Comments:_____	
	Physician notified of discharge:_____
	Spoke to:_____ Date/Time:_____
	Nurse's Signature: Date:

Assessment Visit # 1 Date:	Assessment Visit # 2 Date:
1. Vital signs: Temperature_____	1. Vital signs: Temperature_____
Apical pulse_____	Apical pulse_____
Regular_____	Regular_____
Irregular_____	Irregular_____
Murmur_____ (S1/S2?)	Murmur_____ (S1/S2?)
Respirations_____	Respirations_____
2. STATE: Deep Sleep_____ Light Sleep_____ Drowsy_____ Alert, Eyes Bright_____ Eyes Open, Motor Activity_____ Crying (consolable)_____ Crying (not consolable)_____	2. STATE: Deep Sleep_____ Light Sleep_____ Drowsy_____ Alert, Eyes Bright_____ Eyes Open, Motor Activity_____ Crying (consolable)_____ Crying (not consolable)_____
3. Presence of NB reflexes: Moro_____ TN_____ Root_____ Suck_____ Grasp_____ Plantar_____	3. Presence of NB reflexes: Moro_____ TN_____ Root_____ Suck_____ Grasp_____ Plantar_____
4. Fontanels: Flat _____ Depressed_____ Bulging_____	4. Fontanels: Flat _____ Depressed_____ Bulging_____
5. Skin color, including which areas of the skin area jaundiced:_____	5. Skin color, including which areas of the skin area jaundiced:_____
Skin turgor:_____	Skin turgor:_____
Areas of pressure/ skin breakdown:_____	Areas of pressure/ skin breakdown:_____
Signs of birth trauma (describe and measure):_____	Signs of birth trauma (describe and measure):_____
6. Current weight (Calibrate scale using known weight measure prior to weighing newborn):_____	6. Current weight (Calibrate scale using known weight measure prior to weighing newborn):_____
_____weight loss over_____(hours, days) _____weight gain over_____ (hours, days)	_____weight loss over_____(hours, days) _____weight gain over_____ (hours, days)
Nurse's Signature:	**Nurse's Signature:**
Print Name: **Initial:**	**Print Name:** **Initial:**

Courtesy of Christiana Care Visiting Nurse Association, New Castle, DE

Page 2 of 5
Newborn Hyperbilirubinemia
Home Care Pathway

Christiana Care
Visiting Nurse Association

Client Name:_____
ID #:_____

Assessment Visit # 1 Date:	**Assessment Vist #2 Date:**

7. Feeding
    Breastfeeding:_____minutes, q._____hour(s)
    Do breast(s) feel lighter after feeding?Yes____No__
    Is suck strong and coordinated? Yes____No____
    Formula Type:_____
       Amount and frequency:_____
 	
 8. Elimination
    Diapers wet:____(over_____hours)
      Soiled:____(over_____hours)
 	
 9. Circumcision? Yes_____ No_____ N/A_____
 	
 Goals:
 ☐   **Newborn is normothermic.**
 ☐   **Adequate # wet/soiled diapers (If BF: 2 wet, 2 soiled on day 2).**
 ☐   **Vital signs wnl.**
 ☐   **Newborn is alert and responsive.**
 ☐   **Skin is intact.**
 ☐   **No S/Sx of dehydration.**
 ☐   **Newborn is feeding well.**
 	
 Comments:_____
	7. Feeding
	    Breastfeeding:_____minutes, q._____hour(s)
	    Do breast(s) feel lighter after feeding?Yes____No__
	    Is suck strong and coordinated? Yes____No____
	    Formula Type:_____
	       Amount and frequency:_____
	
	 8. Elimination
	    Diapers wet:____(over_____hours)
	      Soiled:____(over_____hours)
	
	 9. Circumcision? Yes_____ No_____ N/A_____
	
	 Goals:
	 ☐ **Newborn is normothermic.**
	 ☐ **Adequate # wet/soiled diapers (If BF: 2 wet, 2 soiled on day 2).**
	 ☐ **Vital signs wnl.**
	 ☐ **Newborn is alert and responsive.**
	 ☐ **Skin is intact.**
	 ☐ **No S/Sx of dehydration.**
	 ☐ **Newborn is feeding well.**
	
	 Comments:_____

Treatment Visit	**Treatment Visit**

1.   Heelstick for serum bilirubin level=_____
      Area: L heel____ R heel____
         Medial____ Lateral____
 2.   Laboratory should call physician with results.
 3.   Home care nurse should communicate with physician for further
     orders (Record communication with MD office here: Name of
     person spoken to, date/time):_____
 4.   Phototherapy unit placed in accordance with manufacturer's
     guidelines. Intensity selected is HIGH.
     Single_____ or Double_____ Phototherapy
 Goals:
 ☐ **Bilirubin level is decreasing.**
 ☐ **Skin is intact at heelstick site(s).**
 ☐ **Phototherapy unit is correctly placed.**
 	
 Comments:_____
	1. Heelstick for serum bilirubin level=_____
	      Area: L heel____ R heel____
	         Medial____ Lateral____
	 2. Laboratory should call physician with results.
	 3. Home care nurse should communicate with physician for further orders
	     (Record communication with MD office here: Name of person spoken to,
	     date/time):_____
	 4. Phototherapy unit placed in accordance with manufacturer's guidelines.
	     Intensity selected is HIGH.
	     Single_____ or Double_____ Phototherapy
	 Goals:
	 ☐ **Bilirubin level is decreasing.**
	 ☐ **Skin is intact at heelstick site(s).**
	 ☐ **Phototherapy unit is correctly placed.**
	
	 Comments:_____

Medications	**Medications**
Record on Medication List. Untoward side effects of medications:_____ **Goal:** ☐ **Medications given by caregiver as directed.**	Document changes on Medication List. Untoward side effects of medications:_____ **Goal:** ☐ **Medications given by caregiver as directed.**
Nurse's Signature:	**Nurse's Signature:**
Print Name: **Initial:**	**Print Name:** **Initial:**

Courtesy of Christiana Care Visiting Nurse Association, New Castle, DE

Christiana Care
Visiting Nurse Association

Page 3 of 5
Newborn Hyperbilirubinemia
Home Care Pathway

Client Name:_____
ID#:_____

Instruction Visit 1 Date:	Instruction Visit 2 Date:

1.   Instruct caregiver in the following:
   • Cause of newborn hyperbilirubinemia
   • Normal breakdown mechanism of hemoglobin and excretion (urobilinogen in urine: dark urine; stercobilinogen in stool: brown stool)
   • Record-keeping: Axillary temperature
      Oral intake
      Elimination
	1. Instruct caregiver in the following:
	   • Cause of newborn hyperbilirubinemia
	   • Normal breakdown mechanism of hemoglobin and excretion (urobilinogen in urine: dark urine; stercobilinogen in stool: brown stool)
	   • Record-keeping: Axillary temperature
	      Oral intake
	      Elimination

2.   Instruct on use of phototherapy unit(s):
   • Keep newborn on phototherapy 23 out of 24 hours
   • Phototherapy unit should be on highest intensity
   • Changing light bulb
   • Unit should be placed so ventilation is not obstructed
	2. Instruct on use of phototherapy unit(s):
	   • Keep newborn on phototherapy 23 out of 24 hours
	   • Phototherapy unit should be on highest intensity
	   • Changing light bulb
	   • Unit should be placed so ventilation is not obstructed

3.   Instruct caregiver on skin care:
   • Avoidance of skin lotion
   • Appearance of maculopapular rash is common and disappears spontaneously
   • Reporting extreme skin erythema, dryness, and blistering
	3. Instruct caregiver on skin care:
	   • Avoidance of skin lotion
	   • Appearance of maculopapular rash is common and disappears spontaneously
	   • Reporting extreme skin erythema, dryness, and blistering

4.   Instruct caregiver to do the following:
   • Check axillary temperature qid
   • Report 97.4 <T>99.4F to VNA nurse
   • Offer frequent feedings
   • If breastfeeding, encourage at least 8 feedings daily
   • Positioning
   • Report decreased intake or urine output or projectile vomiting to VNA nurse
	4. Instruct caregiver to do the following:
	   • Check axillary temperature qid
	   • Report 97.4 <T>99.4F to VNA nurse
	   • Offer frequent feedings
	   • If breastfeeding, encourage at least 8 feedings daily
	   • Positioning
	   • Report decreased intake or urine output or projectile vomiting to VNA nurse

Patient education materials provided/used:_____ 	Patient education materials provided/used:_____
Goals: ❑ Newborn is properly placed on phototherapy unit(s). ❑ Caregiver demonstrates ability to assemble and use phototherapy unit(s). ❑ Caregiver verbalizes knowledge of disease, purpose, and phototherapy procedure. Comments:_____	**Goals:** ❑ Newborn is properly placed on phototherapy unit(s). ❑ Caregiver demonstrates ability to assemble and use phototherapy unit(s). ❑ Caregiver verbalizes knowledge of disease, purpose, and phototherapy procedure. Comments:_____
Nurse's Signature:	**Nurse's Signature:**
Print Name: **Initial**	**Print Name:** **Initial:**

Courtesy of Christiana Care Visiting Nurse Association, New Castle, DE

Christiana Care
Visiting Nurse Association

Page 4 of 5
Newborn Hyperbilirubinemia
Home Care Pathway

Client Name:_____
ID#:_____

Psychosocial Visit 1 Date:	Psychosocial Visit 2 Date:

Psychosocial Visit 1 — Date:

1. Comprehension (Ability to grasp concepts and respond to?)
   Exhibits: High _____ Medium _____ Low _____
2. Motivation Level (Code: F=Family/Caregiver C=Client)
   _____ Asks questions   _____ Eager to learn
   _____ Extremely anxious   _____ Uncooperative
   _____ Seems uninterested   _____ Denies educational need
3. Language barrier:_____ Yes _____ No
4. Literate:_____ Yes _____ No

Comments:_____
_____
_____
_____
_____
_____
_____
_____

Goal:
❑ Caregiver is comfortable using phototherapy unit(s)

Referrals / Interdisciplinary Services
1. Smoking cessation for caregiver/ family
2. MSW
3. Lactation Consultant
4. La Leche League International: 1(800)La Leche (525-3243)
5. Nursing Mother's, Inc.: (302)733-0973
6. The Warm Line: (302)762-8938
7. Other:_____
_____
_____

Goal:
❑ Client / Family can list resources available.

Comments:_____
_____
_____
_____
_____
_____
_____
_____
_____

Nurse's Signature_____

Print Name: _____ **Initial:** _____

Psychosocial Visit 2 — Date:

1. Family Relationships:
_____
_____
_____
_____
_____
_____
_____

2. Family Stressors:
_____
_____
_____
_____

3. Financial Problems:
_____
_____
_____

4. Other:
_____
_____

Goal:
❑ Caregiver / Family gaining increasing sense of control over treatment of hyperbilirubinemia.

Referrals / Interdisciplinary Services
1. Smoking cessation for caregiver/ family
2. MSW
3. Lactation Consultant
4. La Leche League International: 1(800)La Leche (525-3243)
5. Nursing Mother's, Inc.: (302)733-0973
6. The Warm Line: (302)762-8938
7. Other:_____
_____

Goal:
❑ Client / Family can list resources available.

Comments:_____
_____
_____
_____
_____
_____
_____
_____

Nurses's Signature:_____

Print Name: _____ **Initial:** _____

Courtesy of Christiana Care Visiting Nurse Association, New Castle, DE

Christiana Care
Visiting Nurse Association

Page 5 of 5
Clinical Pathway for Home Care: Hyperbilirubinemia
Outcome Record

Client Name:_____
Admission #:_____
ID #:_____

ICD9 Code:_____

Pathway Start Date:_____   Pathway Stop Date:_____
# of Home Visits:_____

Client Variance

❑ A1 Readmitted to hospital   ❑ A5 Other_____
❑ A2 Death
❑ A3 Caregiver noncompliance
❑ A4 Continues home care r/t_____

System Variance
Internal

❑ B1 Equipment not available
❑ B2 Visit delay impending progress or treatment

System Variance
External

❑ B3 Insurance problem
❑ B4 Transportation problem

Nurse's Initials	Date	Visit Day	Variance Code	Variance/Explanation/Comments	Variance Caused Delay (Y/N)	Action Taken

Note: Y= Yes, N= No

Nurse's Signature:	Initials:	Nurse's Signature:	Initials:
Print Name:		Print Name:	
Nurse's Signature:	Initials:	Nurse's Signature:	Initials:
Print Name:		Print Name:	
Nurse's Signature:	Initials:	Nurse's Signature:	Initials:
Print Name:		Print Name:	

Hyperout 698 Gale

Courtesy of Christiana Care Visiting Nurse Association, New Castle, DE

Clinical Pathway - | **DRAFT** | CONGESTIVE HEART FAILURE

***ACUTE PHASE* - EMERGENCY DEPARTMENT**   DATE ____ / ____ / _____

Disclaimer for Pathways and Guidelines: Clinical Pathways and Guidelines are developed by a multidisciplinary team. They are guidelines for care. They are not compulsory or mandatory plans of treatment or standards of care. When considering individual patient needs, alternative independent clinical assessments and judgements may be necessary.

		BELOW: SELECT SHIFT & INITIAL		
		0700-1500	1500-2300	2300-0700
Assessment	H&P per ED Protocol.	☐ _____	☐ _____	☐ _____
	Vital signs & multisystem assessment per ED protocol	☐ _____	☐ _____	☐ _____
	Advanced directives addressed	☐ _____	☐ _____	☐ _____
	Guideline I: S&S Diagnosis of CHF	☐ _____	☐ _____	☐ _____
	Guideline II: CHF Pathway/Risk Stratification.	☐ _____	☐ _____	☐ _____
	Guideline VI: Level of Care for CHF Patients	☐ _____	☐ _____	☐ _____
Treatments	Continuous cardiac monitoring	☐ _____	☐ _____	☐ _____
	Weight prior to diuresis (if appropriate)	☐ _____	☐ _____	☐ _____
	Foley catheter as indicated	☐ _____	☐ _____	☐ _____
Tests/Labs	**Guideline III / IV: Diagnostic Procedures in New Onset/Established CHF** (EKG,CXR,CBC, complete chemistry profile, Mg, thyroid function, other as indicated)	☐ _____	☐ _____	☐ _____
	Pulse Oximetry per protocol	☐ _____	☐ _____	☐ _____
Medications/IVs	IV access	☐ _____	☐ _____	☐ _____
	Oxygen therapy per protocol	☐ _____	☐ _____	☐ _____
	Guideline IX: Diuresis	☐ _____	☐ _____	☐ _____
	Evaluate patient's routine medications	☐ _____	☐ _____	☐ _____
Consults	Cardiology consult as indicated	☐ _____	☐ _____	☐ _____
Nutrition	NPO except for medications	☐ _____	☐ _____	☐ _____
Activity/Safety	Bedrest	☐ _____	☐ _____	☐ _____
	High Fowlers position	☐ _____	☐ _____	☐ _____
Discharge Planning	Responsible support person identified	☐ _____	☐ _____	☐ _____
	Residence prior to admission identified	☐ _____	☐ _____	☐ _____
Patient/Family Teaching Outcomes	Verbalizes understanding of: Treatment plan and need for admission. . .	☐ _____	☐ _____	☐ _____
	Importance of notifying the staff when experiencing SOB or chest pain	☐ _____	☐ _____	☐ _____
	Need for limited activity.	☐ _____	☐ _____	☐ _____
Clinical Processes/ Outcomes	If patient meets criteria, meds given in ED:			
	• Furosemide	☐ _____	☐ _____	☐ _____
	• Bumetanide.	☐ _____	☐ _____	☐ _____
	• Morphine.	☐ _____	☐ _____	☐ _____
	• Nitrates	☐ _____	☐ _____	☐ _____
	• Heparin	☐ _____	☐ _____	☐ _____
	Documentation of support person on record. Residence and telephone documented on record	☐ _____	☐ _____	☐ _____

INITIAL	SIGNATURE	TITLE	INITIAL	SIGNATURE	TITLE

PHYSICIAN SIGNATURE: _____

Courtesy of St. Francis Hospital, Wilmington, Delaware

Clinical Pathway - | **DRAFT** | **CONGESTIVE HEART FAILURE**

| *ACUTE PHASE* - DAY 1 | (ICU/TELEMETRY/MS UNIT) | DATE ___/___/___ |

(ADMISSION DAY or OBSERVATION DAY [0-24 hrs])

Disclaimer for Pathways and Guidelines: Clinical Pathways and Guidelines are developed by a multidisciplinary team. They are guidelines for care. They are not compulsory or mandatory plans of treatment or standards of care. When considering individual patient needs, alternative independent clinical assessments and judgements may be necessary.

		BELOW: SELECT SHIFT & INITIAL		
		0700-1500	1500-2300	2300-0700
Assessment	Vital signs & systems assessment per unit protocol	□ ____	□ ____	□ ____
	Advanced directives addressed	□ ____	□ ____	□ ____
	Monitor for signs & symptoms of SOB, JVD, rales, peripheral edema, S3,S4, murmur, arrhythmias .	□ ____	□ ____	□ ____
	Guideline VI: Level of Care for CHF Patients . . .	□ ____	□ ____	□ ____
Treatments	Continuous cardiac monitoring as indicated	□ ____	□ ____	□ ____
	Weight q AM	□ ____	□ ____	□ ____
	Intake & output	□ ____	□ ____	□ ____
Tests/Labs	Pulse Oximetry per protocol	□ ____	□ ____	□ ____
	Guideline III: Diagnostic Procedures in New Onset CHF.	□ ____	□ ____	□ ____
	Guideline IV: Diagnostic Procedures in Established CHF.	□ ____	□ ____	□ ____
	GuidelineV: Assessment of LV Function in CHF	□ ____	□ ____	□ ____
Medications/IVs	IV access	□ ____	□ ____	□ ____
	Oxygen therapy per protocol	□ ____	□ ____	□ ____
	Guideline IX: Diuresis	□ ____	□ ____	□ ____
	Guideline X: ACE Inhibitors	□ ____	□ ____	□ ____
	Guideline XII: Digoxin	□ ____	□ ____	□ ____
	Guideline XIII: Indications for Anticoagulation .	□ ____	□ ____	□ ____
	Guideline XIV, XV, XVI, and XVII.	□ ____	□ ____	□ ____
	Patient's routine medications as indicated	□ ____	□ ____	□ ____
Consults	Cardiology consult as indicated	□ ____	□ ____	□ ____
Nutrition	Cardiac diet as tolerated (additional Na and fluid restrictions as indicated)	□ ____	□ ____	□ ____
	Nutrition screen, Diet Teaching Needs Assessment	□ ____	□ ____	□ ____
Activity/Safety	Bedrest with BRP/bedside commode	□ ____	□ ____	□ ____
	Fall risk assessment completed	□ ____	□ ____	□ ____
	Maintain semi-Fowlers position	□ ____	□ ____	□ ____
Discharge Planning	Care management assessment:			
	• Evaluation of support system and discharge needs	□ ____	□ ____	□ ____
	• Preadmission compliance with diet and medication evaluated	□ ____	□ ____	□ ____
	• Initial discharge plan addressed, with patient and caregiver.	□ ____	□ ____	□ ____
	• Need for DME and home weight scale identified.	□ ____	□ ____	□ ____
Patient/Family Teaching Outcomes	• Verbalizes basic understanding of disease process (reason for SOB and decreased activity level, etc.)	□ ____	□ ____	□ ____
Clinical Processes/ Outcomes	• Decreasing SOB	□ ____	□ ____	□ ____
	• JVD decreasing	□ ____	□ ____	□ ____
	• Improved breath sounds	□ ____	□ ____	□ ____
	• Negative fluid balance >500(8hr), 750(12hr) . . .	□ ____	□ ____	□ ____
	• LV Function ordered or documented in record (as appropriate).	□ ____	□ ____	□ ____
	• O₂ Sat maintained > 92%	□ ____	□ ____	□ ____

INITIAL SIGNATURE	TITLE	INITIAL SIGNATURE	TITLE

PHYSICIAN SIGNATURE: _____

Courtesy of St. Francis Hospital, Wilmington, Delaware

Clinical Pathway -   **DRAFT**   CONGESTIVE HEART FAILURE

| IMPROVING PHASE - DAY 2 ICU/TELEMETRY/MS Unit | | DATE ____ / ____ / ____ |

Disclaimer for Pathways and Guidelines: Clinical Pathways and Guidelines are developed by a multidisciplinary team. They are guidelines for care. They are not compulsory or mandatory plans of treatment or standards of care. When considering individual patient needs, alternative independent clinical assessments and judgements may be necessary.

		BELOW: SELECT SHIFT & INITIAL		
		0700-1500	1500-2300	2300-0700
Assessment	Vital signs & multisystem assessment per unit protocol	☐ _____	☐ _____	☐ _____
	Monitor for signs & symptoms of SOB, JVD, rales, peripheral edema	☐ _____	☐ _____	☐ _____
	Guideline VI: Level of Care for CHF Patients . . .	☐ _____	☐ _____	☐ _____
Treatments	Continuous cardiac monitoring as indicated	☐ _____	☐ _____	☐ _____
	Weight q AM	☐ _____	☐ _____	☐ _____
	Intake & output q 8 hours	☐ _____	☐ _____	☐ _____
	D/C foley if indicated	☐ _____	☐ _____	☐ _____
Tests/Labs	**Guideline III: Diagnostic Procedures in New Onset CHF**	☐ _____	☐ _____	☐ _____
	Guideline IV: Diagnostic Procedures in Established CHF	☐ _____	☐ _____	☐ _____
	Guideline V: Assessment of LV Function in CHF	☐ _____	☐ _____	☐ _____
	Pulse Oximetry per protocol	☐ _____	☐ _____	☐ _____
Medications/IVs	Oxygen therapy per protocol	☐ _____	☐ _____	☐ _____
	Guideline IX: Diuresis	☐ _____	☐ _____	☐ _____
	Guideline X: ACE Inhibitors	☐ _____	☐ _____	☐ _____
	Guideline XII: Digoxin	☐ _____	☐ _____	☐ _____
	Guideline XIII: Anticoagulation in CHF	☐ _____	☐ _____	☐ _____
	Guideline XIV, XV, XVI, and XVII.	☐ _____	☐ _____	☐ _____
	Patient's routine medications as indicated	☐ _____	☐ _____	☐ _____
Consults	Nutrition for Level 4 Malnutrition Risk and diet teaching.	☐ _____	☐ _____	☐ _____
Nutrition	Cardiac diet (additional Na and fluid restrictions as indicated)	☐ _____	☐ _____	☐ _____
Activity/Safety	OOB X 3 with assistance (meals in chair, remain up for 30 minutes)	☐ _____	☐ _____	☐ _____
	Encourage high to semi-Fowlers position when in bed and during meals	☐ _____	☐ _____	☐ _____
Discharge Planning	• Care manager reassessment of discharge plan, assess needs for Home O₂ and refer as indicated.	☐ _____	☐ _____	☐ _____
	• Assess need for Home Health, Telemanagement, Cardiac Rehab referral.	☐ _____	☐ _____	☐ _____
Patient/Family Teaching Outcomes	• Demonstrates understanding of activity level. . . .	☐ _____	☐ _____	☐ _____
	• Medication instructions initiated.	☐ _____	☐ _____	☐ _____
	• Verbalizes understanding of relationship of increased Na and fluid intake with SOB, weight gain, and peripheral edema.	☐ _____	☐ _____	☐ _____
	• Verbalizes rationale for daily weight monitoring. .	☐ _____	☐ _____	☐ _____
Clinical Processes/ Outcomes	• Decreased weight	☐ _____	☐ _____	☐ _____
	• Increased activity without increased SOB.	☐ _____	☐ _____	☐ _____
	• Negative fluid balance.	☐ _____	☐ _____	☐ _____
	• ECHO completed.	☐ _____	☐ _____	☐ _____
	• Receiving Ace inhibitors.	☐ _____	☐ _____	☐ _____
	• Receiving digoxin.	☐ _____	☐ _____	☐ _____
	• Receiving diuretics.			

INITIAL	SIGNATURE	TITLE	INITIAL	SIGNATURE	TITLE

PHYSICIAN SIGNATURE: _____

COPYRIGHT 1998 St. Francis Hospital, INC   1/98   H:\ceu\Pathways\CHF\pathway.doc

Courtesy of St. Francis Hospital, Wilmington, Delaware

Clinical Pathway - | **DRAFT** | **CONGESTIVE HEART FAILURE**

DISCHARGE PHASE - DAY 3, 4, ___ (TELEMETRY/MS UNIT) DATE ___/___/___

Disclaimer for Pathways and Guidelines: Clinical Pathways and Guidelines are developed by a multidisciplinary team. They are guidelines for care. They are not compulsory or mandatory plans of treatment or standards of care. When considering individual patient needs, alternative independent clinical assessments and judgements may be necessary.

		BELOW: SELECT SHIFT & INITIAL		
		0700-1500	1500-2300	2300-0700
Assessment	Vital signs & system assessment per unit protocol..........................	...□ _____	□ _____	□ _____
	Advanced directives addressed.............	...□ _____	□ _____	□ _____
	Guideline VI: Level of Care for CHF Patients	...□ _____	□ _____	□ _____
	Guideline VIII: NYHA Classification Circle - I , II , III, IV)..................	...□ _____	□ _____	□ _____
Treatments	Continuous cardiac monitoring as indicated ...	...□ _____	□ _____	□ _____
	Weight q AM..........................	...□ _____	□ _____	□ _____
	Intake and output q 8 hours................	...□ _____	□ _____	□ _____
Tests/Labs	Pulse Oximetry per protocol..............	...□ _____	□ _____	□ _____
Medications/IVs	Oxygen Therapy per protocol..............	...□ _____	□ _____	□ _____
	Guideline IX: Diuresis...................	...□ _____	□ _____	□ _____
	Guideline X: Ace Inhibitors...............	...□ _____	□ _____	□ _____
	Guideline XII: Digoxin...................	...□ _____	□ _____	□ _____
	Guideline XIII: Anticoagulation in CHF.....	...□ _____	□ _____	□ _____
	Guideline XIV, XV, XVI, and XVII..........	...□ _____	□ _____	□ _____
	Patient's routine medications as indicated	...□ _____	□ _____	□ _____
Consults	High-risk patients meeting nutrition needs.....	...□ _____	□ _____	□ _____
	Diet education completed..................	...□ _____	□ _____	□ _____
Nutrition	Cardiac diet (additional Na and fluid restrictions as indicated)	...□ _____	□ _____	□ _____
Activity/Safety	OOB and ambulating as tolerated...........	...□ _____	□ _____	□ _____
	Meals in chair, remain up for 30 minutes	...□ _____	□ _____	□ _____
	Encourage self care......................	...□ _____	□ _____	□ _____
Discharge Planning	Discharge resources identified and referrals made as indicated:			
	• Smoking cessation program.............	...□ _____	□ _____	□ _____
	• Home Health referral...................	...□ _____	□ _____	□ _____
	• Cardiac Rehabilitation.................			
Patient/Family Teaching Outcomes	Verbalizes understanding of:			
	• Discharge medication regimen, action, side effects, drug and food interaction..........	...□ _____	□ _____	□ _____
	• Importance of monitoring daily wt - notify MD with increase of 3lbs in weight and/or increasing SOB......................	...□ _____	□ _____	□ _____
	• Cardiac diet as indicated................	...□ _____	□ _____	□ _____
Clinical Processes/ Outcomes	Resp. rate at baseline with increased activity. ..	...□ _____	□ _____	□ _____
	Stable rate, rhythm, & BP with increased activity...............................	...□ _____	□ _____	□ _____
	• Receiving ACE inhibitors...............	...□ _____	□ _____	□ _____
	• Receiving digoxin.....................	...□ _____	□ _____	□ _____
	• Receiving diuretics....................	...□ _____	□ _____	□ _____
	• **Guideline VII: Discharge Criteria met :** (Y = D/C) (N= reapply next day)........	...□ _____	□ _____	□ _____

INITIAL	SIGNATURE	TITLE	INITIAL	SIGNATURE	TITLE

PHYSICIAN SIGNATURE: _____

Courtesy of St. Francis Hospital, Wilmington, Delaware

References/
Bibliography

Abraham, W. T., & Schriert, R. W. (1994). Body fluid volume regulation in health and disease: *Advances in Internal Medicine, 39.* St: Louis: Mosby-Year Book Inc., pp. 23–43.

Acid-base tutorial. Tulane University School of Medicine, Department of Anesthesiology. (2002). Available at http://www.acid-base.com

Adroque, H. J., & Madias, N. E. (2000). Hyponatremia. *New England Journal of Medicine, 342*(21), 1581–1589.

Ahrns, K. S., & Harkins, D. R. (1999). Initial resuscitation after burn injury: Therapies, strategies, and controversies. *AACN Clinical Issues in Advanced Practice and Critical Care Nursing, 10*(1), 46–60.

American College of Surgeons Committee on Trauma. (1997). *Advanced trauma life support course.* Chicago: Author.

American College of Surgeons Committee on Trauma. (1999). *Resources for optimal care of the injured patient.* Chicago: Author.

American Diabetes Association. (2002). Hyperglycemic crises in patients with diabetes mellitus. *Diabetes Care, 25*(1), S100–S108.

American Nurses Association. (1991). *Standards of clinical nursing practice.* Kansas City: Author.

American Thoracic Society. (1995). Standards for the diagnosis and care of patients with chronic obstructive pulmonary disease. *American Journal of Respiratory Critical Care Medicine, 152,* S77–S120.

Aminoff, M. J. (2001). Nervous system. In L. M. Tierney, S. J. McPhee, & M. A. Papadakis (Eds.), *Current medical diagnosis and treatment* (pp. 969–1027). New York: McGraw-Hill.

Ball, J., & Binder, R. (1995). *Pediatric nursing: Caring for children.* Norwalk, CT: Appleton & Lange.

Barnett, M. L. (1999). Hypercalcemia. *Seminars in Oncology Nursing, 15*(3), 190–201.

Barone, M. A. (Ed.). (1996). *The Harriet Lane handbook* (14th ed.). St. Louis: Mosby.

Bartley, M. K., & Laskowski-Jones, L. (1995). Postsplenectomy sepsis syndrome. *American Journal of Nursing, 95*(1), 56A–56D.

Baum, G. L., Crapo, J. D., Celli, B. R., & Karlinsky, J. B. (1998). *Textbook of pulmonary diseases* (6th ed.). Philadelphia: Lippincott-Raven.

Bayley, E., & Turke, S. (1999). *A comprehensive curriculum for trauma nursing.* Boston: Jones & Bartlett.

Behrman, R. E., Kliegman, R. M., & Arvin, A. M. (1996). *Nelson textbook of pediatrics* (15th ed.). Philadelphia: W. B. Saunders.

Bezerra, J. A., Stathos, T. H., Duncan, B., Gaines, J. A., & Udall, J. N. (1992). Treatment of infants with acute diarrhea: What's recommended and what's practiced. *Pediatrics, 90,* 1–4.

Birney, M. H., & Penney, D. G. (1990). Atrial natriuretic peptide: A hormone with implications for clinical practice. *Heart and Lung, 19*(2), 174–182.

Black, J. M., & Matassarin-Jacobs, E. (2002). *Medical-surgical nursing* (6th ed.). Philadelphia: W. B. Saunders.

Body, J. J. (2000). Current and future directions in medical therapy: Hypercalcemia. *Cancer, 88* (Supple. 12), 3054–3058.

Bordow, R. A., Ries, A. L., & Morris, T. A. (2000). *Manual of clinical problems in pulmonary medicine* (5th ed.). Philadelphia: Lippincott, Williams & Wilkins.

Bove, L. A. (1994). How fluids and electrolytes shift after surgery. *Nursing 1994, 24*(8), 34–39.

Brensilver, J. M., & Goldberger, E. (1996). *A primer of water, electrolyte, and acid-base syndromes* (8th ed.). Philadelphia: Davis.

Brown, R. G. (1993). Disorders of water *and* sodium balance. *Postgraduate Medicine, 93*(4), 227, 228, 231–234, 239–244.

Burn Foundation. (2001). *Nursing care of the patient with a burn injury: An introductory seminar for student nurses.* Symposium conducted at the Crozier-Chester Burn Center, Chester, PA.

Carlstedt, F., & Lind, L. (2001). Hypocalcemic syndromes. *Critical Care Clinics, 17*(1), 139–153.

Carpentito, L. J. (2001). *Nursing diagnosis application to clinical practice* (8th ed.). Philadelphia: Lippincott.

Cefalu, W. T. (1991). Diabetic ketoacidosis. *Critical Care Clinics, 7*(1), 89–107.

Chen, C., Paxton, P., & Williams-Burgess, C. (1996). Feeding tube placement verification: Using gastric pH measurement. *The Online Journal of Knowledge Synthesis for Nursing, 3*(10).

Chernow, B., Bamberger, E., & Stoiko, M. (1989). Hypomagnesemia in patients in postoperative intensive care. *Chest, 95*(2), 391–396.

Clark, B. A., & Brown, R. S. (1995). Potassium homeostasis and hyperkalemic syndromes. *Endocrinology and Metabolism Clinics of North America, 24*(3), 573–591.

Cohn, J. N., Kowey, P. R., Whelton, P. K., & Prisant, M. (2000, Sept. 11). New guidelines for potassium replacement in clinical practice. *Archives of Internal Medicine, 160,* 2429–2436.

Cornell, S. (1997). Maintaining a fluid balance. *Advances for Nurse Practitioners, 5*(12), 43–44.

Crensaw, J., & Winslow, E. (2002). Preoperative fasting: Old habits die hard. *American Journal of Nursing, 102*(5), 36–43.

D'Avella, D., & Tomei, G. (2001). Guidelines for medical and surgical management in head trauma patients in the United States and Europe. In L. P. Miller & R. L. Hayes (Eds.), *Head trauma: Basic, preclinical and clinical directions* (pp. 385–415). New York: Wiley-Liss.

Davis, K. D., & Attie, M. F. (1991). Management of severe hypercalcemia. *Critical Care Clinics, 7*(1), 175–189.

Des Jardins, T., & Burton, G. G. (2000). *Clinical manifestations and assessment of respiratory diseases* (4th ed.). St. Louis: Mosby.

Doran, A. (1992). S.I.A.D.D.: Is your patient at risk? *Nursing 1992, 22*(6); 60–63.

Dorland's illustrated medical dictionary (28th ed.). (1994). Philadelphia: W. B. Saunders.

Dunbar, S., Jacobson, L., & Deaton, C. (1998). Heart failure: Strategies to enhance patient self management. *AACN Clinical Issues in Advanced Practice and Critical Care Nursing, 9*(2), 244–256.

Ebersole, P., & Hess, P. (1998). *Toward healthy aging: Human needs and nursing response* (5th ed.). Baltimore, MD: Mosby.

Eliopoulos, C. (2001). *Gerontological nursing* (5th ed.). New York: Lippincott.

Emergency Nurses Association. (2000). *Trauma nursing core course* (5th ed.). Park Ridge, IL: Author.

Ezzone, S. A. (1999). Tumor lysis syndrome. *Seminars in Oncology Nursing, 15*(3), 202–208.

Fall, P. J. (2000). Hyponatremia and hypernatremia. *Postgraduate Medicine, 107* (5), 75–82.

Fishman, A. P. (Ed.). (1998). *Pulmonary diseases and disorders* (3rd ed.). New York: McGraw-Hill.

Foster, E. E., & Lefor, A. T. (1996). General management of gastrointestinal fistulas. *Surgical Clinics of North America, 76*(5), 1019–1033.

Freeman, B. I., & Burkart, J. M. (1991). Hypokalemia. *Critical Care Clinics, 7*(1), 143–153.

Gennan, F. J. (1998). Hypokalemia. *New England Journal of Medicine, 352,* 135–140.

Gershan, J. A., Freeman, C. M., Ross, M. C., & members of the Research committee, Greater Milwaukee area chapter of the American Association of Critical Care Nurses. (1990). *Heart and Lung, 19*(2), 152–156.

Giesecke, A. H., Grande, C. M., & Whitten, C. W. (1990). Fluid therapy and the resuscitation of traumatic shock. *Critical Care Clinics, 6*(1), 61–71.

Global strategy for the diagnosis, management, and prevention of chronic obstructive pulmonary disease. (2001). NHLBI/WHO workshop report. Retrieved on March 29, 2002, from http://www.goldcopd.com/exec_summary/summary_2001

Greenfield, E. (1999). Burns. In L. Bucher & S. Melander (Eds.), *Critical care nursing* (pp. 1036–1069). Philadelphia: W. B. Saunders.

Gross, P. (2001). Correction of hyponatremia. *Seminars in Nephrology, 21*(3), 269–272.

Guell, R., Casan, P., Belda, J., Sangenis, M., Morante, F., Guyatt, G. H., et al. (2000). Long-term effects of outpatient rehabilitation of COPD: A randomized trial. *Chest, 117,* 976–983.

Gura, M. (2001). Heart failure: Pathophysiology, therapeutic strategies, and assessment of treatment outcomes. *Medscape Nursing.* Retrieved November 19, 2001, from http://nurses.medscape.com/Medscape/nurse/journal/2001/v01.no3/mns1105.01.gura.html

Guyton, A. C., & Hall, J. (1995). *Textbook of medical physiology* (9th ed.). Philadelphia: Saunders.

Held, J. L. (1995). Correcting fluid and electrolyte imbalance. *Nursing 1995, 25*(4), 71.

Hilton, G. (2001). Emergency: Thermal burns. *American Journal of Nursing, 101*(11), 32–34.

Iggulden, H. (1999). Dehydration and electrolyte disturbance. *Nursing Standard, 12*(19), 48–54.

Ignatavicius, D. D., & Workman, M. L. (2002). *Medical-surgical nursing: Critical thinking for collaborative care* (4th ed.). Philadelphia: W. B. Saunders.

Innerarity, S., & Stark, J. (1997). *Fluid and electrolytes.* Springhouse, PA: Springhouse.

Intravenous Nursing Society. (2000). Intravenous standards. *Infusion Nursing 23*(65).

Jones, A. M., Moseley, M. J., Halfmann, S. J., Health, A. H., & Henkelman, N. J. (1991). Fluid volume dynamics. *Critical Care Nurse, 11*(4), 74–76.

Jones, A., & Rowe, B. (2000). Bronchopulmonary hygiene physical therapy and chronic obstructive lung disease: A systematic review. *Heart and Lung, 29,* 125–135.

Jones, D. H. (1991). Fluid therapy in the PACU. *Critical Care Nursing Clinics of North America, 3*(1), 109–130.

Josephson, D. L. (1999). *Intravenous infusion therapy for nurses: Principles and practice.* Clifton Park, NY: Delmar Learning.

Kamel, K. S., Ethier, J. H., & Richardson, M. A. (1990). Urine electrolytes and osmolality: When and how to use them. *American Journal of Nephrology, 10*(2), 89–102.

Kapoor, M., & Chan, G. Z. (2001). Fluid and electrolyte abnormalities. *Critical Care Clinics, 17*(3), 503–529.

Karch, A. (1998). *Nursing Drug Guide.* Philadelphia: Lippincott.

Kee, J. L. (2002). *Laboratory and diagnostic tests with nursing implications* (6th ed.) East Rutherford: Prentice Hall Health.

Kee, J. L., & Boyda, E. K. (1998). Knowledge base for patients with fluid, electrolyte, and acid-base imbalances. In F. D. Monahan & M. Neighbors (Eds.), *Medical surgical nursing* (2nd ed., pp. 75–112). Philadelphia: Saunders.

Keenan, A. M. (1999). Syndrome of inappropriate secretion of antidiuretic hormone in malignancy. *Seminars in Oncology Nursing, 15*(3), 160–167.

Klemm, P. (1992). *Total nutritional admixture (TNA): Programmed instruction.* Baltimore: Johns Hopkins Hospital Department of Nursing.

Knebel, A. R., Bentz, E., & Barnes, P. (2000). Brief report. Dyspnea management of alpha-1 antitrypsin deficiency: Effect of oxygen administration. *Nursing Research, 49,* 333–338.

Kokko, J. P., & Tanner, R. L. (1995). *Fluids and electrolytes* (3rd ed.). Philadelphia: Saunders.

Kositzke, J. A. (1990). A question of balance, dehydration in the elderly. *Journal of Gerontologic Nursing, 16*(5), 4–11, 40–41.

Kugler, J. P., & Hustead, T. (2000, June 15). Hyponatremia and hypernatremia in the elderly. *American Family Physician, 61,* 3623–3634.

Laskowski-Jones, L. (1993). Acute SCI: How to minimize the damage. *American Journal of Nursing, 93*(12), 22–32.

Laskowski-Jones, L. (1995). Meeting the challenge of chest trauma. *American Journal of Nursing, 95*(9), 22–30.

Laskowski-Jones, L. (1997). Managing hemorrhage. *American Journal of Nursing, 97*(9), 36–41.

Laskowski-Jones, L. (1999). Multisystem problems: Trauma. In L. Bucher & S. D. Melander (Eds.), *Critical care nursing* (pp. 1088–1119). Philadelphia: W. B. Saunders.

Latifi, R., Merrell J., Itano, J., & Taoka, K. N. (1998). *Core curriculum for oncology nursing.* (3rd ed.). Philadelphia: Saunders.

Latifi, R., & Merrell, R. C. (Eds.). (2002). *Nutritional support of cancer and transplant patients.* Austin, TX: Eurekah.com.

Lebovitz, H. E. (1998). Diabetic ketoacidosis. *The Lancet, 345* (8952), 767–772.

Levy, D. B., & Peppers, M. P. (1991). IV fluids used in shock. *Emergency, 23*(4), 22–26.

Lewis, S., Heitkempe, M., & Dirksen, S. (2000). *Medical-surgical nursing assessment and management of clinical practice* (5th ed.). Philadelphia: Mosby.

Lorenz, J. M. (1997). Assessing fluid and electrolyte status in the newborn. *Clinical Chemistry, 43*(1), 205–210.

Lueckenotte, A. (1996). *Gerontologic nursing.* St. Louis: Mosby.

Mandal, A. K. (1997). Hypokalemia and hyperkalemia. *Critical Care Nursing Clinics of North America, 81,* 611–639.

Mange, K., Matsuura, D., Cizman, B., Soto, H., Ziyadeh, F., Goldfarb, S., et al. (1997). Language guiding therapy: The case of dehydration versus volume depletion. *Annals of Internal Medicine, 127*(9), 848–853.

March, K. (1999). Acute head injury. In L. Bucher & S. Melander (Eds.), *Critical care nursing* (pp. 843–867). Philadelphia: W. B. Saunders.

Marik, P. E. (2001). *Handbook of evidence-based critical care.* New York: Springer.

Martin, R. Y., & Schrier, R. W. (1995). Renal sodium excretion and edematous disorders. *Endocrinology and Metabolism Clinics of North America, 24*(3), 459–475.

Matheny, N. (1996). *Fluid and electrolyte balance* (3rd ed.). Philadelphia: Lippincott.

Matheny, N., Wehrle, M., Wierssema, L., & Clark, J. (1998). Testing feeding tube placement: Auscultation vs. pH method. *American Journal of Nursing, 98*(5), 37–42.

Mattox, K., Feliciano, D., & Moore, E. (2000). *Trauma* (4th ed.). Stamford, CT: Appleton & Lange.

Matz, R. (1994). Parallels between treated uncontrolled diabetes and the refeeding syndrome with emphasis on fluid and electrolyte abnormalities. *Diabetes Care, 17*(10), 1209–1213.

McCance, K., & Huether, S. (1990). *Pathophysiology: The biologic basis for disease in adults and children.* St. Louis: Mosby.

McDermott, K. C., Almadrones, L. A., & Bajorunas, D. R. (1991). The diagnosis and management of hypomagnesemia: A unique treatment approach and case report. *Oncology Nursing Forum, 18,* 1145–1152.

McFadden, M. E., & Gatoricos, S. E. (1992). Multiple systems organ failure in the patient with cancer, Part 1: Pathophysiologic perspectives. *Oncology Nursing Forum, 19,* 719–727.

Medical Center of Delaware. (1992). *Calculating infusion rate.* Newark, DE: Medical Center Orientation Materials.

Meighan-Davies, J., & Parnell, H. (2000). Management of COPD. *Journal of Community Nursing, 14,* 10, 22, 24.

Merrill, P. (2000). Oncologic emergencies. *Primary Care Practitioner, 4*(4), 400–409.

Millam, D. (1991). Myths and facts . . . About IV therapy. *Nursing 1991, 21*(6), 75–76.

Miller, J. (1999). Management of diabetic ketoacidosis. *Journal of Emergency Nursing, 25*(6), 514–519.

Moiser, L. C. (1991). Anaphylaxis: A preventable complication of home infusion therapy. *Journal of Intravenous Nursing, 14*(2), 108–112.

Mueller, K. D., & Boisen, A. M. (1989). Keeping your patient's water level up. *RN, 52*(7), 65–68.

Murphy, R., Driscoll, P., & O'Driscoll, R. (2001). Emergency oxygen therapy for the COPD patient. *Emergency Medical Journal, 18,* 333–339.

NANDA. (2001). *Nursing diagnoses: Definitions and classification.* Philadelphia: North American Nursing Diagnosis Association.

Novartis Foundation Symposium. (2001). *Chronic obstructive pulmonary disease: Pathogenesis to treatment.* Chichester, UK: John Wiley & Sons.

O'Donnell, M. E. (1995). Assessing fluid and electrolyte balance in elders. *American Journal of Nursing, 95*(11), 40–45.

Olinger, M. L. (1989). Disorders of calcium and magnesium metabolism. *Emergency Medicine Clinics of North America, 7*(4), 795–819.

Oski, F. A. (1994). *Principles and practice of pediatrics.* Philadelphia: Lippincott.

Oskvig, R. M. (1999). Special problems in the elderly. *Chest, 115*(5), 158–164.

Oster, J. R. Reston, R. A., & Materson, B. J. (1994). Fluid and electrolyte disorders in congestive heart failure. *Seminars in Nephrology, 14*(5), 485–505.

Peppers, M. P., Geheb, M., & Desai, T. (1991). Hypophosphatemia and hyperphosphatemia. *Critical Care Clinics, 7*(1), 201–213.

Perazella, M. A. (2000). Drug-induced hyperkalemia: Old culprits and new offenders. *American Journal of Medicine, 109*(9), 307–314.

Pereira, N., & Cooper, G. (2000). Systolic heart failure: Practical implementation of standard guidelines. *Clinical Cornerstone.* Retrieved July 16, 2001, from http://nurses.medscape.com/excerptaMed/clincornerstne/2000/v03.n02/clc03.02.pere.html

Perry, A. G., & Potter, P. A. (2002). *Clinical nursing skills and techniques* (5th ed.). St. Louis: Mosby.

Phillips, L. D. (2001). *Manual of I.V. therapeutics* (3rd ed.). Philadelphia: F. A. Davis.

Piano, M., Bondmass, M., & Schwertz, D. (1998). The molecular and cellular pathophysiology of heart failure. *Heart and Lung, 27*(1), 3–17.

Pillitteri, A. (1999). *Child health nursing: Care of the child and family.* Philadelphia: Lippincott.

Porth, C. M. (2002). *Pathophysiology: Concepts of altered health states* (6th ed.). Philadelphia: Lippincott, Williams & Wilkins.

Powers, F. (1999). The role of chloride in acid-base balance. *Journal of Intravenous Nursing, 22*(5), 286–291.

Practice parameter: The management of acute gastroenteritis in young children. (1996). *Pediatrics, 97,* 424–436.

Ragland, G. (1990). Electrolyte abnormalities in the alcoholic patient. *Emergency Medicine Clinics of North America, 8*(4), 761–771.

R. C. (Eds.). (2002). *Nutritional support of cancer and transplant patients.* Austin, TX: Eurekah.com.

Redden, M., & Wotton, K. (2001). Clinical decision making by nursing when faced with third-spacing fluid shift: How well do they fare? *Gastroenterology Nursing, 24*(4), 182–191.

Riera, H. S., Rubio, T. M., Ruiz, F. O., Ramos, P. J., Otero, D. D. C., Hernandez, T. E., et al. (2001). Inspiratory muscle training in patients with COPD. *Chest, 120,* 748–757.

Robson, A. (1997). Parenteral fluid therapy. In R. Behrman (Ed.), *Nelson textbook of pediatrics* (14th ed., pp. 171–211). Philadelphia: Saunders.

Rose, B. D. (1997). *Clinical physiology of acid-base and electrolyte disorders* (3rd ed.). New York: McGraw-Hill.

Rosenberger, K. (1998). Management of electrolyte abnormalities: Hypocalcemia, hypomagnesemia, and hypokalemia. *Journal of American Academy of Nurse Practitioners, 10*(5), 209–217.

Ross Roundtable Report, 12th. (1992). Enteral nutrition support for the 1990's: Innovations in nutrition, technology and techniques. Columbus, OH: Ross Laboratories (Division of Abbott Laboratories).

Sadovsky, R. (2002). Managing dyspnea in patients with advanced COPD. *American Family Physician, 65,* 935.

Salem, M., Munoz, R., & Chernow, B. (1991). Hypomagnesemia in critical illness. *Critical Care Clinics, 7*(1), 225–247.

Samson, L. F., & Ouzts, K. M. (1996). Fluid and electrolyte regulation. In M. Curley, J. Smith, & P. Moloney-Harmon (Eds.), *Critical care nursing of infants and children* (pp. 385–409). Philadelphia: Saunders.

Savoy, A., Palant, C. E., Patchin, G., & Graellinger, W. F. (1998). Losartan effects on serum potassium in an elderly population. *Journal of American Society of Nephrology, 9,* 111A.

Schrler, R. W. (1997). *Renal and electrolyte disorders* (3rd ed.). Boston: Little, Brown.

Selekman, J., Scofield, S., & Swenson-Brousell, C. (1999). Diabetes update in the pediatric population. *Pediatric Nursing, 25*(6), 666–669.

Shakir, K. M. M., & Amin, R. M. (1991). Hypoglycemia. *Critical Care Clinics, 7*(1), 75–87.

Siberry, G. K., & Iannone, R. (Eds.). (2000). *The Harriet Lane handbook* (15th ed.). St. Louis: Mosby.

Smith, Z. H., & VanGeilick, A. J. (1992). Management of neutropenic enterocolitis in the patient with cancer. *Oncology Nursing Forum, 19,* 1337–1342.

Snow, V., Lascher, S., & Mottur-Pilson, C. (2001). The evidence base for management of acute exacerbations of COPD: Clinical practice guideline (Pt. 1). *Chest, 110,* 1185–1189.

Snyder, J. (1994). *Seminars in pediatric infectious disease* (5th ed., P. 231). Oxford England, Oxford University Press.

Sommers, M. (1990). Rapid fluid resuscitation: How to correct dangerous deficits. *Nursing 1990, 20*(1), 52–60.

Sommers, M. S., & Johnson, S. A. (Eds.). (2002). *Diseases and disorders* (pp. 176–181). Philadelphia: F. A. Davis.

Sterns, R. H. (1991). The management of hyponatremic emergencies. *Critical Care Clinics, 7*(1), 127–141.

Szerlip, H., & Goldfarb, S. (1993). *Fluid and electrolyte disorders.* New York: Churchill Livingstone.

Taccetta-Chapnick, M. (2002). Using Carvedilol to treat heart failure. *Critical Care Nurse, 22*(2), 36–58.

Terry, J. (1994). The major electrolytes. *Journal of Intravenous Nursing, 17*(5), 240–247.

The Merck manual. (2002). Acid-base balance (chap. 138). Available at http://www.merck.com/pubs/mmanual_home/sec 12/138.htm

Truesdell, S. (2000). Helping patients with COPD manage episodes of acute shortness of breath. *MEDSURG Nursing, 9,* 178–182.

VanHook, J. W. (1991). Hypermagnesemia. *Critical Care Clinics, 7*(1), 215–223.

Votey, S. R., Peters, A. L., & Hoffman, J. R. (1989). Disorders of water metabolism: Hyponatremia and hypernatremia. *Emergency Medicine Clinics of North America, 7*(4), 749–765.

Watkins, S. L. (1995). The basics of fluid and electrolyte therapy. *Pediatric Annals, 24*(1), 16–22.

Whedon, M. B., & Wujcik, D. (1997). *Blood and marrow stem cell transplantation* (2nd ed.). Sudbury, MA: Jones & Bartlett.

Wiebelhaus, P., & Hansen, S. L. (2001). Burn emergencies. *Nursing Management, 32*(7), 29–36.

Wong, D. (1998). *Essentials of pediatric nursing* (4th ed.). Philadelphia: Mosby-Year Book.

Wu, C., Lee, Y. Y., Bain, K., & Wichaikhum, O. (2001). Coping behaviors of individuals with chronic obstructive pulmonary disease. *MEDSURG Nursing, 10,* 315–321.

Yarbro, C. H., Frogge, M. H., & Goodman, M. (Eds.). (1999). *Cancer symptom management* (2nd ed.). Boston: Jones & Bartlett.

Yarbro, C., Goodman, M., & Frogge, M. H. (2000). *Cancer nursing: Principles and practice* (5th ed.). Sudbury, MA: Jones & Bartlett.

Zalaga, G. P. (1991). Hypocalcemic crisis. *Critical Care Clinics, 7*(1), 191–199.

Index